Taking Charge of Your Stroke Recovery:

A Personal Recovery Workbook

**How to Pick Up When Rehab Ends,
Complete Your Recovery and
Be Better than You Ever Were Before!**

Taking Charge
of Your **Stroke Recovery:**
A Personal Recovery Workbook

How to Pick Up When Rehab Ends, Complete Your Recovery and Be Better than You Ever Were Before!

ROGER MAXWELL, KATHY MAXWELL and DAVEDA LAMONT

Taking Charge Books, Inc.
Dallas, Texas

TAKING CHARGE OF YOUR STROKE RECOVERY: A PERSONAL RECOVERY WORKBOOK.
Copyright © 2008 by Roger Maxwell, Kathy Maxwell and Daveda Lamont. All rights reserved.

First Edition: September 2008

ISBN 978-0-615-24916-2

TAKING CHARGE BOOKS, INC.
3221 Amherst Avenue,
Dallas, TX 75225
Telephone: 214-363-4929
Fax: 214-363-4942
www.takingchargebooks.com

Special thanks to Clay Fredrickson, C.S.C.S., Health Director of Infiniti Health in Dallas, Texas, for his review and contributions to the exercise workouts, and to Robin Rinearson, O.D., of Bailey's Crossroads, Virginia, for her helpful comments and suggestions. Grateful thanks to Brian Peskin, B.Sc. (B.S.E.E.), Founder, *Life-Systems* Engineering Science, for his helpful suggestions and permission to include his recommendations about EFAs.

Information and concepts from *Survival of the Fattest: The Key to Human Brain Evolution* used with the kind permission of Stephen C. Cunnane and World Scientific Publishing Co. Ptd. Ltd., Singapore.

Information and statistics from *The Better Brain Book* used with the kind permission of David Perlmutter, M.D.

Quotations from *Becoming a True Champion: A Handbook for Young Athletes Aiming for Greatness* prepublication manuscript used with permission of Kirk Mango and Daveda Lamont.

Cover Design and Illustrations by Daveda Lamont
Recovery Tree Logo Design by Maggy Graham
Interior Book Design by Daveda Lamont and Maggy Graham
Interior and Cover Book Production by Maggy Graham

NOTE TO READERS

Contents

Part 1: What You Need to Know to Get Started

Part 2: Stroke Recovery Plans

Part 3: Worksheets to Keep Track of Your Recovery Progress

Part 4: Retest Yourself!

Special Note for Stroke Survivors

*T*he authors are delighted that you are interested in taking charge of your stroke recovery. Doing so is the best thing you could do for yourself to enable you to return to a full, active life.

Your safety is of the utmost concern to us. The walking plans are intended for stroke survivors who can at least walk with a walker or cane. If you cannot yet walk assisted by a walker or cane, you should not attempt any of the walking recovery plans. However, you may still benefit from the plans included for recovery of other abilities and functions. Additionally, the plans for recovery of various physical functions and the plan to remedy single-sided weakness are intended for those who have at least some movement in the affected body parts, even if there is numbness or tingling. These plans are not designed to remedy complete paralysis.

We also want to clarify that we have not included a separate recovery plan to remedy balance problems because all of the walking plans contain components designed to improve balance. One of the most important of these is yoga classes. If you are suffering from poor balance, be sure to include the yoga lessons that are recommended in each walking plan. Yoga is an extremely effective way to improve your balance and the practice of yoga was the chief means by which Roger eliminated the severe balance problems resulting from his stroke.

Most of the walking plans involve exercising at a gym or health club and doing work with weight machines. We suggest that all beginning walkers (who can walk assisted) start with Recovery Plan 1, which is done under the supervision of a personal athletic trainer who can guide you and ensure you are doing the exercises properly and safely. Your trainer will ensure that you start exercising at a level appropriate for your physical capabilities, thus setting the stage for further progress.

Then read chapters 1-8 and do the introductory steps contained in them. Read each plan you are interested in to find out its prerequisites and to assess whether you will be able to carry it out. Be sure to get your doctor's approval for the recovery plans you want to undertake. Do not attempt to begin any recovery plan whose exercises you don't think you can do safely (because of your individual physical limitations), or that your doctor does not think you should do. On the other hand, you should expect to challenge yourself physically and mentally, so don't shy away from a plan that looks like it will be hard work.

While the recovery plans are designed to be intensive, aggressive, and repetitive, *they should not cause injury* if the instructions are followed and the exercises are done correctly. Nonetheless, you should use your discretion and common sense when exercising, because everyone's body and physical condition is different. Do not continue an exercise if you feel pain that increases if you continue. Also do not continue exercising if you are unable to maintain proper form with each exercise— if pain or fatigue prevents you from holding your body in the correct position for the exercise, don't continue it. Proper form is important: if your body is not in the right position for an exercise, the muscles and joints may be positioned wrongly as you stress them and that can invite injury, even for someone very fit. It goes without saying that you will recover faster from stroke if you don't have to stop to recover from an injury!

The 13-week length of each plan is not intended to be an estimate or guarantee of the total recovery time that will be needed for each ability or function. The time needed to achieve satisfactory results will vary, depending upon each individual's physical and medical status. But if your progress isn't as rapid as you expected, please don't be concerned about it! Doing these plans will enable you to recover at the rate that your body is able and it doesn't matter how long it takes. What *does* matter is that you are doing something about it and improving. Many stroke survivors will want to continue their plans for as long as necessary until they have achieved the level of recovery they desire.

After the 13-week period is over, you can perform an informal "Self-Test and Abilities Assessment," located in Part 4, which will help you gauge your recovery progress. You can repeat any recovery plan as many times as you want or begin another plan.

We wish you the very best success with your stroke recovery!

Contact Information

Personal Recovery Workbook of:

_____

Workbook No. _____

Date Started: _____   Date Finished: _____

My Contact Information:

My Name:_____

Address:_____

Phone Number:_____

Alternate Phone Number:_____

Email Address:_____

Emergency Contact Person/Close Family Member:

Name: _____

Address:_____

Phone Number:_____

Alternate Phone Number:_____

Email Address:_____

Emergency Contact Person/Close Family Member:

Name: _____

Address:_____

Phone Number:_____

Alternate Phone Number:_____

Email Address:_____

Doctor or Primary Care Physician Contact Information:

Name:_____

Address:_____

Phone Number:_____

Alternate Phone Number:_____

Email Address:_____

Personal Athletic Trainer Contact Information:

Name:_____

Address:_____

Phone Number:_____

Alternate Phone Number:_____

Email Address:_____

Yoga Instructor Contact Information:

Name:_____

Address:_____

Phone Number:_____

Alternate Phone Number:_____

Email Address:_____

Contact Information for _____:

Name:_____

Address:_____

Phone Number:_____

Alternate Phone Number:_____

Email Address:_____

Contact Information for _____:

Name:_____

Address:_____

Phone Number:_____

Alternate Phone Number:_____

Email Address:_____

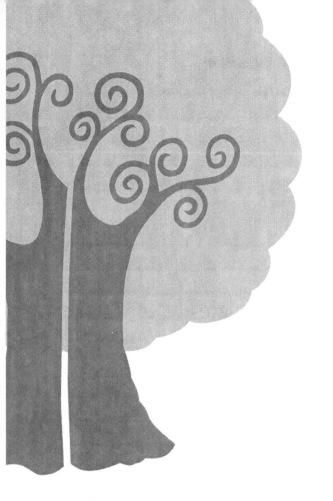

Introduction

How Can This Workbook Help You?

Taking Charge of Your Stroke Recovery: A Personal Recovery Workbook was created to provide you with a clear roadmap to recovery from the losses of physical and mental functions suffered as the result of a stroke. The workbook contains two important parts to help you recover:

(1) Ready-to-use, complete recovery plans designed to help you rehabilitate particular functions such as walking, speaking, hand function and swallowing, and

(2) A workbook section with specially designed pages on which you can keep track of your progress. You will be able to record the exercises you do, your nutritional regimen, your successes, and more.

The recovery plans in this workbook were developed by three people—a stroke survivor, a stroke caregiver, and a professional writer—and were reviewed by a qualified rehabilitation specialist. The instructions and plans have been written in clear, simple language so that you don't have the additional hurdle of trying to understand technical terms before you can get to work. They were designed to be used by a wide range of stroke survivors with differing physical capabilities and lifestyles. Because stroke survivors don't all have the same functional losses, we have included plans for recovery of a variety of skills and functions.

I, Roger Maxwell, am a stroke survivor. I lived through the tremendous difficulties, both physical and mental, that accompany having a stroke. I was told by medical professionals after my stroke that I had a 5% chance of living and would be permanently disabled. I couldn't walk, speak or swallow and my vision was severely affected. When my insurance coverage ended, I found myself stranded, with apparently no options. My doctor told me there was nothing I could do but cross my fingers—I just had to "wait and see" whether I would get better.

I decided I could never accept that and I was going to do whatever it took to recover fully. I researched which recovery techniques worked the best, and then, with the help of my wife Kathy, I began doing the kinds of exercises we've included in this workbook. Despite my condition and those daunting predictions, I successfully and fully recovered from my stroke. Today, five years later, I am a marathon runner and full-time patent attorney—and I *don't* use a cane! And I *know* from my personal experience that stroke survivors can recover completely and be even better than they were before, *if they do the right things.*

The thing that most stroke survivors probably don't realize is that if they find themselves in the situation I did and *don't* do anything, they run a substantial risk of not recovering. Dr. David Perlmutter, in *The Better Brain Book,* reports that only 10% of stroke survivors return to their normal lives fully recovered. In contrast, 40% of stroke survivors remain mildly disabled, 40% severely disabled, and 10% so disabled that they require nursing home care for the rest of their lives.[i]

Why do so many stroke patients fail to recover fully? As nearly as we can determine, there are two main reasons. The first is that stroke recovery is usually a lengthy process, and insurance-paid rehabilitation in this country ends too soon to permit full recovery for most. As a result, the rehabilitation that is administered in the hospital is designed mainly to restore basic patient self-sufficiency, *not* to bring about full recovery. So after their insurance coverage ends, most stroke survivors find themselves at home, still disabled, with no way to continue their rehabilitation. Often they have the mistaken idea that they can't, or won't, recover further.

The second reason for this discouraging failure rate is that, as hard as it may be to believe, many of the stroke rehabilitation techniques still in use today were developed before scientists learned about the compensatory healing characteristics of the human brain. Based on outdated and discounted principles, the older treatment and rehabilitation methods are still frequently used although they often produce unsatisfactory results.

We bring these facts to your attention to help you understand that you *need to take charge of your own recovery* and *do something about it!* If you don't, nobody else will. The recovery plans and methods contained in this workbook *give you the right things to do* to recover from your stroke, because they are based upon the proven best stroke recovery techniques.

Before you begin your exercise plans, make sure you've gone through all the information presented in Chapters 1 through 8.

Please Contact Us with Your Successes, Suggestions and Stories! We are eager to hear from you. Please let us know if you have good luck in implementing these stroke recovery plans, or if any problem areas crop up you have questions or comments about. We'd also like to know about any other recovery exercises or techniques you have found particularly useful that may not have been included here.

Please email your comments, suggestions and/or stories to strokerecovery@ takingchargebooks.com. Good luck and good recovery!

Part 1:

What You
Need to Know
to Get Started

Chapter 1

Why You Should Take Charge of Your Stroke Recovery

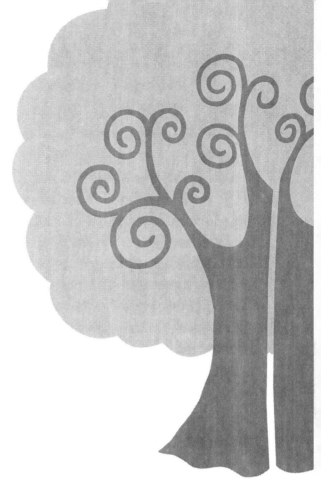

*T*aking charge of your recovery is the best thing you can do. It does not matter how long ago the stroke occurred, how disabled you became, or even whether you feel that you may never recover fully from your stroke—*none* of these things really matter. Anyone CAN recover fully—and that includes YOU. What it takes is your simple decision that you will, and then adopting and sticking with your recovery plans. Follow your recovery plans with dedication and the intention to succeed.

Our Plans are Supported by Scientific Research. Many studies have shown that even people with extensive physical brain damage, whether from disease, injury or surgery, can still function normally with no reduction in their physical or mental abilities.[ii] These people are able to make effective use of their remaining brain structures as well as form new brain pathways to take the place of missing or damaged areas. Scientists call this resilience of the brain "cognitive reserve." The higher someone's cognitive reserve, the better they can function despite brain injury.

This workbook shows how stroke survivors can make the best use of their cognitive reserve—and, we believe, optimize it—through using what have been proven to be the most effective methods of rehabilitation from stroke. A 2003 article in *ScienceDaily* reported on a research study led by Pamela Duncan, Ph.D., then director of the Brooks Center for Rehabilitation Studies in Gainesville, Florida. Dr. Duncan's study consisted of a comprehensive stroke recovery program that concentrated on walking, balance and cardiovascular endurance, plus upper extremity function, supervised by a physical therapist. Dr. Duncan stated, "We demonstrated that by providing a home-based exercise program that's much more aggressive than what is typically prescribed, stroke survivors can improve their walking ability, balance and cardiovascular endurance."[iii]

While *Taking Charge of Your Stroke Recovery: A Personal Recovery Workbook* does not utilize exercises from Dr. Duncan's study, the principle upon which our recovery plans are based is the same. When you do what this workbook suggests, you can expect to begin functioning better as you progress with these recovery plans.

Don't Set Any Limits on Your Recovery. It is important that you not set any limits on how long it will take you to recover or how fully you will be able to recover. (This is one special case where you should not believe *anyone* if they attempt to tell you that you will only be able to recover partway, or that you have a limited time within which to recover.) When you set limits (or accept limits that someone else sets), problems can arise. For example, a woman Roger heard about lost much of her field of vision because of a stroke, and a doctor told her that she had three months to recover her vision or likely would not ever. In three months, her vision hadn't returned, so she became depressed and went on antidepressant drugs. Then, in six months, her normal field of vision came back—which was wonderful—but in the meantime she had become dependent on the antidepressants and it was very hard for her to get off them.

That was an example of how people can make things worse by imposing or accepting limits on their recovery. It is nearly impossible for anyone—even doctors— to forecast or determine how long any individual's recovery will take or how fully they will recover. It takes a different amount of time for each person to recover—so just work at it until you have succeeded.

Take Action Toward Your Recovery. We believe that it is far better to *take action toward your recovery* than to take medications, many of which have very bad side effects. Because we cannot dispense medical advice, however, be sure to consult with your doctors if you are taking medications that you feel may not be necessary or are affecting you negatively, and ask them to help you ease off the drugs safely.

Intention and Recovery. Experts in various healthcare and self-improvement fields believe that human intention and determination can positively affect bodily injuries. Everyone has heard of a seriously ill person who never gave up their determination to get better and who did finally recover in spite of all odds against them. By adopting these stroke recovery plans and working intensively on them, you are telling your body and brain what you want them to do, and *making* them do it with practice and exercise. That is how you will restore your body's capabilities.

As you work on your recovery plans with strong determination to successfully recover, you *will* start to recover, just as Roger did. You will be turning the tide on what might otherwise have been ever-decreasing activity and function. By deciding to adopt these recovery plans and working on them, you should feel yourself becoming more energetic, happier and more "alive." You should experience increasing satisfaction and enjoyment in life as you progress.

Expenses. To make the stroke recovery plans in this workbook as effective and convenient as possible, some plans have been designed to take advantage of the skills and expertise of professionals, as well as the health club and gym facilities that are available in nearly every community. This will require that you incur some expenses. Because taking charge of your stroke recovery is one of the most worthwhile things you can do for yourself, we encourage you to find a way to afford these expenses so you can move forward with your stroke recovery—even if it stretches your budget somewhat! Here are the main items of stroke recovery expense you can expect to incur through adopting these recovery plans:

Expenses for Walking Plans (Recovery Plans 1-5)

1. Health Club. All of the walking plans require you to join a health club or gym. Membership fees vary a great deal and some clubs offer monthly rates or monthly payment plans if you don't want to purchase an entire year's membership in advance. Often you can find a local health club with very reasonable membership fees.

---

2. Personal Athletic Trainer. Beginning walkers will need to hire a personal athletic trainer for two sessions a week. While several walking plans don't require you to hire a trainer, those are for more independent stroke survivors. We suggest that all stroke survivors complete Recovery Plan 1 with a personal trainer before attempting a more advanced walking recovery plan on their own.

3. Yoga Class or Instructor. If your health club does not offer yoga classes that are included in the membership fee, you will need to locate a yoga facility where you can sign up for one class a week. (Many if not most health clubs do offer yoga classes, however, so try to find such a club.)

Expenses for Other Plans

1. Speech Therapist. Those who undertake the speaking recovery plan will need to hire a speech therapist for two sessions a week. Additionally, those who undertake the swallowing recovery plan have the option of hiring a speech therapist to help them improve their swallowing in conjunction with doing the exercises in the plan. Speak with your selected therapist to determine the most appropriate schedule and times per week for swallowing work.

We feel the expertise that a speech therapist can exercise on your behalf is very much worth the expense. We also understand that many stroke survivors have limited budgets. It is very possible that you'll be able to locate a speech therapy student at a local college or university who will work with you for a reduced fee or even just for the experience. Check with your local colleges. (A benefit to finding a student is that he or she will likely be working with the latest materials and theories.) You might also be able to find a speech therapist just returning to practice after an extended break who is eager to do good work to reestablish herself; such a therapist might be willing to work with you for less than the going rate.

Also, if you worked with a speech therapist while in the hospital, he or she likely provided you with printed hand-outs, forms and exercises—sounds and words to practice, and specially written paragraphs to read. If you have such materials, work with them as well as doing what is suggested in our speech recovery plan.

2. Household, Craft and Athletic Items. Other recovery plans require that you use or purchase inexpensive household items, craft supplies, or simple sports or athletic devices such as balls, a hand gripper, and a metronome (for pacing yourself as you walk). Check the plans you expect to undertake to see what items you'll need to get. You won't have to buy everything at once—just what you need so you can work on your current recovery plans.

3. Nutritional Supplements. Finally, you will need to purchase nutritional supplements based on the nutrients you select for your Nutritional Improvement Plan.

An Expensive Option—Hyperbaric Oxygen Treatments

If you have ample money to devote to your stroke recovery, you may want to try this technique. Many scientists have observed that people experience remarkable recovery from stroke (and other ailments) by flooding their cells with oxygen in a hyperbaric chamber. We don't recommend this technique across the board because hyperbaric chambers are not easy to locate and the cost for their use is high. However, if you are willing and able to spend more than a few thousand dollars on your stroke recovery, hyperbaric oxygen treatments may be worth looking into.

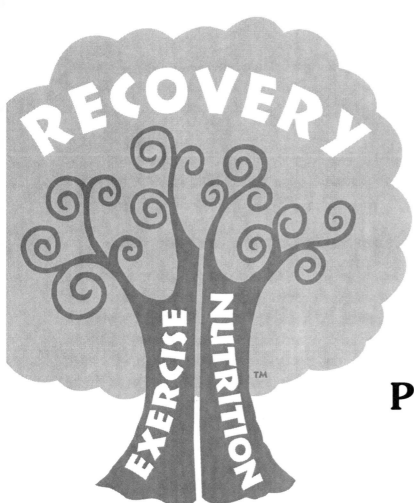

Chapter 2

The Main Parts of Your Recovery Program

Our Recovery Workbook tree logo illustrates the process of recovery—that is, the simple actions that lead to recovery. Your overall stroke recovery program needs to have two parts—EXERCISE and NUTRITION. The exercise part can consist of one or more of the recovery plans presented in this workbook to help you improve physical and mental abilities and functions—or it could include a special recovery plan you develop yourself, or one which has been given to you by a health advisor. The nutrition part is the nutrition plan presented in this book.

1. Exercise. The exercise part of your recovery plans aims to help you become able to again do physical things such as walk, talk and see, and to rehabilitate mental abilities such as comprehension and thinking. Just as you have always developed and improved your ability to do things by "practicing" them—getting better at doing things each time you do them—the same principle applies here. *You get better at doing things by actually doing them.* Also, the exercise recovery plans provided in this workbook require that you work on all aspects of the desired ability so that nothing is missed. When you break down each function or ability into its parts and practice each one, you end up being able to do the entire function too.

2. Nutrition. The nutrition part is designed to make sure that you have everything your body needs to recover. It would not make sense for you to make recovery harder (or impossible) by depriving yourself of some helpful (or critical) nutrient. Good nutrition for your brain is overwhelmingly helpful. Scientists say that your brain can make 100 trillion decisions every second! Good nutrition allows you to think clearly and use your brain to make good decisions. Also, your brain is incredibly sensitive. Just as cutting off oxygen to your brain for 10 seconds can cause you to lose consciousness, the absence—or presence—of certain nutrients has a virtually instantaneous effect on your brain. In fact, some nutrients measurably increase the oxygenation ability of all your cells, including your brain cells. When you implement the nutrition plan in this workbook, you will immediately affect your brain for the better!

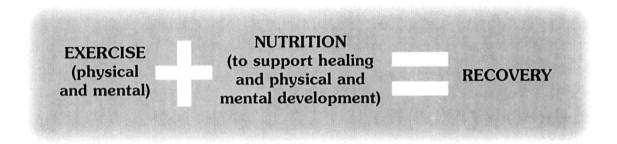

EXERCISE (physical and mental) **+** **NUTRITION** (to support healing and physical and mental development) **=** **RECOVERY**

Stroke Recovery Basics. You can make sure your recovery plans work by carrying out your exercises according to the general guidelines given below. We call them "Stroke Recovery Basics." These recovery basics tell you *how* to do your exercises so they are most effective.

Exercising **intensively**, **aggressively** and **repetitively**, with **increasing difficulty** has been proven to be the most successful method for stroke patients in recovery and rehabilitation programs.[iv] In fact, if people don't push themselves to do their recovery exercises intensively, aggressively and repetitively, they increase the risk of becoming part of the large statistic of stroke patients who fail to recover fully.

The First Recovery Basic

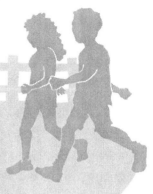

All your work must be INTENSIVE, AGGRESSIVE and REPETITIVE, with INCREASING DIFFICULTY

Hundreds of thousands of years of evolutionary experience have shown humans what kind of practice is successful in allowing us to improve ourselves and gain new skills. When we practice something—whether it be to learn the piano, to learn to walk as a baby, or to learn to figure-skate professionally—we are most successful when we practice intensively, aggressively and repetitively. Since you want to improve and recover from your stroke, you've got to work intensively, aggressively, and repetitively on your recovery exercises, and do them with increasing difficulty. In this recovery workbook, this principle applies mainly to your physical exercises, but it is a valid principle for mental exercises and tasks that use a combination of mental and physical skills as well.

Here is what we mean by these words:

INTENSIVE means **thorough, concentrated, rigorous, performed with constant attention,** and **done consistently.** For your exercises, it would mean that you adhere to your exercise schedule, so you are doing every exercise you are supposed to be doing, on the days and at the times it is scheduled. It is this consistency of doing your exercises as often as each plan's schedule requires that will eventually retrain your body to operate the way you want it to. Also, while you are doing your exercises, you should concentrate on what you are doing. Focus your attention on the exercise (don't daydream), and endeavor to control your motions so they are as normal as you can make them. Do them as well as you possibly can—perfectly if possible. Ultimately you will be able to do each action without giving it much thought, but for now, always *concentrate on the exercise you are doing and try to do it right.*

In contrast to that, *nonintensive* exercise would mean that you would do it randomly, irregularly, or whenever you felt like it. It would also be doing it lazily or slowly, uncaring

---

whether you did it well or not. You wouldn't even bother to maintain the proper form (position of your body) for each exercise while you exercised. You would probably injure yourself pretty fast and your stroke recovery would slow or stop!

AGGRESSIVE means **with energy, forcefully, pushing vigorously to accomplish something, self-assertive**. For your exercises, it means that you push yourself and muster the energy to make every movement as perfectly and completely as you can. Never stop trying to perform a certain movement or action just because you encounter pain or resistance, or feel somewhat tired. Many people, if they encounter pain when exercising, stop dead and don't persist in spite of it. Unfortunately, recovering from stroke can be an unavoidably painful experience in many ways—so can retraining your body! Don't push so hard that you injure yourself, but do try to go further than just the point when you begin to feel some discomfort. As you exercise, force your body to do MORE than it currently can! That's the only way you will INCREASE your strength, range of movement and flexibility.

Aggressive also means that you **never skip an exercise session because your energy is low**. Force yourself to exercise regularly, and perform all the movements as well as you can. This is how you will eventually increase your strength and endurance, and become able to perform movements better and better while encountering fewer and fewer limitations. So never let any limitations stop you from continuing to practice what you need to practice to become 100% normal.

Also, a word to the wise—never become satisfied or complacent because you have developed so-called "compensatory movements"—this is where you become good at using an alternative means of doing something to avoid doing something else that is hard to do. (An example is using your left hand more because it is so difficult to use your right hand, or becoming good with a wheelchair to avoid walking). If you keep relying on compensatory movements, they will become crutches that prevent you from regaining the normal use of your body!

**Effective Exercise to Recover Lost Functions
Consists of Work That is
INTENSIVE + AGGRESSIVE + REPETITIVE
+ INCREASES IN DIFFICULTY**

REPETITIVE means that you **practice the exercise again and again so that eventually each motion and function becomes second nature to you once more.** Doing your exercises repetitively causes your brain, your muscles and your nerves all to absorb and learn and create new paths to do all the jobs and functions you need them to do. Repetitive exercise works hand-in-hand with intensive, consistent exercise as described above. If your daily exercise periods are too short, if you are not focused on what you are doing, or if your exercise days are too far apart, you will receive less benefit because you won't be repeating the exercises often enough to benefit yourself. It is the repetition of desired movements (through exercises) in combination with the consistency of exercise, day after day and week after week, that retrains your body to do what you want it to.

WORKING WITH INCREASING DIFFICULTY means that **as you improve, you should increase the difficulty of the exercise so that your body is forced to improve even more.** Research has shown that increasing the demand of performance, such as increasing treadmill speed, increases the effectiveness of the exercise therapy.[v] This principle was also covered under the "Aggressive" heading above: as you exercise, force your body to do MORE than it currently can. That's the only way you will INCREASE your strength, range of movement and flexibility.

Examples of increasing the difficulty include increasing the speed of the treadmill every day or week, and increasing the length of time you walk on the treadmill. It means increasing the weight on a weight machine when the exercise begins to seem easy at the current weight you are using. Work with your personal trainer to make sure that you continue to increase the difficulty of your exercises as you progress.

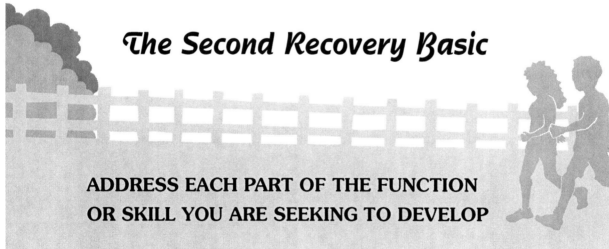

The Second Recovery Basic

ADDRESS EACH PART OF THE FUNCTION OR SKILL YOU ARE SEEKING TO DEVELOP

The second requirement for a good stroke recovery plan is for you to **ADDRESS EACH PART OF THE FUNCTION YOU ARE SEEKING TO DEVELOP**. Prior to your stroke, you were used to performing all kinds of actions smoothly and easily, without thought. Breaking down each function into its component parts can seem slow or monotonous in contrast. But addressing each part of a function directly is the most effective method and makes the most sense.

A good example of practicing components of a skill is the way a beginning guitarist learns to play: first she practices playing single notes. Then she practices simple chords (combinations of notes) over and over again. Then she learns and practices playing more notes and more difficult chords repetitively. By practicing them over and over again, these movements become very smooth and natural. Eventually the guitarist is able to combine whatever chords and notes are necessary to play complex or difficult songs.

The recovery plans you find in this workbook break down many important functions and abilities into their component parts so each part can be practiced separately.

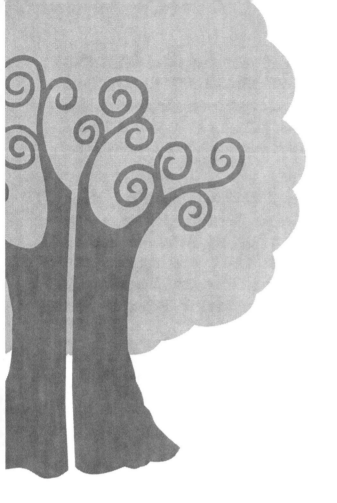

Chapter 3

How to Select and Use the Recovery Plans and the Weekly and Daily Worksheets

This workbook is designed to allow you to organize your stroke recovery by selecting the plan or plans you want to adopt and keeping records of all your recovery work. You can also write down your progress, improvements and successes on the Start of Week Worksheets and Daily Worksheets. Each Daily Worksheet has space for you to record progress on up to four recovery plans at a time (one walking plan, two other plans, and the nutrition plan), for three months (13 weeks) of work. Each recovery plan is self-contained, meaning that it contains all the information you will need to complete that plan without referring to other recovery plans.

Here are the steps you should follow to get going with your stroke recovery plans.

---

1. Finish Reading Part I (Chapters 1 through 8).

Be sure to read all information and instructions before beginning your recovery plans.

2. Read the Following Guidelines for Selecting a Walking Plan.

Walking is a skill that can take many months to rehabilitate, and initial insurance-paid rehabilitation normally does not last long enough to allow the average person to fully recover his or her walking ability. For personal freedom and independence, walking is essential, so if you lost the ability to walk after your stroke, you are going to need and want to take charge of your stroke recovery to get it back. These plans will tell you exactly what to do. If you want to become a marathon runner like Roger, you can do that, or you may just want to be able to walk anywhere you want without falling. You can do that too. You can do whatever seems like the best choice for yourself.

This book contains five different walking recovery plans (Recovery Plans 1-5). Each plan is designed to rehabilitate your ability to walk independently. The more advanced plans improve your walking skills even further. These walking plans suit people of differing capabilities and exercise tolerances, so no matter what your individual abilities and preferences, there should be one you can do. Plans 1 and 2 are easier than 3, 4 and 5.

There may be more than one walking plan that is appropriate for you because there is some built-in overlap in who can do them. So if, for example, you are a average or moderately active woman (or were before your stroke), you should look through the plans themselves to see which one seems best for you. The Recovery Plan Selection Chart which follows Chapter 8 shows the main differences between the plans, the prerequisites for each one and who it is for.

Walking Plans 2, 3 and 5 each contain several separate resistance training (weight training) workout sections for people of differing physical strength. If you are doing one of these walking plans, be sure you start with the resistance training workout most suited to your capabilities and strength and don't select one that is too difficult. As explained further below, we strongly recommend that everyone begin with Recovery Plan 1 so you can work out at a gym or health club with a personal trainer to get you going, guide you and ensure your safety as you exercise. And if you are a senior with limited physical strength, you should certainly select Recovery Plan 1.

**WE RECOMMEND THAT ALL BEGINNING
WALKERS START WITH
WALKING RECOVERY PLAN 1**

3. Select Your Recovery Plans.

a. Complete the Initial Self-Test and Abilities Assessment. Chapter 6 consists of an informal, practical "Initial Self-Test and Abilities Assessment" that you can use to help determine your current status in the skills of walking, use of your hands, speaking, thinking, vision, and swallowing. This assessment can help you determine which recovery plans you want to adopt. Completing this self-test is optional. If you don't wish to use it, you may just skip to step (b) below.

b. Review the "Selection Chart of Stroke Recovery Plans" in Chapter 7. This chart shows you what recovery plans are available and the main features and requirements of each one. Use the chart to find and select those plans that seem best for you to start with. Most people will begin by picking a walking plan and the nutrition plan. Those stroke survivors who feel more energetic or who wish to progress more rapidly may pick one or two additional plans so they can work on rehabilitating additional skills at the same time. Place a checkmark in the checkbox in the left-hand column of the Selection Chart next to each plan you are interested in starting. (As you go through the Selection Chart, refer, if necessary, to the checkmarks and answers in your Initial Abilities Assessment that indicate the skills and abilities you want to work on.)

Recovery plans 13 and 14 are blank plans—essentially "blank slates"—where you can develop and insert your own custom recovery plans if you wish. Recovery plans 15 and 16 are also blank plans into which you can insert exercises and workout programs that may be given to you by your health advisors. After you write down the exercises on the blank forms provided, you will be able to utilize these plans exactly like the exercise plans already provided in this workbook.

4. Select and Purchase Your Supplements for Your Nutrition Plan.

Review the information in the "Detailed Stroke Recovery Nutrient Information and Selection Table" starting on page 154 and check off which supplements you will purchase and begin taking. If you are taking medications, consult with your doctor to avoid any conflicts between supplements and medicines. (Also find out from your doctor or healthcare advisor what your weight should be, so if you are overweight, you can plan to lose weight while you do your recovery plans). Purchase your supplements at a good health food store or over the Internet (which frequently has better prices than regular stores) and look for the highest quality available. And, of course, purchase high-nutrition foods and groceries as recommended in the Nutrient Selection Table.

Try to find fish oil supplements that have been distilled or purified to remove contaminants like mercury and other toxins, or are made from fish wild caught and certified to be low in mercury and other contaminants. ①

Each day, on your Daily Worksheet, record what nutritional supplements you take and what nutrient-rich foods you eat. You can compare your daily record to the nutrition chart to make sure that you are getting every nutrient you need. If you find you missed selecting a nutrient you need, add it to your nutrition plan.

5. Get Ready to Start.

a. See Your Doctor for Approval of Your Exercise Plan. If you have not already done so, have an appointment with your doctor and bring along your Workbook. Get the doctor's approval for all physical exercises you will be doing. Be sure to find out if there is a maximum heart rate you shouldn't exceed as you do your walking and cardio exercises.

b. Equipment and Supplies. Get organized by obtaining any equipment and supplies you will need, as noted in your selected plans under "Equipment or Supplies to Buy." (If you will be working at a health club or gym, you will not need to purchase very much equipment.) For all walking plans you will need a scale to monitor your

---

① NutriWest makes such products and they can be ordered online from various websites. Also, though not an absolute requirement for this plan, many health advisers consider vitamins, minerals and other nutrients that have been extracted or derived from whole food sources to be more effective than vitamins synthesized in a laboratory (USP), so you may want to look for them. NutriWest, available online at www.Bayho.com, also offers such supplements.

weight and a blood pressure cuff to monitor your blood pressure. A variety of blood pressure cuffs are available that fit onto your arm or wrist and inflate automatically, making them very easy to use. At the first opportunity, compare the reading of your blood pressure cuff to the reading of the equipment at your doctor's office to make sure your own cuff's reading is the same as your doctor's. If it is not, calibrate it according to instructions, or if it contains no calibration feature, add or subtract the appropriate numbers from each reading you do to compensate for the difference between it and your doctor's device.

If your doctor requires it, you will also need to monitor your heart rate during the cardiovascular exercises in each walking recovery plan. Most treadmills, elliptical machines and stair-steppers have heart-rate monitors built in—to use them you just grasp special handlebars containing sensors while you are exercising. However, you may wish to purchase your own heart-rate monitor. While sophisticated and expensive

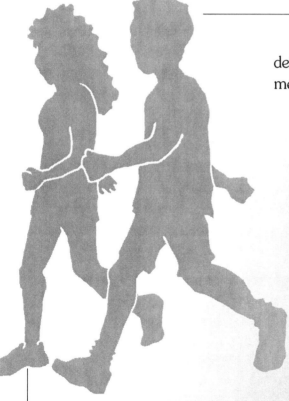

Joining a health club or gym will definitely be worth the extra effort and arrangements you have to make, for these reasons:

- A gym, health club and yoga facility will have much more equipment, of better quality, than most people can afford in their home workout rooms.

- Having to travel to a facility is good practice—it requires you to go places. The ability to travel and move from place to place is one of the attributes and necessities of a good and full life for most people.

- You will be forced to interact with different people at these facilities—interaction that cannot be done alone at home. This interaction makes the brain stronger and gets you using your social skills again.

monitors are available that use a strap fastened around your chest that communicates with a special watch, you can also find small inexpensive electronic pedometers that contain a simple fingertip heart-rate monitor. Refer to the sidebar titled "Measuring Your Heart Rate" on page 24-25 for more information on monitoring your heart rate.

c. Join a Health Club or Gym for Workouts. All of the walking recovery plans, including Recovery Plan 1, the easiest, require you to travel regularly to a gym or health club. With some plans, you work out there with your own personal trainer. With others, you work out on your own. Most communities have smaller health clubs with membership fees that are quite a bit lower than the big-name chain health clubs. However, if you cannot afford any of the clubs in your area, investigate your local YMCA or YWCA. These organizations often have excellent facilities available for very reasonable fees, and they are not limited to use by youth.

d. Hire a Personal Athletic Trainer for Your Workout Sessions. While you could hire a stroke rehabilitation therapist rather than a personal athletic trainer, that can be very expensive. Instead, you should be able to find an excellent personal trainer for much less money who can still provide all the assistance and help you will need. Your health club or gym should have a list of personal trainers affiliated with the club or a list of private trainers they can refer you to. (Most health clubs have exercise staff available who can show you how to use the machines, but they cannot stay with you during your entire workout. You should definitely hire someone who will be dedicated to you and your workout for the entire session.)

While we have included several advanced walking plans for those who can't or don't want to hire a personal trainer, we do suggest that everyone begin with Recovery Plan 1, which requires you to work with a personal trainer. Having a personal trainer to guide your workout offers many immediate advantages. Not only can a trainer teach you how to perform all the exercises correctly, he or she can tailor various exercises for you according to your condition and capabilities. The trainer will make sure you do everything safely, and give you prompt feedback on how you are doing. This will enable you to progress more rapidly and confidently, as well as help you learn to exercise by yourself later when you are ready. You probably already worked with a rehab therapist in the hospital after your stroke—working with a personal athletic trainer is very similar.

When you talk to personal trainers, let them know you are doing a stroke recovery exercise plan and ask if they are interested in and able to help you with your stroke

---

rehabilitation exercises. The trainer you select should understand how to work with and help someone with limited mobility and physical functions.

e. Sign Up for a Yoga Class. We have included yoga classes in all five walking plans. As a stroke survivor, it is important that you work with a certified yoga instructor rather than with a DVD or video, because a DVD cannot offer the personal instruction, instant feedback and safety that a live yoga instructor provides. Yoga provides excellent benefits in improving balance and flexibility and it is available widely (including group classes at most gyms and health clubs). Group classes will work fine as long as the instructor understands you are a stroke survivor and is interested in assisting you. If your health club doesn't have yoga classes, you'll need to locate a yoga facility. **②**

We recommend the type called "Iyengar" yoga, because it is more accessible to more people—it is known for being suitable for anyone, and helps improve the structural alignment of the body by using "props" of various kinds (objects) to help beginners more easily assume the positions. Many of its postures involve standing, which can help you develop strong legs and improve circulation, coordination and balance. However, other forms of yoga are also excellent; it is your choice which kind you select. Speak to the instructor of the class about your needs before enrolling.

f. Find an Athletic Track. The more advanced walking plans involve walking at an athletic track. If your walking plan includes it, locate a track that you can easily get to. Often local high schools make their tracks available to the community after school hours or in the evenings, or on weekend days when no sports events are being held. Also, some YMCAs and the larger health clubs have running tracks. If there is absolutely no track available to you in your area, you may walk on a running path, street or sidewalk. Walking on a track is much preferable, though, because your walking lane will be smooth and there will be no interruptions or other reasons to stop, as there may be on a street or sidewalk.

---

② Yoga originated in India as a group of ancient spiritual practices, but today in the United States yoga is mainly used as a form of exercise to improve balance, strength and flexibility. It consists of the practice of assuming postures (positions) called "asanas." In including yoga in your recovery plans, we have no intention to impose a spiritual belief or practice in place of your own, and you are not required to meditate or adhere to any spiritual practice unless you want to. There are actually different types of yoga you could practice that are also excellent (like "Hatha" yoga, "Power" yoga, and "Bikram" yoga). However, if you prefer not to do yoga, you may perform some other exercise for increasing balance and flexibility, like Tai Chi.

---

6. Get Started!

Your Plan. Fill out the "Date Begun" box at the top of your chosen recovery plan(s). Then write down any personal goals you have for the plan in the box provided. Each recovery plan has a 7-day daily schedule that you will follow each week, Monday through Sunday. Each day, do the exercises indicated in the schedule for that day. Each type of exercise in the plan schedule is followed by a bold circled number which corresponds to numbered instructions below it that you can follow.

Start of Week Worksheet. At the start of each week, take your measurements and record your weight and blood pressure on the Start of Week Worksheet, then fill out the rest of the page. (Women will measure and record their waist, hips, upper leg and upper arm; men will measure their waist, chest, upper leg and upper arm.)

Daily Worksheets. Seven Daily Worksheets per week are provided (Monday through Sunday). Look over a blank Daily Worksheet to familiarize yourself with how it is laid out. At the beginning of every day, record your morning weight and blood pressure at the top. (If your blood pressure measures higher than 120 over 80, be sure your doctor knows.) Also write down your maximum heart rate if your doctor has given it to you. If your weight or blood pressure is too high when you begin your recovery plans, you'll be able to watch the numbers improve as you progress with your recovery. If you want to reduce your weight, you can eat less and exercise more, or follow a diet plan of your own choosing—whether given to you by your doctor or published in a diet book.

Each page has room for recording progress on one walking plan, two other recovery plans, and the nutrition plan. Keep in mind your Recovery Basics as you work out and check off which ones you adhered to that day in the box at the bottom left side of your Daily Worksheet. As you work out, write down in the "Walking Plan" column what exercises you did, how many repetitions you completed in each set, what weight was used, and any other statistics the worksheet requests.

As each day progresses, briefly record your meals and snacks, what you drink, and the nutritional supplements and medicines you take, in the appropriate spaces. Writing down your meals and drinks will help to remind you to include in your diet the brain-healthy nutrients suggested in your nutrition plan. These daily records may also prove helpful to your doctor if he or she is monitoring your health. At the top of the sheet there are also circles you can check off to count the glasses of water you drink each day.

Bring Your Workbook With You! Whenever you work out at the health club or track, bring your Recovery Workbook with you so you can record your exercises immediately. That will save you time and also save you from forgetting what you did before you have a chance to write it down. Your workbook will become a complete record of everything you did in your recovery plan. Whenever you want, you can look back on the information entered to see where you were at any past point, or even to remind yourself of what you did recently or on the previous day. Depending on your progress, you will be able to see if you should change or improve anything. You can also use this information to pick or develop future recovery plans.

Record Your Successes and Progress. Be sure to write down, day by day, successes and breakthroughs you experience, as well as other observations that you feel should be recorded. Use the extra notesheet space provided at the back of the workbook if you don't have enough room on the worksheet itself. If you cannot yet write legibly enough to make your workbook entries, have your caregiver or your personal trainer make the notations for you, as it is important that your progress is recorded in your Recovery Workbook. But try to write them yourself, if at all possible, because it will help give you a very real sense of what you are accomplishing each day.

After Thirteen Weeks. Your recovery workbook will take you through approximately three months of work (a total of 13 weeks). In Part 4, at the end of the 13 weeks of Daily Worksheets, you will find the "13-Week Self-Test and Abilities Assessment." This Self-Test will help you evaluate your progress, determine whether you are ready to begin new plans, or whether you want to repeat the same plan or plans so you can make further progress with them. If you have not met your goals for a plan at the end of 13 weeks, you can repeat it for another 13 weeks—or as many times as you wish. Or, if you feel ready, you can graduate up to a more strenuous walking recovery plan.

Chapter 4

Additional Tips and Guidelines

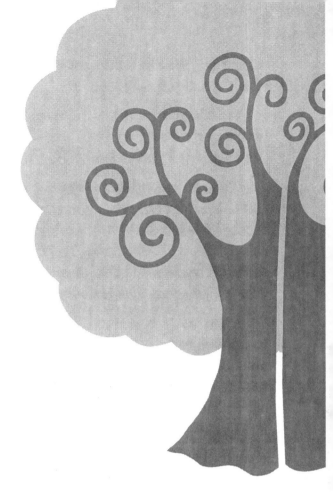

Daily Expectations. Here's an attitude Roger maintained during his recovery which helped him stay upbeat and positive. Even though you know that you will ultimately recover completely, you should maintain fairly low *daily* expectations. Then, regularly, your *actual* progress will exceed your expectations and, as we know, when your experiences are better than your expectations, you feel good about it, rather than stressed or disappointed. Feeling good about your progress and minimizing your stress will make it easier for you to recover.

Practically speaking, how would you apply this attitude to an exercise plan? First, you would make sure your daily exercises aren't so tough that you are likely to not always be able to do them. Next, you would ensure that you are regularly making your exercises just a *little bit* harder, or doing them a *little* longer, or in some other way increasing the difficulty (as in the First Recovery Basic)—but not by so much that you can't do it and can't meet your exercise target for that day! Just do a little more, or make it a little harder than the previous few days or the previous week, so you keep

---

improving. In other words, set things up so you have satisfying daily victories as you work toward recovery.

It also helps to remember that recovery is a gradual process, with each day and week building on the previous days' and weeks' work, so there is no point in stressing out if day-to-day progress seems small. It may *seem* small, but *every* bit of it is necessary.

How to Handle Fatigue. Fatigue can be a large problem for stroke survivors. Not only is your body undergoing an extended healing process which can cause excess tiredness, but pushing it to perform strenuous exercises for several hours each day can definitely be very tiring. You should realize that the exercises which tire you out each day, especially those in your walking plan, are most definitely also *increasing* your overall endurance and strength at the same time.

When you are fatigued, you may have the urge to deal with it by reducing the amount of exercise you do (even to the point of stopping it) and stepping up the amount of high calorie foods (like sweets) that you consume. In other words, you may have the urge to abandon a good exercise and nutrition program. In such a case, your instincts would be absolutely 100% wrong.

Do not let daily tiredness discourage you—instead, realize you are pushing your body to both work and heal faster than if you did nothing. Fatigue will be a natural result of that daily effort. First, make sure you are getting a good, full night's sleep each night. Then, if you perform your exercises to the best of your ability, in the manner recommended, and if you make sure that you are eating a balanced diet and taking all the recommended nutrients to help your body and brain heal and become stronger, you will begin steadily increasing in strength and endurance as your physical functions improve. Even very strong people feel fatigue, so do not take it as a bad sign, but a good one that you are actively taking charge of your recovery!

Another good way to deal with fatigue, if and when you encounter it (besides exercising and eating as usual), is to spread out your activities over several days rather than cramming too much into one day. When you don't try to do too much any particular day, you are most likely to do your best at those things you do undertake. And that—doing the best you can—should be one of your major goals.

A nutritionist may be able to suggest other special nutrients to give you extra support and energy. If at all possible, try to avoid having to take further medicines or drugs (as differentiated from nutritional supplements) because, even though they might eliminate certain symptoms, as a rule they frequently cause *extra* stress and wear on your body, not to mention unwelcome side effects.

The only exception to these suggestions would be if you experience extreme fatigue that does not improve from day to day, even with a full night's rest. A full night's sleep should leave you feeling refreshed and ready to begin again, but if this isn't the case, we suggest you consult your doctor, who can check for the cause. It could be a metabolic or endocrine condition causing extreme fatigue. As an example, low thyroid function, which has become widespread, can lead to a myriad of symptoms and eventual illnesses that are often mistakenly attributed to other causes when the correct diagnosis is missed.[vii] These include chronic fatigue, atherosclerosis, high blood pressure, heart attacks, and diabetes type 2, among others.[viii] ③

Proper Form. To use "proper form" with an exercise means you perform it like it was designed to be performed, with your arms, legs and torso in the exact positions the exercise requires. In addition, make sure the correct muscles being exercised are doing all the work. In other words, don't "cheat yourself" by letting another part of your body do some of the work when it's not supposed to.

To Use Proper Form In Your Resistance Training

- Follow the instructions and diagrams on the exercise machines precisely—they show you how to perform the exercise correctly.

- By doing a warm-up set with a low weight first, you will learn how it feels to perform the exercise correctly. When you increase the weight, do the exercise the exact same way so it feels right.

- If you have any questions about how to use any machine correctly, ask one of the staff in the gym to show you.

---

③ For well-presented information on the often-missed condition of subclinical hypothyroidism, read the book, *Hypothyroidism Type 2: The Epidemic,* by Mark Starr, M.D., or visit Dr. Starr's website at http://www.type2hypothyroidism.com/. Also visit the Broda O. Barnes M.D. Research Foundation Inc. website at http://www.brodabarnes.org.

Measuring Your Heart Rate

Target Heart Rates

Most exercise experts recommend that people doing cardiovascular exercise keep their heart rates within certain limits, called target heart rates, so they can achieve the optimum conditioning results and cardiovascular benefits from their exercises. Target heart rates vary depending on individual factors including age and resting heart rate, and do include minimum heart rates as well as maximum. The minimum value guarantees the person is exercising vigorously enough, and the maximum value ensures the person doesn't exercise too vigorously to be safe.

Heart Rate Measurement for Rehabilitative Exercise

In contrast to the above, stroke survivors such as yourself will be performing cardio-style exercises on the treadmill, elliptical machine, stair-stepper and athletic track primarily for rehabilitative purposes (to regain function in the legs—balance, strength and movement), rather than for pure cardiovascular conditioning. Because of this different purpose, and because

Using proper form, you would make sure the muscles being exercised move through the entire range of movement required by the exercise. (That means you would not stop short or only do a partial version of the exercise by moving less than you are supposed to). Using proper form also means you remain in complete control by always moving smoothly, at the same speed, and not "lurching" through part of the movement or going so fast that momentum makes the weights easier to move. Breathe regularly while exercising, fueling your body with oxygen and warding off fatigue.

If you don't use proper form, you increase your risk of injury and you won't get maximum benefit from your exercises!

Putting it All Together. Being able to perform the complex actions and activities of normal life requires you to be able to perform each of the individual skills that go into each activity. The recovery plans in this workbook will help you

you will be working intentionally at slow speeds for a good part of your cardio workout, it is not necessary or advisable to try to adhere to the standard cardiovascular target heart rate range (usually calculated using a special formula called the Karvonen Formula), unless your doctor advises you to.

Your doctor may, however, want to give you individualized directions for a maximum heart rate, or have you adhere to other guidelines or limits when doing your cardiovascular exercises, due to your current physical or medical condition. Therefore, as recommended elsewhere in this book, you should check with your doctor before beginning your walking plan. If your doctor recommends that you not raise your heart rate above a certain level while exercising, you can monitor it using either the built-in monitors on the equipment or by purchasing a heart-rate monitor, as discussed in Chapter 3 under "Equipment and Supplies."

Advanced Walkers

When your walking has improved markedly and you are capable of walking at greater speeds (as well as with perfect control at slower speeds), you should again have your doctor examine you and provide you with a target heart rate range and/or other guidelines to use during more vigorous cardio exercise.

develop and recover some vital individual skills and functions. As you return to normal functioning, you'll find that you are going to have to use a combination of these individual skills for almost any activity you participate in. We don't just walk, talk, eat, look, think or swallow as separate individual tasks—rather, we use a variety of these skills simultaneously or in rapid succession to perform all kinds of activities. Driving, working, cleaning house, socializing and participating in sports are just a few out of many complex or combination activities that comprise "normal operation." Undertaking these recovery plans is the necessary step that will eventually enable you to put it all together!

Alternatives. Virtually everything about the recovery plans in this book can be modified to best serve your needs. As you work on your plans, ideas and sources for new exercises may come your way that you will want to add to your plans—go for it! You may run into people who recommend different exercises. Those people may be right—or what they say may be OK for them, but not for you. You are the one best equipped to figure out the optimum recovery plan for yourself. Provided you exercise intensively, aggressively, and repetitively, and provided you exercise each component of the skill or function you are seeking to recover, you will recover.

How to Handle Unexpected Events that Take You Off Your Set Recovery Schedule. From time to time something will occur that will prevent you from following your desired exercise and nutrition routine. You may go on a trip and not be able to exercise. You may be ill. You may be at a party where there are no good nutritional choices. In such instances you should recognize that there is also great value in variety and change and you should wholeheartedly embrace its value and not for a minute regret that you aren't following your schedule. When you can, resume your recovery schedule. New, different experiences make you better and stronger.

Chapter 5

Special Tips for Caregivers

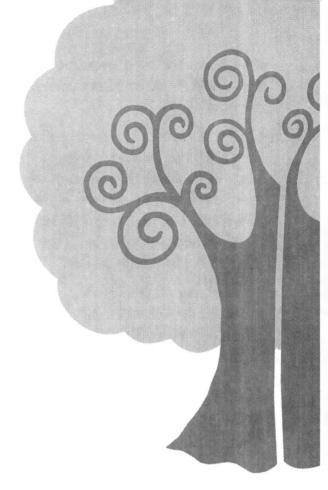

*T*his chapter is for your caregiver(s), whose part in your recovery cannot be underestimated. Your caregiver plays an important role in helping you complete your recovery plans—not only will he or she take you to the health club or gym, the doctor, and the other places you will go during your recovery, but this person will be present and help you during many of your recovery plan exercises and activities. If your caregiver is a spouse or member of your family, he or she will be helping you out of a personal desire to see you improve, but may also be more subject to frustration from not knowing how to deal with various situations they've never had to confront before. Whoever your caregivers are, they can benefit from the tips and suggestions offered here. This chapter is addressed directly to them.

Communication with Your Stroke Survivor. Be patient in your efforts to understand the stroke survivor's communication. You should realize that in many, perhaps most cases, his or her garbled speech is NOT an indication that he or she can no longer think clearly or rationally. It only means that the "connections" between their brain and their speaking muscles have not been reestablished yet. They are very likely *thinking* pretty clearly and have lost none of their intelligence or real personality.

Do whatever you can to allow and help them to get their communications across to you. Don't get angry with them if you can't understand them—just work out a way to help them communicate. And once you understand them, cheerfully acknowledge them so they know you understood what they said! This will bring immense relief and help alleviate the isolation and feeling of being "cut off" that many stroke survivors feel after the loss of their faculties, senses, mobility and their ability to communicate.

Also, you have probably already learned this, but try not to speak "baby talk" to the stroke survivor! People sometimes do this without thinking in their efforts to make themselves understood, but it's not necessary and can feel demeaning to the stroke survivor or give them the idea that you think they have lost their wits. Speak in your normal tone of voice. If your stroke survivor has a diminished sense of hearing, you may need to speak louder to make yourself understood (unless a hearing aid has restored their hearing)—but still make it sound normal, from equal to equal.

Don't Create Increasing Dependence. As your stroke survivor improves, gradually lessen the amount you are doing for them so they don't become more and more dependent. Without outright cruelty, do the minimum to help them so they will come to rely less and less on you. Kathy didn't realize it, but she was hindering Roger's ability to be independent by getting all of his clothes out of the closet to wear each day. The occupational therapist said *he* needed to do that so she could monitor his progress level—and Kathy had thought she was being so helpful! One goal of the stroke survivor is to be able to function as independently as possible, so sometimes you need to show "tough love" and let them try to accomplish something that may be very difficult for them to do (and very easy for you to do for them). But let them try—it will get easier for them, the more times they do it.

Tips for Caregiver Spouses and Family Members. Don't try to "do it all." Caregiving can be very exhausting and you need to set limits for yourself so you don't wear yourself out. You are no good to anyone if you are not feeling yourself. Always give yourself a break. Try to have a friend, family member or a hired sitter come in every week or two to relieve you from your caregiver duties for a while. You need time for yourself to do something simple, yet pleasurable, in order to recharge

For example, for women, satisfying activities can be going to the movies or shopping, gardening or reading a few chapters of a good novel. Treat yourself to a cup of coffee or tea at a coffeehouse; take a long walk in the neighborhood. Try to resume your regular routines of getting out into the community. For the men, do whatever will help you relax—a favorite hobby or sport, a movie, gardening, lunch with a buddy, going to your own health club for a workout, taking the dog for a run, spending an hour at the seashore if it is nearby.

Also take some quiet time for yourself every day to enjoy the "stillness." You can meditate, listen to a relaxation CD, enjoy a beautiful view or vista, pray, sit mindfully, or whatever else you find helps rejuvenate your mind and spirit.

For some people, it works best to keep your attention in the present and focus on getting through the current day only—not to look too far out into the future. For others, it is sustaining to renew your own goals and determination for the recovery of your partner. In any case, remember to realize that you *have* achieved something if you got through the day "pretty well." Each day is one step further on the road to recovery.

Keeping Up Worksheets/Keeping a Journal. Help ensure that your partner keeps up his or her Daily and Start of Week Worksheets in this workbook. It will form a complete record of his or her progress, and it's always reassuring for you as well to look back and see how far they have come in their recovery. You may also want to keep your own journal, in which you can write down your thoughts and feelings, whether positive or negative. Many people find doing this helps them let off steam and renew their purpose to keep going and keep helping the stroke survivor to recover.

Get Assistance. Allow friends and family who offer support to help in whatever ways they can. Do not hesitate to give them suggestions of things they can do that would be helpful to you—most people want to help, but sometimes they don't know exactly what to do. Also, do not hesitate to call your doctor or physical therapists for advice or to talk about a problem you may be having at home. It is better to be safe than sorry!

Disability Parking Placard or License Plates for the Car.

Finally, remember to get the proper disability placard for your car, so it is easier for the stroke survivor to go places with you in the initial stages of recovery. You'll have to research which agency in your area issues them.

Feel free to email us if you have any questions about the recovery plans. Our email address is **strokerecovery@takingchargebooks.com**.

Chapter 6

Initial Self-Test and Abilities Assessment

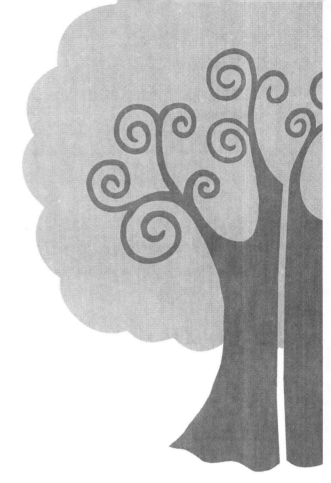

Take these informal, practical self-tests and answer these questions to get an idea of the skills and functions you want to improve. Check the box at the end of each question if you decide you want to work on that skill.

MEASUREMENTS— MEN:	MEASUREMENTS— WOMEN:	WEIGHT:
Waist:_____	Waist:_____	
Chest:_____	Hips:_____	BLOOD PRESSURE:
Upper Leg: _____	Upper Leg:_____	
Upper Arm:_____	Upper Arm:_____	_____ over _____

1. Walking

How far I can walk or run in 10 minutes (on a treadmill or a track or the sidewalk):

_____

How far (or for how long) I can walk without any support: _____

☐ *I want to adopt (or continue with) a walking recovery plan so I can improve on this!*

2. Use of Hands

Paragraph copying:

a. Copy the following paragraph in longhand on the next page.

Taking Charge Books thinks people ARE strong enough to do just about anything and they often need to take charge of things in order to succeed. We collect all the hard-to-track-down information and put everything in one place. Taking Charge Books refuses to accept that something is a "fact" when it has not been proven to be true and we defy "authority" when it is wrong. We show you how to do something even when others have maintained it is impossible. A Taking Charge Book is practical, not theoretical. It tells the reader exactly what to do. Its plans fit into normal budgets and schedules. Taking Charge Books' recovery workbooks are written by people who have successfully recovered. *Taking Charge of Your Stroke Recovery* was designed to help stroke survivors recover even if they thought they had no other options.

My copy of this paragraph:

_____

_____

_____

_____

_____

_____

_____

_____

_____

_____

_____

_____

_____

_____

b.   Now assign your ability to write AND the appearance of the handwriting an overall rating:

O Outstanding   O Very good   O Good   O Fair   O Poor

☐ *I want to adopt an "Improvement of Hand Function" recovery plan so I can write better.*

---

3. Speaking

Answer the following questions:

a.   Has anyone ever commented that some part of my speech is bad or needs improving?

O Yes   O No

If so, what did they say? _____

_____

_____

b.   Have I ever tried to say something (since the stroke) and had difficulty or failed?

O Yes   O No

If so, what sounds, words, phrases or sentences are hard for me to say?

_____

_____

_____

_____

_____

c. Are there certain circumstances that consistently make it hard for me to speak?

_____

_____

_____

d. Can I control my rate of speaking?

      O Yes O Somewhat O No

e. Can I control how loudly and softly I speak?

      O Yes O Somewhat O No

f. Can I vary the pitch of sounds?

      O Yes O Somewhat O No

□ *I want to adopt a speaking recovery plan so I can speak better.*

4. Thinking

Read an article in a newspaper or magazine. A few hours later the same day or the next day, using your recall, tell your caregiver or family member about what you read so they can understand you and use the information you impart.

Am I able to understand things I read and see?	O Yes O Somewhat O No
Can I evaluate the information I obtain?	O Yes O Somewhat O No
Can I use information that I read and see?	O Yes O Somewhat O No
Can I convey information to others?	O Yes O Somewhat O No

☐ *I want to adopt a thinking recovery plan so I can think better!*

5. Vision

a. Go outside with a book to a place where you can see a street sign that is some distance away from you. Hold the book. Look at the book. Look at the street sign.

Am I satisfied with my ability to detect details?　　　O Yes　　O No

Am I satisfied with the rate at which my eyes focus on things?

O Yes　　O No

b. Stare at the street sign. See how far around it you can see things without moving your eyes from it.

Are you satisfied with your field of vision?　　　O Yes　　O No

c. Go to a fairly busy intersection. Look at the moving traffic. Imagine how you would react to that traffic and test yourself with two possible responses: (1) Each time a car moving in one direction passes a specific point you select beforehand, try to immediately close your hand. (2) At the same time, watch for each time a car passes a second point, and immediately make a *different* small movement of your hand. Do this test for about 5 minutes, then answer these questions:

Are you satisfied with how quickly you can react to something you see?

O Yes　　O No

Are you certain that you would react "properly" to it?

O Yes　　O No

☐ *I want to adopt a vision recovery plan so I can see better!*

6. Eating, Drinking and Swallowing

a. General eating and drinking difficulties I have:

O Not being able to chew items well

O Not being able to move things back and down the right "pipe"

O Not being able to keep food down

b. Foods and drinks I have difficulty with:

Difficult foods	
Difficult drinks	

[ ] *I want to adopt a swallowing recovery plan so I can swallow better!*

7. Single-Sided Weakness

Which areas of my body have single-sided weakness, numbness or tingling?

_____

_____

_____

_____

_____

☐ *I want to adopt a single-sided weakness recovery plan to reduce my single-sided weakness and improve my function in those areas of my body!*

8. Other Functions/Skills I Want to Improve (Optional)

Write down the additional functions and skills you want to improve in blank Recovery Plans 13 and 14. Locate or develop exercises you will undertake to work on these abilities and write them into your plans and the weekly schedule. Photocopy the blank plan form if you need more space or additional blank Self-selected Recovery Plans.

9. Functions/Skills My Therapist or Healthcare Advisor Suggests I Need to Work On (Optional)

In blank Recovery Plans 15 and 16, write down the additional functions and skills your healthcare advisor has suggested you work on. Then write out the exercises and weekly schedule you will adopt to work on these abilities. Photocopy a blank plan if you need more space.

Chapter 7

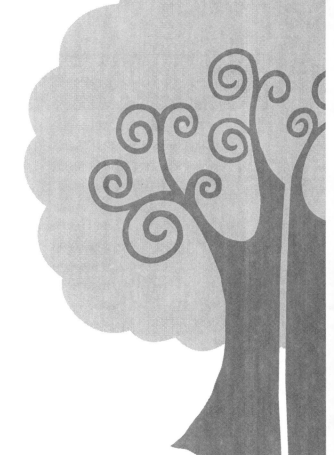

Selection Chart of Stroke Recovery Plans

*I*n the left-hand column, mark the checkbox of each plan as you select it. We recommend that everyone select and do Plan 12—Improvement of Nutrition.

PLAN NO.	GOAL	WHO IT'S FOR	MAIN PREREQUISITES	SPECIAL FEATURES
WALKING PLANS 1 THROUGH 5				
1 PAGE 53	To recover ability to walk without any mechanical aid	Complete beginners: Inactive or nonathletic men and women; Average or moderately active men and women; Seniors	Capable of walking with a walker Note: This plan is suggested for all stroke survivors just home from the hospital as the best beginner walking recovery plan.	Hire personal trainer Must travel to health club 2x week (and to yoga facility 1x week)

PLAN NO.	GOAL	WHO IT'S FOR	MAIN PREREQUISITES	SPECIAL FEATURES
2 PAGE 58	To recover ability to walk without any mechanical aid	More independent beginners: Inactive, nonathletic men and women, or Average, moderately active men and women; or Active, strong or athletic men and women; or someone who has completed Walking Plan 1	Capable of walking with a walker Must be able to work out by oneself at gym/health club: move from one fixed-weight machine to another and set and adjust weight machines by oneself	No personal trainer For someone who would like to do all the strength training on his or her own but still be as safe as possible Must travel to health club 2x week (and to yoga facility 1x week)
3 PAGE 72	To recover ability to walk without any mechanical aid	Independent advanced beginners: Average or moderately active men and women, Active, athletic men and women; or Someone who has completed Walking Plan 1 or 2	Capable of walking with a walker Must be able to work out by oneself at gym/health club: move from one fixed-weight machine to another and set and adjust weight machines by oneself	No personal trainer For someone would like to do strength training on his or her own but still be as safe as possible Must travel to health club and yoga facility regularly Cardio workouts in health club 3 ways: on treadmill, elliptical and stair-stepper machines Person interested in becoming able to perform yoga on their own.

PLAN NO.	GOAL	WHO IT'S FOR	MAIN PREREQUISITES	SPECIAL FEATURES
4 PAGE 85	To recover ability to walk without any mechanical aid	Independent Active or Athletic Person: An active or athletic person; or Someone who has completed Walking Plan 3	Capable of walking with a cane Must be able to work out by oneself at gym/ health club: move from one fixed-weight machine to another and set and adjust weight machines by oneself Able to get to athletic track and walk there on one's own	Hire personal trainer Cardio workouts in health club on elliptical and stair-stepping machines Resistance/weight training 4x week Cardio walking at an athletic track
5 PAGE 92	To walk perfectly without any mechanical aid whatsoever— in fact, better than virtually anyone else	Strong, Active, Athletic and Independent Person: Very strong, athletic person who wants to do all strength training on his or her own, or Has graduated from having a personal trainer on hand to watch him or her exercise, or Has completed Walking Plan 4	Capable of walking without mechanical aid Must be able to work out by oneself at gym/ health club Must be able to move from one fixed-weight machine to another and set and adjust weight machines by oneself Able to get to athletic track and walk there on one's own	Introduces the person to special exercises to spur greater and faster improvement in walking functionality. This plan is very intensive and aggressive. Resistance/weight training 3x week Eclectic workout 1x week Cardio walking at an athletic track 5x week Designed to also help someone begin to become able to perform yoga on their own.

PLAN NO.	GOAL	WHO IT'S FOR	MAIN PREREQUISITES	SPECIAL FEATURES
RECOVERY PLAN 6—IMPROVEMENT OF HAND FUNCTION				
6 PAGE 102	To use the hands perfectly	Anyone who wants to use their hands better (writing, pressing buttons, typing, etc.)	No special requirements except desire to be able to use one's hands for anything one wishes, normally and proficiently	No trainer or assistant needed Trains for strength (strong muscles to function); positioning control (able to put one's hands and body in place to accomplish a task); balance (able to hold objects for use); and perceptual skill (hand-eye coordination)
RECOVERY PLAN 7—ABILITY TO SPEAK WELL				
7 PAGE 109	To become fluent in speaking so you can speak perfectly normally	Anyone who wants to improve their speaking ability and become fluent with their speech	Anyone who is capable of making sounds Anyone who wants to recover their ability to speak clearly and naturally and to be able to easily make himself or herself understood	Hire a speech therapist Trains articulation (ability to form word sounds); intonation (to vary pitch); rate (to speak at varying speeds); and intensity (to vary loudness) Note: If you also have swallowing difficulties, you can ask your speech therapist to help you improve your swallowing too, as that is one of a speech therapist's special skills and they *(continued, p. 43)*

PLAN NO.	GOAL	WHO IT'S FOR	MAIN PREREQUISITES	SPECIAL FEATURES
				(cont.'d from p. 42) have many ways to help. You may want to do this instead of undertaking Plan 10.

RECOVERY PLAN 8—THINKING SKILLS

PLAN NO.	GOAL	WHO IT'S FOR	MAIN PREREQUISITES	SPECIAL FEATURES
8 PAGE 115	To think more clearly, improve memory; improve ability to recall, compare, classify, infer, generalize, evaluate, experiment, and analyze	Anyone who wants to think better	Time available to do these exercises and drills uninterrupted	No hired instructor needed

RECOVERY PLAN 9—VISION AND ABILITY TO USE YOUR EYES BETTER

PLAN NO.	GOAL	WHO IT'S FOR	MAIN PREREQUISITES	SPECIAL FEATURES
9 PAGE 123	To see better, to perceive details both near and far better	Anyone who wants to see better	Make sure you have up-to-date prescription eyeglasses, if you need them, for both close and distance vision Make sure you have other vision aids, such as prisms to correct double vision, if your doctor has recommended them	No hired instructor needed Components trained are those involved with hand-eye coordination; visual reaction time; focusing and peripheral vision

PLAN NO.	GOAL	WHO IT'S FOR	MAIN PREREQUISITES	SPECIAL FEATURES
RECOVERY PLAN 10—ABILITY TO EAT, DRINK AND SWALLOW NORMALLY				
10 PAGE 128	To swallow better	Anyone who needs and wants to improve their ability to swallow	Make sure that you always have someone around you, watching you when you eat or drink anything. If you have a swallowing problem, it is critical that you swallow safely. If a problem develops that you cannot deal with, that person can act immediately. You must not have anything restricting or blocking your food passage that will interfere with swallowing, such as a food tube.	Unnecessary to hire a therapist to do this plan, but you should know that speech therapists are trained to deal with swallowing problems, so you may wish to hire one or use the speech therapist you are hiring for Plan 7, Speaking. Important: must have a caregiver or other assistant present when eating or drinking anything. You will need to have food and drink of varying consistencies available for these exercises.
RECOVERY PLAN 11—SINGLE-SIDED WEAKNESS				
11 PAGE 135	To eliminate single-sided weakness	Anyone who has a weak face, arm, or leg One side of your body – perhaps an arm, a leg, or your face – "tingles," is	None.	Alleviates single-sided weakness of the face, hand, arm or leg – trains components of facial muscle strengthening; hand, arm and leg strength training; hand

PLAN NO.	GOAL	WHO IT'S FOR	MAIN PREREQUISITES	SPECIAL FEATURES
		numb, or doesn't act or respond like you want it to		positioning control; hand-eye coordination; cardio walking; resistance training; balance. Hire personal trainer. Depending on what function you are working on, some must travel to health club, to yoga facility, or to athletic track.
RECOVERY PLAN 12—IMPROVEMENT OF NUTRITION				
12 PAGE 149	To get every nutrient needed to support brain function	Anyone who wants to improve brain health and function as well as overall health	Every stroke survivor. Have no conflicting food or nutrient allergies. Have no drug conflicts (see Special Features column).	Go through the Supplement Quick Selection List first to pinpoint the areas in which you want to improve your nutrition. Go to the Detailed Stroke Recovery Nutrient Information & Selection Table to look up the nutrients you want detailed information about. Take the checked list to your doctor and get his or her approval of each nutrient you want

PLAN NO.	GOAL	WHO IT'S FOR	MAIN PREREQUISITES	SPECIAL FEATURES
				to take. When you have your doctor's approval, put a check in the appropriate boxes (and mark "no" if your doctor disapproves any, so you have a record of which ones not to get). Purchase your supplements from a good health food store or an internet vendor such as www.vitacost.com. As time passes, monitor your supplies and don't let yourself run out. Follow the instructions listed in the nutrition plan itself.

Chapter 8

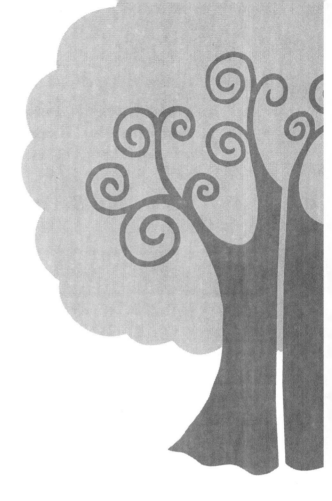

Recovery Affirmations

An affirmation is a statement of desirable intention or condition about yourself, your family, friends, or any aspect of the world. When Roger was in the hospital, Kathy wrote out affirmative statements that she read to him every day—for example, "You are able to run around White Rock Lake" (a 10-mile run), and "You can eat or drink anything you want." This was when he was in hospital rehab and not able to walk or swallow. In the authors' experience, when affirmations are deliberately contemplated and/or repeated, they more easily become firm intentions that you fix in your mind and consciousness. Affirmations mobilize your inner resources. Affirmations become fact. Affirmations are an effective way to utilize and realize the power of positive intention.

A good affirmation is phrased in the first person and the present tense (I am) rather than the future tense (I will). For example, "I have the strength and willpower to do what I need to do to completely recover from stroke." However, until you can state your own affirmations, your caregiver may say them to you using "you" just as Kathy did for Roger.

Here are some of the affirmations Kathy used with Roger, and which you should feel free to use, in addition to writing out your own in the space below:

"I am in perfect health in mind, body and soul."

"I choose joy and abundance at all times."

"I freely forgive everyone, including myself."

My Recovery Affirmations

_____

_____

_____

_____

_____

_____

_____

_____

_____

_____

_____

My Recovery Affirmations (continued)

_____

_____

_____

_____

_____

_____

_____

_____

_____

_____

_____

_____

_____

Part 2:

Stroke Recovery Plans

Recovery Plan 1

Ability to Walk Without Mechanical Aid

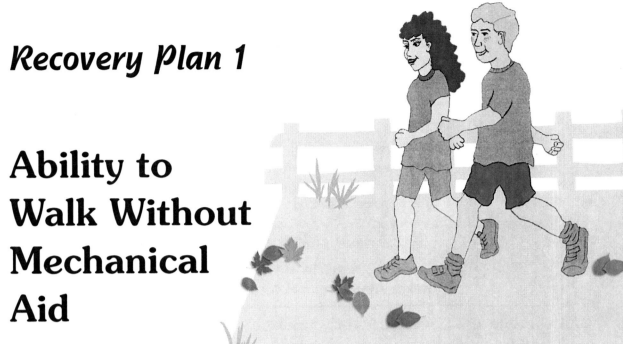

(For Beginners)

Date Begun:	Date Finished:	Repeat Dates:	Start:	Finish:
Goal:	To recover the ability to walk without using any mechanical aid (like a walker or a cane).			
My Personal Goals for this Plan:				
Who Plan is For:	**Complete beginners.** Anyone who can walk with a walker: average or nonathletic men and women; senior stroke survivors.			
Location:	A health club or gym for resistance training and access to a treadmill; a yoga facility for yoga (or group yoga class held at the same health club).			

People to Hire:	(1) A personal trainer (for two sessions a week). This person should be capable of and interested in working with a stroke survivor and able to design an appropriate workout for people of varying physical abilities.
	(2) A certified yoga instructor (for one session a week), or a group yoga class at your health club. The yoga instructor should be capable of and interested in working with a stroke survivor.
Special Requirements, Information or Features:	This plan requires you to travel regularly to a gym or health club (and a yoga facility if no classes at your health club), and to work with your personal trainer (and yoga instructor).
	Important Note: To ensure your safety, your personal trainer should remain with you during all your exercises.
Components Trained:	Strength, flexibility, balance, and endurance.
Exercises Performed:	Resistance training exercises for strength; yoga for flexibility and balance; cardio walking for endurance.
Equipment or Supplies to Buy:	A heart-rate monitor if required by your doctor (if your health club's cardio equipment does not incorporate heart-rate monitors).
Facility Equipment/ Supplies Used:	Machine weights, free weights, weighted balls, mats, tilt boards, etc., at a gym where you meet with the personal trainer; yoga props at a yoga studio where you meet with the yoga instructor; a treadmill.

13-Week Training Plan

This plan is a perfect starting point for your own "intensive, aggressive, and repetitive" walking recovery program. Many stroke survivors underwent hospital rehab for about three hours a day, five or six days a week. This plan requires less time than that (1-2 hours a day, five days a week), yet it is extremely effective.

Each week, follow the workout schedule below. The numbers which appear after an exercise category in the schedule refer to the numbered instructions below.

Weeks	Mon	Tue	Wed	Thu	Fri	Sat	Sun
Weeks 1 - 13	Resistance Training ❶ Cardio Walking ❷ (20 min. to 1 hr)	Cardio Walking (20 min. to 1 hr)	Off	Resistance Training (1 hr) Cardio Walking (20 min. to 1 hr)	Cardio Walking (20 min. to 1 hr)	Yoga ❸ (1 hr)	Off

Instructions

 Resistance Training (muscle resistance) is done under the guidance and supervision of a personal trainer, who will help you determine which fixed-weight machines to use, how much weight to begin with and how many repetitions of each movement to make (called "reps"), depending upon your present strength and mobility. Specific resistance training exercise workouts are presented in Walking Plan 2 that your personal trainer can use in designing your exercise plan if he or she wishes (see pages 66-71).

This walking plan features upper and lower body resistance training. You need both upper and lower body strength to walk well. A strong upper body keeps you balanced and allows you to support yourself when walking or when you need to grab hold of something to regain balance, or support yourself to keep from falling. It also enables you to smoothly carry loads that might be unevenly distributed when you hold them. Additionally, you need to strengthen both your upper and lower body to completely remedy any single-sided weakness you might have.

Each resistance training session lasts about an hour. On days with both resistance training and cardio walking, try to perform resistance training *before* cardio walking. Your personal trainer should make sure you warm up appropriately during each exercise session. This is important so as to *avoid injury*.

Core Training. Your personal trainer will also likely understand the importance of "core training"—exercises that strengthen and stabilize the spine and pelvis. Many fitness specialists think that having a well-trained core is the KEY to being able to walk well. Your personal trainer should guide you through appropriate core training exercises. However, if your trainer doesn't mention it, be sure to ask that core training be included in your workout. (Core exercises are included in Walking Plan 2 on pages 62-64 that you can adopt for use in this plan if you wish.)

Daily Worksheet Entry. A standard worksheet entry for the resistance training workouts might appear as follows (the first number is the weight used, the slashes show the number of repetitions in each of three sets). Change the exercise names or amounts based on your actual workouts. (If it's easier for you while you're just getting started, ask your personal trainer to make the entries in your workbook for you as you work out.)

> **Core Work – 10 minutes**
> **Lateral Raise – 25 – 8/8/8**
> **Pull down – 50 – 8/8/8**
> **Seated Squat – 80 – 8/8/8**
> **Triceps Overhead Press – 40 – 8/8/8**
> **Seated Biceps Incline Curl – 35 – 8/8/8**

 Cardio Walking is done on a treadmill with the help of your personal trainer. The treadmill is somewhat like a walker—if you can use a walker, you can use a treadmill. Each cardio walking session should last as long as you can continue to walk on the treadmill with proper form, up to one hour maximum. If you are very weak or out of shape, start at 20 or 30 minutes and push yourself to increase your time every week, as you are able. Proper form would consist of moving straight forward, holding your body erect. Move smoothly, getting all the balance you need from the act of walking. Keep one of your feet firmly planted on the ground (or treadmill platform) at all times, "vaulting" your body directly over your forward leg. (This means try not to rock side to side as you walk, as can happen if you keep your feet too far apart in an effort to balance yourself).

If your doctor has requested that you not exceed a certain maximum heart rate during cardio exercise, have your personal trainer show you how to monitor this using your heart rate monitor or the sensors on the cardio machines.

There are two variations you can perform on the treadmill:

a. **Walk at different speeds:** Begin with slower speeds until you gain sufficient strength and endurance to increase the speed. As soon as possible, begin varying and alternating your speeds from slower to faster, then slower again *within the same workout session,* so you are raising the demand on your muscles.

Note that walking at a *slower* speed, such as 0.5 miles per hour (or the slowest speed that the treadmill permits) is just as important for improving your ability to walk as the faster speeds. This is because it is more difficult to maintain your balance and proper form at slower speeds—it requires more muscle control. So even as you become able to walk faster, always include at least half your time walking at the slowest speed.

b. **Walk with different levels of support:** (1) holding on with both hands; (2) holding on with one hand; (3) only grasping or leaning against the treadmill handrail if you feel yourself losing your balance, but otherwise walking without support.

Your goal is to become able to walk without using any support at all (without holding the handrails or handlebars).

Daily Worksheet Entry. A standard worksheet entry for this could be:

> **Treadmill –**
> **Distance – 2 miles**
> **Time – 1 hour**
> **Speed – 1.6–2.4 mph** (shown on treadmill panel)
> **Time walked without support – 1 min. 15 seconds**
> (time measured by treadmill)

❸ **Yoga** is done under the guidance and supervision of a certified yoga instructor in your health club or at a yoga facility. Each yoga session should last about an hour.

Daily Worksheet Entry. A standard worksheet entry for this is:

> **Yoga as directed by my yoga Instructor**
> (or name the individual postures you assumed)

Recovery Plan 2

Ability to Walk Without Mechanical Aid

(For More Independent Beginners)

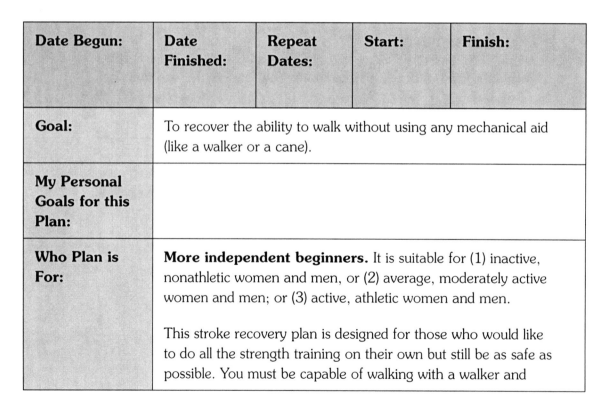

Date Begun:	Date Finished:	Repeat Dates:	Start:	Finish:
Goal:	To recover the ability to walk without using any mechanical aid (like a walker or a cane).			
My Personal Goals for this Plan:				
Who Plan is For:	**More independent beginners.** It is suitable for (1) inactive, nonathletic women and men, or (2) average, moderately active women and men; or (3) active, athletic women and men. This stroke recovery plan is designed for those who would like to do all the strength training on their own but still be as safe as possible. You must be capable of walking with a walker and			

	moving from one piece of fixed weight equipment to another in a gym, and adjusting the weights and positions on your own.
Location:	A health club or gym for resistance training and for access to a treadmill; a yoga facility (or your health club) for yoga.
People to Hire:	A certified yoga instructor (for one session a week) who is capable of and interested in working with a stroke survivor. No personal trainer is required.
Special Requirements, Information or Features:	**This recovery plan requires you to work out independently at a health club or gym.** No personal trainer is required. You will travel to a health club or gym and to a yoga facility regularly (unless your health club gives yoga classes). **Only use fixed-weight machines** (resistance training machines that allow you to select the weight you will work out with by placing a pin into a hole in a stack of weights). Fixed-weight machines provide the support you need and ensure that your movements are done correctly. Do not use free weights (such as adjustable barbells and dumbbells), because they are not safe for a stroke survivor to use. **Important Note: To ensure your safety, your caregiver or another person should remain with you during all your exercises.**
Components Trained:	Strength, flexibility, balance, and endurance.
Exercises Performed:	Resistance training exercises for strength; yoga for flexibility and balance; cardio walking on treadmill for endurance.
Equipment or Supplies to Buy:	A heart-rate monitor if required by your doctor (if your health club's cardio equipment does not incorporate heart-rate monitors).
Facility Equipment/ Supplies Used:	Fixed-weight machines and mats at a gym; yoga props at a yoga studio where you meet with the yoga instructor; a treadmill (at the gym).

13-Week Training Plan

Each week follow the workout schedule below. When a number appears after an exercise, refer to the numbered explanation below this exercise schedule for instructions.

Weeks	Mon	Tue	Wed	Thu	Fri	Sat	Sun
Weeks 1 - 13	Resistance Training❶ (1 hr) Cardio Walking❷ (20 min. to 1 hr)	Cardio Walking (20 min. to 1 hr)	Off	Resistance Training (1 hr) Cardio Walking (20 min. to 1 hr)	Cardio Walking (20 min. to 1 hr)	Yoga❸ (1 hr)	Off

Instructions

 This plan features upper and lower body resistance training, done unsupervised (no personal trainer) on fixed-weight machines at the health club or gym. You need both upper and lower body strength to walk well. A strong upper body keeps you balanced and allows you to support yourself when walking or when you need to grab hold of something to regain balance or to keep from falling. It likewise enables you to smoothly carry loads, which may be heavy or of odd size or shape, with unevenly distributed weight. Additionally, you need to strengthen both your upper and lower body to completely remedy any single-sided weakness you may have. You will perform two resistance training sessions a week.

During each resistance training session, you will train all the important body parts with the fixed-weight machines. Every session uses five types of machines:

- A machine for **shoulders or chest** (like a lateral raise machine or a bench press machine);

- A machine for the **back** (like a rowing machine or a pull down machine);

- A machine for the **triceps** – the muscle on the back upper arm (like a push down or overhead pull machine);

- A machine for the **biceps** – the muscle on the front upper arm (like a standard curl or a preacher curl machine);

- A machine for the **legs** (like a seated leg press machine). Do NOT use a standing leg press machine because it is too easy to injure yourself on!

Resistance Training Workouts for People of Six Varying Exercise Capabilities and Tolerances

After your core training exercises, do resistance training with the fixed-weight machines for the remainder of the session. Each resistance training session should last as long as it takes for you to perform all the prescribed exercises. On days with both resistance training and cardio walking, try to perform resistance training *before* cardio walking.

At the end of Walking Recovery Plan 2 you'll find the suggested resistance training workouts:

Workout 1—for inactive or nonathletic women

Workout 2—for inactive or nonathletic men

Workout 3—for average or moderately active women

Workout 4—for average or moderately active men

Workout 5—for active athletic women

Workout 6—for active athletic men

Select the workout for the category most appropriate for you. Note: Many stroke survivors will have necessarily been inactive during their hospital recuperation. If you expect and want to return to your former physical activity and strength level after recovery, begin one or two levels down, then work up to the next level as your strength increases. As you improve and grow stronger, make adjustments to the weights, number of repetitions and sets as needed.

Get a staff member or athletic trainer at the health club/gym to show you exactly how to use the machines before you begin. The fixed-weight machines have pictures and instructions mounted on them. Refer to these instructions if you forget how to use any machine. Do NOT use the dumbbells or other free weights at your gym, as you would need someone (a spotter) with you constantly to watch and guard against accidents.

Resistance Training Warm-up. If you lift weights without first making sure that your body is ready for the stress, you run a risk of injuring yourself. An injury can disrupt and delay your efforts to recover from stroke. The best warm-up method is to first perform one set of each resistance exercise at a reduced weight (half the weight or even less). This gets your muscles warmed and ready to exercise with the full weight. Do this on each fixed-weight machine prior to your usual sets.

Setting the Proper Weight on the Fixed-Weight Machines. Each workout chart below contains the suggested starting weights to use with each machine. If an exercise is too difficult for you to do with proper form at the listed weight, reduce the weight an increment or two (usually 5 or 10 pounds per increment, depending on the machine). On the other hand, if the listed weight for any machine makes the exercise seem easy, you should increase the weight an increment or two.

Core Training. Every resistance-training workout begins with 10 minutes of core training exercises. The core muscles include those in the abdomen (stomach) and back, as well as muscles in the pelvis and hips. Many of these core muscles lie beneath other muscles. Core training exercises help strengthen and stabilize your spine, increase your ability to stand stably, walk well, and maintain stability as you move your extremities. Fitness specialists say that core training is essential for any stroke survivor who wants to recover the full ability to walk and move well. The benefits of a well-trained core include:

- Greater efficiency of movement
- Improved body control
- Reduced risk of injury (the core is a "shock absorber")
- Improved balance
- Improved stability

Here are four prime core training exercises. It is not necessary to complete all four of the core exercises in each session, but do at least 10 minutes worth of core exercises before each resistance training session.

a.   **The Prone Bridge:** The position you are aiming for in the Prone Bridge is to be balancing on your elbows and toes, facing the floor, with your back as straight as possible (as if you were holding the "up" position of a push-up, but on your *elbows* instead of your hands). You can rest your forearms and elbows on a pad if you wish. If you find it difficult to raise yourself into this position, you can assume it in three stages:

(1) Lie flat on the floor on your stomach. (2) Lift yourself so you are supported on your elbows and knees. Put your feet at right angles to your body so your toes contact the floor. (3) Raise your knees off the floor so you are balancing on your elbows and toes.

Attempt to keep your back as straight as possible. Maintain this "bridge" position as long as you can, one minute maximum. If you lose your balance and fall out of position, get back into position and resume the exercise.

b.   **The Lateral Bridge:** Lie on your side, supporting yourself on one elbow with your forearm flat on the floor (at a right angle to your body for balance), and with one leg and foot resting on top of the other. Lift your hips up off the floor so that you are balanced only on your elbow/lower arm and the edge of your foot. Attempt to stay in this side bridge position for a minute at a time, then repeat on the other side.

c.   **The Supine (or Back) Bridge:** Lie on your back on the floor with your knees bent. Raise your hips so only your head, shoulders, and feet support you. Attempt to stay in this position a minute.

d.   **Pelvic Thrusts: Version 1 (easier):** Lie on your back with your knees bent and feet flat on the floor. Slowly lift your hips off the floor and towards the ceiling so only your head, shoulders, and feet support you. Lower your hips to the floor slowly. Repeat 10 times.

Version 2 (more difficult): Lie on your back with your legs bent 90 degrees at the hips, your feet aimed at the ceiling, and your arms flat on the floor right by your sides. Bracing yourself with your arms, slowly lift your hips off the floor and towards the ceiling, then slowly lower your hips to the floor again. Repeat 10 times.

Daily Worksheet Entry. A standard worksheet entry for these resistance training workouts could appear as follows (the first number is the weight used, the slashes show the number of repetitions in each of three sets—change the amounts based on your own workout):

> **Core Work**
> **Bench Press – 20 – 8/8/8**
> **Rowing – 30 – 8/8/8**
> **Seated Squat – 60 – 8/8/8**
> **Triceps Press Down – 20 – 8/8/8**
> **Seated Biceps Curl – 15 – 8/8/8**

 Cardio Walking is done on a treadmill. Each cardio walking session should last as long as you can continue to walk on the treadmill with proper form—one hour maximum. The treadmill is like a walker in that it has rails you can hold for support—if you can use a walker, you can use a treadmill. If you are very weak or out of shape, start at 20 or 30 minutes and work up from there every week or two as you are able. Proper form would consist of moving straight forward, holding your body erect. Move smoothly, getting all the balance you need from the act of "walking." Keep one of your feet firmly planted on the ground (or treadmill platform) at all times, "vaulting" your body directly over your forward leg. (This means try not to rock side to side as you walk, as can happen if you keep your feet too far apart in an effort to balance yourself).

If your doctor has requested that you not exceed a certain maximum heart rate during cardio exercise, use your heart rate monitor or the sensors on the cardio machines to do so.

There are two variations you can perform on the treadmill:

a. Walk at different speeds. Begin with slower speeds until you gain sufficient strength and endurance to increase the speed. As soon as possible, begin varying and alternating your speeds from slower to faster, then slower again *within the same workout session,* so you are raising the demand on your muscles.

Note that walking at a *slower* speed, such as 0.5 miles per hour (or the slowest speed that the treadmill permits) is just as important for improving your ability to walk as the faster speeds. This is because it is more difficult to maintain your balance and proper form at slower speeds—it requires more muscle control. So even as you become able to walk faster, always include at least half your time walking at the slowest speed.

b. Walk with different levels of support—such as holding on with both hands, holding on with one hand, and holding on by just taking hold of the treadmill handrail briefly when you feel yourself losing your balance.

Your ultimate goal is to be able to walk without having to use your hands for support at all. Each time you walk you should endeavor to go a greater distance and spend less time using your hands for support.

Daily Worksheet Entry. A standard worksheet entry for this would be:

Treadmill –

> **Distance – 2 miles**
> **Time – 1 hour**
> **Speed – 0.5–2.4 mph** (set on the treadmill)
> **Time walked without support – 5 min. 15 seconds**
> (time measured by treadmill)

3 **Yoga** is done under the guidance and supervision of a certified yoga instructor at the health club or a yoga facility. Each yoga session should last about an hour.

Daily Worksheet Entry. A standard worksheet entry for this is:

Yoga as directed by my yoga instructor
(or name the individual postures you assumed)

WORKOUT 1
For Inactive or Nonathletic Women

Monday	Thursday
Core Training	**Core Training**
Bench Press machine [or Seated Chest Press] Weight: 20 lbs. Reps each set: 8 reps/3 sets	**Lateral Raise machine** Weight: 5 lbs. Reps each set: 8 reps/3 sets
Rowing machine Weight: 30 lbs. Reps each set: 8 reps/3 sets	**Pull down machine** Weight: 30 lbs. Reps each set: 8 reps/3 sets
Seated Squat machine Weight: 60 lbs. Reps each set: 8 reps/3 sets	**Seated Squat machine** Weight: 60 lbs. Reps each set: 8 reps/3 sets
Triceps Press Down machine Weight: 20 lbs. Reps each set: 8 reps/3 sets	**Triceps Overhead Press machine** Weight: 20 lbs. Reps each set: 8 reps/3 sets
Seated Biceps Curl machine Weight: 15 lbs. Reps each set: 8 reps/3 sets	**Seated Biceps Incline Curl machine** Weight: 15 lbs. Reps each set: 8 reps/3 sets

WORKOUT 2
For Inactive or Nonathletic Men

Monday	Thursday
Core Training	**Core Training**
Bench Press machine Weight: 40 lbs. Reps each set: 8 reps/3 sets	**Lateral Raise machine** Weight: 25 lbs. Reps each set: 8 reps/3 sets
Rowing machine Weight: 50 lbs. Reps each set: 8 reps/3 sets	**Pull down machine** Weight: 50 lbs. Reps each set: 8 reps/3 sets
Seated Squat machine Weight: 80 lbs. Reps each set: 8 reps/3 sets	**Seated Squat machine** Weight: 80 lbs. Reps each set: 8 reps/3 sets
Triceps Press Down machine Weight: 40 lbs. Reps each set: 8 reps/3 sets	**Triceps Overhead Press machine** Weight: 40 lbs. Reps each set: 8 reps/3 sets
Seated Biceps Curl machine Weight: 35 lbs. Reps each set: 8 reps/3 sets	**Seated Biceps Incline Curl machine** Weight: 35 lbs. Reps each set: 8 reps/3 sets

WORKOUT 3
For Average or Moderately Active Women

Monday	Thursday
Core Training	**Core Training**
Bench Press machine Weight: 25 lbs. Reps each set: 8 reps/4 sets	**Lateral Raise machine** Weight: 10 lbs. Reps each set: 8 reps./4 sets
Rowing machine Weight: 35 lbs. Reps each set: 8 reps/4 sets	**Pull down machine** Weight: 35 lbs. Reps each set: 8 reps/4 sets
Seated Squat machine Weight: 65 lbs. Reps each set: 8 reps/4 sets	**Seated Squat machine** Weight: 65 lbs. Reps each set: 8 reps/4 sets
Triceps Press Down machine Weight: 25 lbs. Reps each set: 8 reps/4 sets	**Triceps Overhead Press machine** Weight: 25 lbs. Reps each set: 8 reps/4 sets
Seated Biceps Curl machine Weight: 20 lbs. Reps each set: 8 reps/4 sets	**Seated Biceps Incline Curl machine** Weight: 20 lbs. Reps each set: 8 reps/4 sets

Taking Charge of Your Stroke Recovery

WORKOUT 4

For Average or Moderately Active Men

Monday	Thursday
Core Training	**Core Training**
Bench Press machine Weight: 45 lbs. Reps each set: 8 reps/4 sets	**Lateral Raise machine** Weight: 30 lbs. Reps each set: 8 reps/4 sets
Rowing machine Weight: 55 lbs. Reps each set: 8 reps/4 sets	**Pull down machine** Weight: 55 lbs. Reps each set: 8 reps/4 sets
Seated Squat machine Weight: 85 lbs. Reps each set: 8 reps/4 sets	**Seated Squat machine** Weight: 85 lbs. Reps each set: 8 reps/4 sets
Triceps Press Down machine Weight: 45 lbs. Reps each set: 8 reps/4 sets	**Triceps Overhead Press machine** Weight: 45 lbs. Reps each set: 8 reps/4 sets
Seated Biceps Curl machine Weight: 40 lbs. Reps each set: 8 reps/4 sets	**Seated Biceps Incline Curl machine** Weight: 40 lbs. Reps each set: 8 reps/4 sets

WORKOUT 5
For Active, Athletic Women

Monday	Thursday
Core Training	**Core Training**
Bench Press machine Weight: 30 lbs. Reps each set: 12 reps/4 sets	**Lateral Raise machine** Weight: 15 lbs. Reps each set: 12 reps/4 sets
Rowing machine Weight: 40 lbs. Reps each set: 12 reps/4 sets	**Pull down machine** Weight: 40 lbs. Reps each set: 12 reps/4 sets
Seated Squat machine Weight: 70 lbs. Reps each set: 12 reps/4 sets	**Seated Squat machine** Weight: 70 lbs. Reps each set: 12 reps/4 sets
Triceps Press Down machine Weight: 30 lbs. Reps each set: 12 reps/4 sets	**Triceps Overhead Press machine** Weight: 30 lbs. Reps each set: 12 reps/4 sets
Seated Biceps Curl machine Weight: 25 lbs. Reps each set: 12 reps/4 sets	**Seated Biceps Incline Curl machine** Weight: 25 lbs. Reps each set: 12 reps/4 sets

WORKOUT 6
For Active, Athletic Men

Monday	Thursday
Core Training	**Core Training**
Bench Press machine Weight: 50 lbs. Reps each set: 12 reps/4 sets	**Lateral Raise machine** Weight: 35 lbs. Reps each set: 12 reps/4 sets
Rowing machine Weight: 60 lbs. Reps each set: 12 reps/4 sets	**Pull down machine** Weight: 60 lbs. Reps each set: 12 reps/4 sets
Seated Squat machine Weight: 90 lbs. Reps each set: 12 reps/4 sets	**Seated Squat machine** Weight: 90 lbs. Reps each set: 12 reps/4 sets
Triceps Press Down machine Weight: 50 lbs. Reps each set: 12 reps/4 sets	**Triceps Overhead Press machine** Weight: 50 lbs. Reps each set: 12 reps/4 sets
Seated Biceps Curl machine Weight: 45 lbs. Reps each set: 12 reps/4 sets	**Seated Biceps Incline Curl machine** Weight: 45 lbs. Reps each set: 12 reps/4 sets

Recovery Plan 3

Ability to Walk Without Mechanical Aid

(For Independent Advanced Beginners)

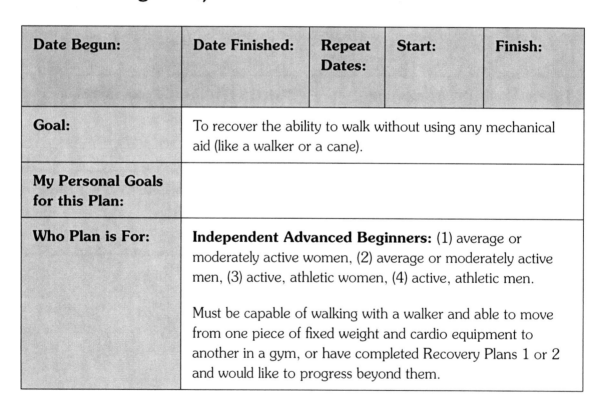

Date Begun:	Date Finished:	Repeat Dates:	Start:	Finish:
Goal:	To recover the ability to walk without using any mechanical aid (like a walker or a cane).			
My Personal Goals for this Plan:				
Who Plan is For:	**Independent Advanced Beginners:** (1) average or moderately active women, (2) average or moderately active men, (3) active, athletic women, (4) active, athletic men. Must be capable of walking with a walker and able to move from one piece of fixed weight and cardio equipment to another in a gym, or have completed Recovery Plans 1 or 2 and would like to progress beyond them.			

Location:	This recovery plan requires you to work out independently at a gym for resistance and cardio training; at a yoga facility for yoga if your health club has no yoga classes.
People to Hire:	No personal trainer is hired. A certified yoga instructor (for one session a week)—this person should be capable of and interested in working with a stroke survivor.
Special Requirements, Information or Features:	This program is designed for an independent advanced beginner—someone who has completed the appropriate workout level in either Recovery Plan 1 or 2, and who would like to do more than that. **This recovery plan requires you to travel to a health club or gym to work out independently.** No personal trainer is required. This stroke recovery plan is designed for people who would like to do strength training on their own but still be as safe as possible, and who would like to develop their walking skills in ways that they cannot accomplish on a treadmill alone. This person is also interested in learning how to perform yoga on their own. This plan also requires you to travel to a health club or yoga facility regularly. All resistance work is done on fixed-weight machines (weight machines that allow you to select the weight you will work out with by placing a pin into a hole in a stack of weights). ONLY USE FIXED WEIGHT MACHINES and not free weights (such as adjustable barbells and dumbbells), which are not safe for a stroke survivor to attempt to use. **Important Note: To ensure your safety, your caregiver or another person should remain with you during all your exercises.**
Components Trained:	Balance, flexibility, strength, and endurance.

Exercises Performed:	Resistance training exercises for strength; yoga for flexibility and balance; cardio walking for endurance.
Equipment or Supplies to Buy:	A heart-rate monitor if required by your doctor (if your health club's cardio equipment does not incorporate heart-rate monitors).
Facility Equipment/ Supplies Used:	At the gym, fixed-weight machines, mats, a treadmill, an elliptical machine, and a stair-stepper machine; yoga props at a yoga studio where you meet with the yoga instructor.

13-Week Training Plan:

Each week follow the workout schedule below. When a number appears after an exercise, refer to the explanation below this exercise schedule for instructions.

Weeks	Mon	Tue	Wed	Thu	Fri	Sat	Sun
1 - 13	Resistance Training ❶ • CHEST & SHOULDERS (1 hr) Cardio Walking ❷ (1 hr)	Cardio Walking (1 hr)	Resistance Training • LEGS & TRICEPS (1 hr) Yoga with instructor ❸ (1 hr)	Cardio Walking (1 hr)	Resistance Training • BACK & BICEPS (1 hr) Cardio Walking (1 hr)	Yoga – individual practice ❹ (1 hr)	Off

Instructions

 Resistance Training. This plan features upper and lower body resistance training, done unsupervised (without a personal trainer) on fixed-weight machines at the health club or gym. You need both upper and lower body strength to walk well. A strong upper body keeps you balanced and allows you to support yourself when walking or when you need to grab hold of something to regain balance or to keep from falling. It likewise enables you to smoothly carry loads that may be heavy or of odd size or shape, with unevenly distributed weight. Additionally, you need to strengthen both your upper and lower body to completely remedy any single-sided weakness you may have.

Resistance Training Workouts for Stroke Survivors of Four Varying Exercise Capabilities and Tolerances

At the end of this plan are typical resistance training workouts appropriate for four different strength and physical activity levels of stroke survivors:

> **Workout 1—average or moderately active women**
>
> **Workout 2—average or moderately active men**
>
> **Workout 3—active, athletic women**
>
> **Workout 4—active, athletic men**

Select the workout for the category you most closely match, or begin one level down if the workout seems too difficult for your current physical condition.

You will perform three resistance training sessions a week with the fixed-weight machines listed in the workout charts below. You should already be familiar with using fixed-weight machines from your previous workout plan(s).

There are three different resistance training sessions per week:

> a. Monday is chest and shoulder day.
>
> b. Wednesday is legs and triceps day (the tricep is the large muscle on the back of your upper arm).
>
> c. Friday is back and biceps day (the bicep is the muscle on the front upper arm).

Each resistance training session consists of four or five exercises, each with between 3 and 4 sets, with between 6 and 12 repetitions a set.

If you are not familiar with the fixed-weight machines at your club, get a staff member at the health club/gym to show you exactly how to use the machines before you begin. (You may only need to be shown any machines you haven't previously used.) Refer to the diagrams and instructions on the machines if necessary. Do NOT use the dumbbells or other free weights at your gym, as you would need someone (a spotter) with you constantly to watch and guard against accidents.

Resistance Training Warm-up. If you lift weights without first making sure that your body is ready for the stress, you run a risk of injuring yourself. An injury can disrupt and delay your efforts to recover from stroke. The best warm-up method is to first perform one set of each resistance exercise at a reduced level (half the weight or even less). This gets your muscles warmed and ready to exercise with the full weight. Do this on each fixed-weight machine prior to your usual sets.

To Set Weights. At this point, you should be able to do an excellent job selecting your own weights, and that is exactly what you need to do. Write your starting weights in the left column of your selected workout chart below. Whatever weights you choose, you should be able to lift them with proper form for at least 6 repetitions per set, but no more than 12 repetitions per set.

Core Training Exercises. Many fitness specialists think that core training is the *single most important thing you can do to walk well*. The core muscles include those deep in the abdomen, back, pelvis and hips. Many of the core muscles lie beneath other muscles. Core training exercises help strengthen and stabilize your spine, increasing your ability to stand stably, walk well, and maintain stability as you move your extremities. A strong core is essential to any stroke survivor who wants to recover full ability to walk and move well.

Spend the first 15 minutes of every resistance training session performing core training. Below are four prime core training exercises. It is not necessary to complete all four of the core exercises in each session, but do at least 15 minutes worth of core exercises before each resistance training session.

Since you are now a more advanced walker, you can and should begin doing things to make the basic core training exercises more challenging and able to help you. You can do this by reducing the amount of support you use during each core training exercise, thereby forcing your body to develop a stronger core. Each exercise contains instructions for increasing the challenge.

a.   **The Prone Bridge:** The position you are aiming for in the prone bridge is to be balancing on your forearms and toes, facing the floor, with your back as straight as possible (as if you were holding the "up" position of a push-up, but on your elbows and forearms instead of your hands). You can rest your forearms on a pad if you wish. If you find it difficult to raise yourself into this position all at once, you can assume it in three stages:

(1) Lie flat on the floor on your stomach.

(2) Lift yourself so you are supported on your forearms and knees. Put your feet at right angles to your body so your toes contact the floor.

(3) Raise your knees off the floor so you are balancing on your forearms and toes.

Attempt to keep your back as straight as possible. Maintain this "bridge" position as long as you can, one minute maximum. If you lose your balance and fall out of position, get back into position and resume the exercise.

To increase the challenge, once you have assumed the prone bridge position:

(1) Raise your right leg from the floor and extend your left arm straight forward so you are balancing entirely on your right forearm and left toe. Maintain this position as long as you can, one minute maximum.

(2) Now reverse the arm and leg you lift. Reassume the full prone bridge position. Raise your left leg from the floor and extend your right arm straight forward so you are balancing on your left forearm and right toe. Maintain this position as long as you can, up to one minute maximum.

b.   **The Lateral Bridge:** Lie on your side, supporting yourself on one elbow with your forearm flat on the floor (at a right angle to your body for balance), and with one leg and foot resting on top of the other. Lift your hips up off the floor so that you are balanced only on your elbow/lower arm and the edge of your foot. Attempt to stay in this side bridge position for a minute at a time, then repeat on the other side.

To increase the challenge, assume the lateral bridge position. Raise your top leg as high as you can, then hold it for as long as possible, up to one minute maximum. This higher center of balance will cause you to work different areas of your core than those exercised in the normal lateral bridge. Repeat this exercise on your opposite side, lifting the other leg.

---

c.   **The Supine (or Back) Bridge:** Lie on your back on the floor with your knees bent. Raise your hips so only your head, shoulders, and feet support you. Attempt to stay in this position a minute.

   To increase the challenge, assume the back bridge position. Raise one of your legs straight up and balance as long as possible, one minute maximum. Balancing in this manner works additional areas of your core. Perform the same exercise but raise the other leg for as long as possible, one minute maximum.

d.   **Pelvic Thrusts:**

   Version 1 (easier): Lie on your back with your knees bent and feet flat on the floor. Slowly lift your hips off the floor and towards the ceiling so only your head, shoulders, and feet support you. Lower your hips to the floor slowly. Repeat 10 times.

   Version 2 (increased challenge): Lie on your back with your legs bent 90 degrees at the hips, your feet aimed at the ceiling, and your arms flat on the floor right by your sides. Bracing yourself with your arms, slowly lift your hips off the floor and towards the ceiling, then slowly lower your hips to the floor again. Repeat 10 times.

Daily Worksheet Entry. A sample standard worksheet entry for this would be:

   Core Work – Bridges

   Bench Press – Weight 60 – Reps 12/10/8

❷   **Cardio Walking** is done four times a week. It is done on three machines at the health club: (1) on a treadmill; (2) on a elliptical machine; and (3) on a stair-stepper machine. You should work out on all three types of machines each day, one after the other—that is, devote one-third of your time (20 minutes) to the treadmill, one-third (20 minutes) to the elliptical machine, and the last 20 minutes to a stair-stepper. Each cardio walking session should last as long as you can continue to exercise with proper form—one hour maximum. Proper form on the treadmill would consist of moving straight forward, holding your body erect. Move smoothly, getting all the balance you need from the act of "walking." Keep one of your feet firmly planted on the ground (or treadmill platform) at all times, "vaulting" your body directly over your forward leg. (This means try not to rock side to side as you walk, as can happen if you keep your feet too far apart in an effort to balance yourself). Proper form on the elliptical and stair-stepper would be keeping your body erect and keeping your movements smooth and evenly paced.

If your doctor has requested that you not exceed a certain maximum heart rate during cardio exercise, use your heart rate monitor or the sensors on the cardio machines to do so.

Each of the three pieces of cardio equipment have hand rails. When using each of them, you should practice using less and less support. Ultimately and ideally, you will be able to use them without using any hand or arm support whatsoever.

On the treadmill, practice walking at different speeds. Since the treadmill automatically measures speed and time, that will be easy to do. For variation, try walking at different inclines (slants). Most treadmills will allow you to vary that easily. As soon as possible, begin varying your speeds from slower to faster and then slower again within the same workout session so you are raising the demand on your muscles. Walking at the slowest speed possible is just as important as the higher speeds, because it forces you to control your muscles more and maintain your balance in order to keep walking smoothly. Always include periods of walking very slowly as well as walking at higher speeds.

On the elliptical machine, walk forward, then after a certain period of time, reverse your direction to go backward. This teaches you to change the direction your legs move upon command. **On the stair-stepper,** you strengthen both your legs as you use each of them to move your body upward and you also learn to balance yourself first on one leg, then the other.

Daily Worksheet Entry. A standard worksheet entry for this is:

> **Treadmill – Distance – 2 miles**
> **Time – 1 hour**
> **Speed – 0.5 to 2.4 mph, set on the treadmill**
> **Time walked without support – 15 min. 15 sec., of that 10 min. at 0.5 mph**

Another could be:

Elliptical – Distance – 1 mile
Time – 1 hr. 15 min.
Reversed direction every minute
Time without support – 1 hr. 15 min.

❸ **Yoga Training** on **Wednesday** is done under the guidance and supervision of a certified yoga instructor at your health club or a yoga facility.

Daily Worksheet Entry. A standard worksheet entry for this is:

> **Yoga as directed by my yoga Instructor**
> (or name the individual postures you assumed)

❹ **Yoga Training** on **Saturday** is done on your own. You should assume the postures you learned on Wednesday that feel most beneficial to you. Each session should last about an hour. Incidentally, a good book on yoga can help you with your individual yoga practice each Saturday. We like *Light on Yoga: The classic guide to yoga from the world's foremost authority,* by B.K.S. Iyengar (Thorsons, 2001, paperback).

Daily Worksheet Entry. A standard worksheet entry for this is:

> **Personal yoga focusing on balancing asanas**
> (or name the individual postures you assumed)

WORKOUT 1

For Average or Moderately Active Women

Monday—Chest and Shoulder Routine:

	Bench Press machine—3 sets/6–12 reps per set
	Pectoral Flye machine—3 sets/6–12 reps per set
	Overhead Press machine—3 sets/6–12 reps per set
	Lateral Raise machine—3 sets/6–12 reps per set

Wednesday—Leg and Triceps Routine:

	Seated Squat machine—3 sets/6–12 reps per set
	Quadriceps Leg Raise machine—3 sets/6–12 reps per set (Quadriceps is the muscle on the front upper part of the leg)
	Triceps Pressdown machine—3 sets/6–12 reps per set
	Seated Overhead Cable Pull machine—3 sets/6–12 reps per set

Friday—Back and Biceps Routine:

	Seated Row machine—3 sets/6–12 reps per set
	Pulldown machine—3 sets/6–12 reps per set
	Biceps Curl machine—3 sets/6–12 reps per set
	Incline Curl machine—3 sets/6–12 reps per set

WORKOUT 2

For Average or Moderately Active Men

Monday—Chest and Shoulder Routine:

	Bench Press machine—3 sets/6–12 reps per set
	Pectoral Flye machine—3 sets/6–12 reps per set
	Overhead Press machine—3 sets/6–12 reps per set
	Lateral Raise machine—3 sets/6–12 reps per set

Wednesday—Leg and Triceps Routine:

	Seated Squat machine—3 sets/6–12 reps per set
	Quadriceps Leg Raise machine—3 sets/6–12 reps per set (Quadriceps is the muscle on the front upper part of the leg)
	Triceps Pressdown machine—3 sets/6–12 reps per set
	Seated Overhead Cable Pull machine—3 sets/6–12 reps per set

Friday—Back and Biceps Routine:

	Seated Row machine—3 sets/6–12 reps per set
	Pulldown machine—3 sets/6–12 reps per set
	Biceps Curl machine—3 sets/6–12 reps per set
	Incline Curl machine—3 sets/6–12 reps per set

Taking Charge of Your Stroke Recovery

WORKOUT 3

For Active, Athletic Women

Monday—Chest and Shoulder Routine:

	Bench Press machine—4 sets/6–12 reps per set
	Pectoral Flye machine—4 sets/6–12 reps per set
	Overhead Press machine—4 sets/6–12 reps per set
	Lateral Raise machine—4 sets/6–12 reps per set

Wednesday—Leg and Triceps Routine:

	Seated Squat machine—4 sets/6–12 reps per set
	Quadriceps Leg Raise machine—4 sets/6–12 reps per set (Quadriceps is the muscle on the front upper part of the leg)
	Lying Hamstring Curl machine—4 sets/6–12 reps per set
	Triceps Pressdown machine—4 sets/6–12 reps per set
	Seated Overhead Cable Pull machine—4 sets/6–12 reps per set

Friday—Back and Biceps Routine:

	Seated Row machine—4 sets/6–12 reps per set
	Pulldown machine—4 sets/6–12 reps per set
	Biceps Curl machine—4 sets/6–12 reps per set
	Incline Curl machine—4 sets/6–12 reps per set

WORKOUT 4

For Active, Athletic Men

Monday—Chest and Shoulder Routine:

	Bench Press machine—4 sets/6–12 reps per set
	Pectoral Flye machine—4 sets/6–12 reps per set
	Overhead Press machine—4 sets/6–12 reps per set
	Lateral Raise machine—4 sets/6–12 reps per set

Wednesday—Leg and Triceps Routine:

	Seated Squat machine—4 sets/6–12 reps per set
	Quadriceps Leg Raise machine—4 sets/6–12 reps per set (Quadriceps is the muscle on the front upper part of the leg)
	Lying Hamstring Curl machine—4 sets/6–12 reps per set
	Triceps Pressdown machine—4 sets/6–12 reps per set
	Seated Overhead Cable Pull machine—4 sets/6–12 reps per set

Friday—Back and Biceps Routine:

	Seated Row machine—4 sets/6–12 reps per set
	Pulldown machine—4 sets/6–12 reps per set
	Biceps Curl machine—4 sets/6–12 reps per set
	Incline Curl machine—4 sets/6–12 reps per set

Taking Charge of Your Stroke Recovery

Recovery Plan 4

Ability to Walk Without Mechanical Aid

(For an Independent Active or Athletic Person)

Date Begun:	Date Finished:	Repeat Dates:	Start:	Finish
Goal:	To recover the ability to walk without using any mechanical aid whatsoever			
My Personal Goals for this Plan:				
Who Plan is For:	**Independent, Active or Athletic Person** who is capable of walking with a cane.			
Location:	This recovery plan requires you to work out at a gym for resistance and cardio training, and at a yoga facility for yoga if your club has no yoga classes.			

People to Hire:	(1) a personal trainer (for two sessions a week)—this person should be capable of and interested in working with a stroke survivor. (2) A certified yoga instructor (for one session a week)—this person should also be capable of and interested in working with a stroke survivor.
Special Requirements, Information or Features:	This stroke recovery plan is designed for a particularly strong participant who is interested in getting help from a personal trainer. **Important Note: To ensure your safety, your personal trainer, caregiver or another person should remain with you during all your exercises.**
Components Trained:	Balance, flexibility, strength, and endurance.
Exercises Performed:	Resistance training exercises for strength; cardio walking for endurance; yoga for flexibility and balance.
Equipment or Supplies to Buy:	A metronome that can hang around your neck for keeping the pace when walking, and a digital watch with a stopwatch function. A heart-rate monitor if required by your doctor (if your health club's cardio equipment does not incorporate heart-rate monitors).
Facility Equipment/ Supplies Used:	Machine weights, free weights, weighted balls, mats, tilt boards, etc., at a gym where you meet with the personal trainer; yoga props at a yoga studio where you meet with the yoga instructor; a treadmill, an elliptical machine, and a stair-stepper machine (at the gym).

13-Week Training Plan:

Each week follow the workout schedule below. When a number appears after an exercise, refer to the explanation below the exercise schedule for instructions.

Weeks	Mon	Tue	Wed	Thu	Fri	Sat	Sun
1 - 13	Resistance Training – with Trainer (1 hr) Cardio Walking – Track❷ (1 hr)	Resistance Training – Individual❸ (1 hr) Cardio Walking – Track (1 hr)	Cardio Workout – Gym/Club❹ (1 hr)	Resistance Training – with Trainer (1 hr) Cardio Walking – Track (1 hr)	Resistance Training – Individual (1 hr) Cardio Walking – Track (1 hr)	Yoga❺ (1 hr)	Off

Instructions

❶ ❸ Resistance Training. This plan features upper and lower body resistance training. You need both upper and lower body strength to walk well. A strong upper body keeps you balanced and allows you to support yourself when walking or when you need to grab hold of something to regain balance or to keep from falling. It also enables you to smoothly carry loads, which may be heavy or of odd size or shape so their weight is unevenly distributed. Additionally, you need to strengthen both your upper and lower body to completely remedy any single-sided weakness you may have.

Schedule. This plan has four resistance training sessions a week. On Monday and Thursday your resistance training sessions are done under the supervision of a personal trainer, who will help you determine the correct weights, number of sets and repetitions on each machine. On Tuesday and Friday, your sessions are done on your own, by repeating exactly the same exercises you did with the personal trainer the preceding day. Each resistance session (whether under the guidance of a personal trainer or done by yourself) will last about a hour. On days with both resistance training and cardio walking, try to complete your resistance training *before* cardio walking.

Before You Begin Resistance Training. On days you work out with a personal trainer, he or she should make sure you do at least 15 minutes of appropriate core training exercises before your resistance training exercises. You should also warm up before each individual resistance exercise on the weight machines by doing one set at half your usual weight (or less) before actually performing the exercise with the full weight.

On the days that you work out alone, make sure you do at least 15 minutes of good core training exercises (instructions below) before beginning your resistance exercises. Also make sure you warm up before each individual resistance exercise as mentioned in the previous paragraph.

Core Training Exercises. Core training exercises help strengthen and stabilize your spine, increasing your ability to stand stably, walk well, and maintain stability as you move your extremities. A strong core is essential to any stroke survivor who wants to recover full ability to walk and move well.

Below are four prime core training exercises. It is not necessary to complete all four of the core exercises in each session, but do at least 15 minutes worth of core exercises before each resistance training session.

Since you are now a more advanced walker, your core training exercises should be more challenging so they can continue to make you stronger. Each exercise contains instructions for increasing the challenge. If you can, you should perform the increased challenge version of each exercise *instead of* doing the exercise the normal way. If necessary, however, you can do the normal version of any exercise until you are able to do the more difficult version.

a. **The Prone Bridge:** The position you are aiming for in the prone bridge is to be balancing on your forearms and toes, facing the floor, with your back as straight as possible (as if you were holding the "up" position of a push-up, but on your elbows and forearms instead of your hands). You can rest your forearms on a pad if you wish. If you find it difficult to raise yourself into this position all at once, you can assume it in three stages:

(1) Lie flat on the floor on your stomach.

(2) Lift yourself so you are supported on your forearms and knees. Put your feet at right angles to your body so your toes contact the floor.

(3) Raise your knees off the floor so you are balancing on your forearms and toes. Attempt to keep your back as straight as possible. Maintain this "bridge" position as long as you can, one minute maximum. If you lose your balance and fall out of position, get back into position and resume the exercise.

To increase the challenge, once you have assumed the prone bridge position:

(1) raise your right leg from the floor and extend your left arm straight forward so you are balancing entirely on your right arm and left toe. Maintain this position as long as you can, one minute maximum.

(2) Now reverse the arm and leg you lift: reassume the full prone bridge position, then raise your left leg from the floor and extend your right arm straight forward so you are balancing on your left elbow and right toe. Maintain this position as long as you can, up to one minute maximum.

b.   **The Lateral Bridge:** Lie on your side, supporting yourself on one elbow with your forearm flat on the floor (at a right angle to your body for balance), and with one leg and foot resting on top of the other. Lift your hips up off the floor so that you are balanced only on your elbow/lower arm and the edge of your foot. Attempt to stay in this side bridge position for a minute at a time, then repeat on the other side.

   To increase the challenge, assume the lateral bridge position. Raise your top leg as high as you can, then hold this position as long as possible, up to one minute maximum. This higher center of balance will cause you to work different areas of your core than those exercised in the normal lateral bridge. Repeat this exercise on your opposite side, lifting the other leg.

c.   **The Supine (or Back) Bridge:** Lie on your back on the floor with your knees bent. Raise your hips so only your head, shoulders, and feet support you. Attempt to stay in this position a full minute.

   To increase the challenge, assume the back bridge position. Raise one of your legs straight up and balance as long as possible, one minute maximum. Balancing in this manner works additional areas of your core. Then perform the same exercise but raise the other leg for as long as possible, one minute maximum.

d.   **Pelvic Thrusts: Version 1** (easier): Lie on your back with your knees bent and feet flat on the floor. Slowly lift your hips off the floor and towards the ceiling so only your head, shoulders, and feet support you. Lower your hips to the floor slowly. Repeat 10 times.

   Version 2 (more difficult): Lie on your back with your legs bent 90 degrees at the hips, your feet aimed at the ceiling, and your arms flat on the floor right by your sides. Bracing yourself with your arms, slowly lift your hips off the floor and towards the ceiling, then slowly lower your hips to the floor again. Repeat 10 times.

Daily Worksheet Entry. A sample standard worksheet entry for this would be:

   Core Work – Bridges

Resistance Training Warm-up. If you lift weights without first making sure that your body is ready for the stress, you run a risk of injuring yourself. An injury can disrupt and delay your efforts to recover from stroke. The best warm-up method is to first perform one set of each resistance exercise at a reduced level (half the weight or even less). This gets your muscles warmed and ready to exercise with the full weight. Do this on each fixed-weight machine prior to your usual sets.

Daily Worksheet Entry. A sample standard worksheet entry for this would be:

Bench Press – Weight 60 – Reps 12/10/8

 Cardio Walking is done at a track, four times a week. Each cardio walking session should last as long as you can continue to exercise with proper form—one hour maximum. Proper form would consist of moving straight forward, holding your body erect. Move smoothly, getting all the balance you need from the act of "walking." Keep one of your feet firmly planted on the ground at all times, "vaulting" your body directly over your forward leg. (This means try not to rock side to side as you walk, as can happen if you keep your feet too far apart in an effort to balance yourself).

If your doctor has requested that you not exceed a certain maximum heart rate during cardio exercise, use a heart rate monitor to do so.

Begin walking with a cane around the track. Set a beat on your metronome and step to the beat. Alternate between slow, then fast, then slow again by varying the beat on your metronome. For example, walk for 2 or 4 minutes at one pace, then the next 2 or 4 minutes at another pace, and so on.

Every so often, and as often as possible, walk without using the cane for support. If you need to use the cane occasionally, do so by setting its tip down.

Once you are strong enough to increase your overall speed, do so, and reset the beat on your metronome to match it. Continue to increase your starting pace periodically as your strength increases.

Daily Worksheet Entry. A standard worksheet entry for this could be:

Distance – 3 miles
Time – 1 hour

Pace – various as set on my metronome
Time walked without support – 1/2 hour
Fastest lap without cane – 4½ min.

❹ **Cardio Workout** at the health club/gym is done on Wednesday:

a.   Work out for 30 minutes on an elliptical machine, reversing your direction of movement (pedaling backwards) every minute.

b.   Then work out for 30 minutes on a stair-stepper machine, having the machine move at different speeds. (Because of the upper thigh strength needed for the stair-stepper, you may need to begin with a 15-minute workout and increase the session length gradually as your strength increases.)

On both the elliptical and stair-stepper machines, use proper form: stand as straight as you can, look to the front, and keep your hands off the handrails as much as possible. It may be more difficult to balance on the elliptical and stepper without support than it was to exercise without support on the treadmill, since your body is going up and down as you pedal. Therefore, exercise without support as much as you can and gradually increase the time as you improve.

Daily Worksheet Entry. A standard worksheet entry for cardio workouts could be:

> **Elliptical –**
> > **Distance – 1 mile**
> > **Time – 30 min.**
> > **Reversed direction every 1 min.**
> > **Time walked without support – entire time except 5 min.**
>
> **Stair-stepper –**
> > **Distance – 2 miles**
> > **Time – 30 min.**
> > **Time walked without support – 15 min.**

❺ **Yoga** is done under the guidance and supervision of a certified yoga instructor at a yoga facility or your health club. Each yoga session should last about an hour.

Daily Worksheet Entry. A standard worksheet entry for this is:

> **1 hr. yoga as instructed by my yoga instructor**

Recovery Plan 5

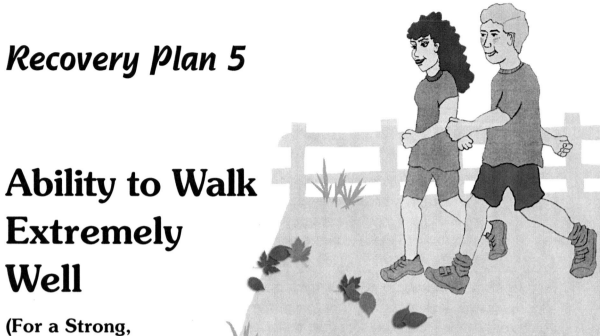

Ability to Walk Extremely Well

(For a Strong, Independent, Active or Athletic Person)

Date Begun:	Date Finished:	Repeat Dates:	Start:	Finish:
Goal:	To walk perfectly—better than virtually anyone I know.			
My Personal Goals for this Plan:				
Who Plan is For:	**Strong, Active or Athletic Independent Person.** Anyone who wants to walk perfectly and has completed Recovery Plan 4.			
Location:	This recovery plan requires you to work out independently at a gym for resistance and cardio training; at a yoga facility for yoga if your health club has no yoga classes; and at an athletic track for cardio walking.			

People to Hire:	A certified yoga instructor (for one session a week)—this person should be capable of and interested in working with a stroke survivor.
Special Requirements, Information or Features:	This advanced stroke recovery walking plan is designed for a particularly strong participant who wants to do all the strength training on his or her own. It is designed for an athletic person who has graduated from having a personal trainer on hand to watch him or her exercise. It is also designed to help you begin to develop your ability to practice yoga on your own. It is further designed to introduce the participant to special exercises to spur greater and faster improvement in walking functionality. This plan is very intensive and aggressive. If a person works out like this, he or she will become a better walker than virtually anyone. **Important Note: To ensure your safety, we recommend that a caregiver or another person should remain with you during all your exercises.**
Components Trained:	Balance, flexibility, strength, and endurance.
Exercises Performed:	Resistance training exercises for strength; yoga for flexibility and balance; cardio walking for endurance.
Equipment or Supplies to Buy:	A heart-rate monitor if required by your doctor (if your health club's cardio equipment does not incorporate heart-rate monitors).
Facility Equipment/ Supplies Used:	Fixed-weight machines and mats at a gym; yoga props at a yoga studio where you meet with the yoga instructor; a treadmill, an elliptical machine, and a stair-stepper machine (at the gym).

13-Week Training Plan:

Each week, follow the workout schedule below. When a number appears after an exercise, refer to the explanation below this exercise schedule for instructions.

Weeks	Mon	Tue	Wed	Thu	Fri	Sat	Sun
1 - 13	Resistance Training❶ -CHEST & SHOULDERS (time: to finish all exercises) Cardio Walking – at Track❷ (1 hr)	Resistance Training -LEG & TRICEPS (time: to finish all exercises) Cardio Walking (1 hr)	Resistance Training -BACK & BICEPS (time: to finish all exercises) Cardio Workout – at Gym❸ (1 hr)	Yoga – with Instructor❹ (1 hr) Cardio Walking (1 hr)	Eclectic Workout❻ (1 hr) Cardio Walking (1 hr)	Yoga – Individual❺ (1 hr) Eclectic Workout (1 hr)	Off

Instructions

 Resistance Training is done unsupervised by a personal trainer, on fixed-weight machines at the gym three times a week. Do not use the dumbbells or other free weights at your gym, as you would need someone (a spotter) with you constantly to watch and guard against accidents. Be sure to follow the instructions and diagrams mounted on the fixed-weight machines describing how they are to be used, or get a staff member or athletic trainer from the health club to show you and answer any questions if you need someone to refresh your knowledge of any machine.

Workout 1 is for strong/athletic men, and Workout 2 is for strong/athletic women. The workouts appear at the end of this walking plan. Each workout consists of three different resistance training sessions that you will do.

- **Monday (number 1) is chest and shoulder day.**

- **Tuesday (number 2) is leg and triceps day.**

- **Wednesday (number 3) is back and biceps day.**

Each resistance training session consists of five exercises, each with 3 sets and between 6 and 12 repetitions a set. Each resistance training session should last long enough for you to perform all your exercises. On days with both resistance training and cardio walking, try to perform resistance training *before* cardio walking.

Resistance Training Warm-up. If you lift weights without first making sure that your body is ready for the stress, you run a risk of injuring yourself. An injury can disrupt and delay your efforts to recover from stroke. The best warm-up method is to first perform one set of each resistance exercise at a reduced level (half the weight or even less). This gets your muscles warmed and ready to exercise with the full weight. Do this on each fixed-weight machine prior to your usual sets.

Setting the Proper Weight on the Fixed-Weight Machines. Each workout chart below contains suggested starting weights to use with each machine. If they are too easy or too difficult, adjust the weight an increment or two up or down (usually 5 or 10 pounds per increment, depending on the machine). To help you determine that you have the right weight, you should be able to complete the listed number of sets and repetitions *with proper form*, but it should be challenging enough that by the end of the last set, you are really working hard to be able to finish.

Core Training. It is so important that it bears repeating: ***Many fitness specialists think that core training is the single most important thing you can do to walk well.*** To make sure you have a strong core, spend the first 20 minutes of every resistance training session performing the four core training exercises given in Recovery Plan 4. As a strong, active, athletic and independent person, you should be able to do the most challenging versions of all four core exercises. Additionally, you can do one or both of the following core exercises:

a.   **Stability Ball Pushups.** A stability ball is one of those big soft balls you see in the gym. They are generally about 32 inches in diameter and made of thermoplastic polymer. Take a stability ball and assume a pushup position with both of your hands resting on the ball. Do ten pushups. Stability ball pushups teach you to maintain your balance with your upper body when moving, and when your primary support is movable. (As a stability ball can rotate, it is definitely movable!)

b.   **Stability Ball Leg Raises.** Place the stability ball next to a wall or in a corner to reduce or eliminate its ability to rotate. Sit on the ball and extend one of your legs straight forward. This will force you to maintain your balance completely with the opposite leg. Maintain this position for as long as you can, one minute maximum. Repeat with your other leg.

Daily Worksheet Entry. A standard worksheet entry could be:

Core Training – 3 bridges/1 rotation/ball crunches

Bench Press – Weight 20 – Reps 6/6/6

(Make an entry for each machine.)

❷ **Cardio Walking** is done at a track. Each cardio walking session should last as long as you can continue to exercise with proper form—one hour maximum.

Begin walking around the track, staying in a particular lane. Set beats on the metronome. Step to the different beats of the metronome. Periodically time yourself for a set distance—like one lap or four laps (a mile). Your goal is to cover more and more distance in less and less time.

Daily Worksheet Entry. A standard worksheet entry for this is:

Distance – 3 miles
Time – 1 hour
Pace – various as set on my metronome
Time walked without support – 1/2 hour
Fastest lap without cane – 4½ min.
Fastest 1/10th of a mile – 2 min.

❸ **Cardio Workouts** at the health club or gym are made up of (a) one thirty minute session on an elliptical machine, reversing direction of movement every minute, and (b) one thirty minute session on a stair-stepper machine, having the machine move at different speeds. On both the elliptical and stair-stepper machines, use proper form: stand as straight as you can, look to the front, and keep your hands off the handrails as much as possible.

Daily Worksheet Entry. Standard workbook entries would be:

Elliptical
> **Distance – 1 mile**
> **Time – 30 min.**
> **Reversed direction every – 1 min.**
> **Time walked without support – entire time**

Stair-stepper
> **Distance – 2 miles**
> **Time – 30 min.**
> **Time walked without support – ½ hour**

❹ **Yoga Training, Supervised.** The Thursday session is done under the guidance and supervision of a certified yoga instructor at a yoga facility (unless your health club has yoga classes).

Daily Worksheet Entry. A standard worksheet entry is:

> **Yoga as directed by my yoga instructor**
> (or name the individual postures you assumed)

❺ **Yoga Training, Individual.** The Saturday session is done on your own. Spend time assuming the postures you learned during previous sessions at the yoga facility, possibly using props you have collected at home. You may find certain books helpful, like *Light on Yoga: The classic guide to yoga from the world's foremost authority,* by B.K.S. Iyengar (Thorsons, 2001, paperback). Assume postures you know are extremely helpful to you, like balancing postures—or postures that you would like to be able to improve on, such as being able to do deeper bends.

Each yoga session will last about an hour.

Daily Worksheet Entry. A standard worksheet entry for this is:

> **Personal yoga focusing on balancing asanas**
> (or name the individual postures you assumed)

❻ **Eclectic Workouts** can be done at the health club/gym, or at home if you have the proper equipment. Eclectic workouts consist of an hour spent doing one or more of the following exercises:

    a. **Medicine Ball Pushups.** Assume a pushup position with one of your hands resting on a heavy medicine ball and the other on the floor. Do a pushup. Staying in the "up" pushup position (arms extended), switch the medicine ball, so that it is now under the other hand. You can do this by moving the hand with no medicine ball in it next to the other hand on the medicine ball, switching the ball, then moving the other hand away from the one on the ball and resting it on the floor. Do another pushup. Switch the medicine ball back so that it is underneath the original hand without getting out of the "up" pushup position. Do another pushup. Switch the ball again, and so on. Do ten pushups this way.

You will notice that during "switches" like this, one of your hands is always going to have to settle down on a movable ball for support. This can prove to be very challenging—and most helpful to ensure you gain strength! You will probably find that the *heavier* the medicine ball is, the easier it is to work with. For variation, use a lighter medicine ball. When you get good at switching a single medicine ball back and forth between your hands while you are doing pushups, you can increase the challenge by putting medicine balls under both your hands.

b. **Dumbbell Step-ups**—Put a low bench that you can comfortably step up onto (about a foot high) in front of you. Hold a lightweight (like 5 lbs.) dumbbell in each hand. Step from the ground up onto the bench, left leg first. Stabilize yourself on top of the bench. Step back off the bench, left leg first. Do the same movement, right leg first. Do 20 steps this way—so each leg has led 10 times. For variation, use various weights of dumbbells.

c. **Dumbbell Shadow Boxing**—Holding lightweight dumbbells in each hand, do boxing movements. With your left leg and hand forward, do jabs, swings and uppercuts.

More specifically, stand in a "boxer" position, with your left leg forward, holding the lightweight dumbbells in each hand, with your left hand slightly forward of the right one. For **jabs**, quickly thrust your left hand straight forward until your arm is extended and withdraw it all in one quick motion. For **swings**, swing your right hand out and across your body in a semi-circle to the left, to where you would connect with an opponent's jaw. For **uppercuts**, drop your rear hand to your stomach and then arc it upward like an upside down "U" as though you were aiming for an opponent's chin. After each movement, return to the starting position.

Then, with your right leg and hand forward, do the same with the opposite hand. Do 10 of each boxing movement with each arm. You can vary the impact of this exercise by resting more or less between each different boxing movement.

d. **Shooting Baskets**—With a basketball and a basketball hoop, practice shooting free throws (from the free-throw line). Between shooting attempts, get the basketball and return to the free-throw line. Force yourself to successfully shoot varying numbers of free throws—like 10, or 15, or 25.

Layups—Alternatively, you can practice shooting layups. A layup is a shot from very near and under the basket, slightly to one side, in which you jump up and lightly throw the ball against the backboard so that it ideally rebounds back and down through the basket. First head into the basket from the left and shoot, then from the right and shoot. (Many people think this is the easiest type of basketball shot to make!)

e.   **Jumping Jacks**—Do jumping jacks. Your goal is to eventually do jumping jacks quicker and more smoothly; however, perform the movement as slowly and as jerkily as necessary to be safe. For example, you may need to move your legs apart, stop, think, then move your legs back together, and so on, at the beginning.

f.   **Yo-yos**—Pick a set distance—like 40 yards or eight houses down the street. Run that distance, there and back. Rest and note how long it took to catch your breath—for example, one minute. Run there and back again. Rest until you catch your breath and note how long it takes. If you can catch your breath in a lesser amount of time, like 45 seconds, do that and then run again. Rest 30 seconds. Run again. Rest 20 seconds. Repeat until you don't rest at all between runs, if possible. But don't worry if you can't improve your rest time between runs right away. Simply do the best you can. Spend no more than 20 minutes at a time doing "yo-yos."

g.   **Tilt Board Bicep Curls**—Stand next to a tilt board with lightweight 5-pound dumbbells in each hand. Step up onto the tilt board. First do one bicep curl, then the other. Step off the tilt board. Repeat, leading with the opposite foot. Do 20 repetitions of this.

h.   **Jump Rope**—Practice jumping rope. Determine that you are going to successfully do a certain number of jumps—like 50—then start. Restart and recount from one if you inadvertently stop. Do this as many times as necessary to jump the total number you have decided to do consecutively without stopping. As you become more fit, increase the number of jumps.

i.   **Dumbbell Lunges**—Holding a 2-pound dumbbell in each hand, take a long step forward with one foot, then bring the trailing leg forward to the front leg and stand up straight. Step forward with the other foot. Again, bring the trailing leg forward. Practice stepping farther and more smoothly as you go. Ideally, your lunges will get so deep that your rear leg will be parallel to the floor in the trailing position. Do lunges for a set distance—like 20 yards— and then do lunges back to where you started.

WORKOUT 1

For Strong/Athletic Men

Chest and Shoulder Routine:

	Core Work	20 minutes
120	Bench Press machine	3 sets/6–12 reps per set
70	Incline Bench Press machine	3 sets/6–12 reps per set
80	Pectoral Flye machine	3 sets/6–12 reps per set
50	Overhead Press machine	3 sets/6–12 reps per set
40	Lateral Raise machine	3 sets/6–12 reps per set

Leg and Triceps Routine:

	Core Work	20 minutes
200	Standing Squat machine	3 sets/6–12 reps per set
240	Seated Squat machine	3 sets/6–12 reps per set
60	Quadriceps Leg Raise machine	3 sets/6–12 reps per set
60	Lying Hamstring Curl machine	3 sets/6–12 reps per set
50	Triceps Pressdown machine	3 sets/6–12 reps per set
50	Seated Overhead Cable Pull machine	3 sets/6–12 reps per set

Back and Biceps Routine:

	Core Work	20 minutes
100	Seated Row machine	3 sets/6–12 reps per set
100	Pulldown machine	3 sets/6–12 reps per set
80	Reverse Flye machine	3 sets/6–12 reps per set
50	Biceps Curl machine	3 sets/6–12 reps per set
40	Incline Curl machine	3 sets/6–12 reps per set

WORKOUT 2
For Strong/Athletic Women

Chest and Shoulder Routine:

	Core Work	20 minutes
50	Bench Press machine	3 sets/6–12 reps per set
40	Incline Bench Press machine	3 sets/6–12 reps per set
40	Pectoral Flye machine	3 sets/6–12 reps per set
30	Overhead Press machine	3 sets/6–12 reps per set
20	Lateral Raise machine	3 sets/6–12 reps per set

Leg and Triceps Routine:

	Core Work	20 minutes
120	Standing Squat machine	3 sets/6–12 reps per set
160	Seated Squat machine	3 sets/6–12 reps per set
50	Quadriceps Leg Raise machine	3 sets/6–12 reps per set
50	Lying Hamstring Curl machine	3 sets/6–12 reps per set
40	Triceps Pressdown machine	3 sets/6–12 reps per set
30	Seated Overhead Cable Pull machine	3 sets/6–12 reps per set

Back and Biceps Routine:

	Core Work	20 minutes
60	Seated Row machine	3 sets/6–12 reps per set
60	Pulldown machine	3 sets/6–12 reps per set
40	Reverse Flye machine	3 sets/6–12 reps per set
30	Biceps Curl machine	3 sets/6–12 reps per set
20	Incline Curl machine	3 sets/6–12 reps per set

Recovery Plan 6

Improvement of Hand Function

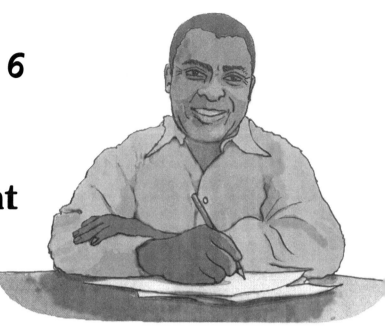

Date Begun:	Date Finished:	Repeat Dates:	Start:	Finish:

Goal:	To be able to use your hands perfectly
My Personal Goals for this Plan:	
Who Plan is For:	Anyone who wants to use their hands better
Location:	At home
People to Hire:	None
Components Trained:	Strength (strong muscles to function); positioning and exertion-of-force control (able to put one's hands and body in place to accomplish a task and exert proper force on objects); fine muscle control (able to use one's hands to grasp, handle, and transfer objects); and perceptual skills (hand-eye coordination)

Exercises Performed:	Light resistance training exercises for hand strength; ball handling for positioning and exertion-of-force control; handling objects for fine muscle control; writing and typing for hand-eye coordination
Equipment and Supplies Needed:	A computer; pen and paper; several dozen coins and small objects (coins will do); about 50 marbles; a small soft rubber ball (like a handball or a tennis ball); a hand gripper; light (1 or 2 lb.) dumbbells. Origami and kirigami books or kits (see "Recommended Books and Other Resources" at end of book). Note that there are two kinds of grippers available. The sport gripper normally has a resistance of about 20-45 pounds. The strength-training gripper has a resistance (tension) of from 60 to 400 pounds and is much more difficult to use. Most stroke survivors will want to begin with a sport gripper with a resistance not so great that you can't close it. Look for one that fits your hand well. Those with smaller hands will want one with a smaller distance between the inside edges of the handles so they can close it properly.

13-Week Training Plan:

Each week follow the exercise schedule below. When a number appears after an exercise, refer to the corresponding explanation below the schedule for instructions.

Weeks	Mon	Tue	Wed	Thu	Fri	Sat	Sun
1 - 13	Strength Training❶ (1 hr) Fine Muscle Control❷ (1 hr)	Hand-Eye Coordina- tion❸ (1 hr) Positioning and Exertion- of-Force Control❹ (1 hr)	Off	Strength Training (1 hr) Fine Muscle Control (1 hr)	Hand-Eye Coordination (1 hr) Positioning and Exertion- of-Force Control (1 hr)	Off	Off

①   **Strength Training for Hand Muscles.** Do the following exercises for periods of 10 minutes each, for a total of one hour of concentrated hand-strength training.

- **Small, Soft Rubber Ball:** squeeze a small, soft rubber ball repetitively, first with one hand, and then the other. This will increase the strength of your hand muscles and your grip.

- **Gripper:** Open and close the gripper repetitively with one hand, then the other, to increase the strength of your grip. See information about grippers in the plan chart above. It is possible that even a sport gripper may be too stiff for some people to close initially, so if this is the case, do the above exercise of squeezing a small soft rubber ball until you are strong enough to begin using the gripper.

- **Soft Rubber Handball (Small) or Tennis Ball:** With your hands close together, change the ball from hand to hand. When you can do that smoothly, toss it from one hand to the other. Widen the distance between your hands every few days as you become more proficient. Also vary the distance between your hands as you toss it from one hand to the other.

- **Small Dumbbell:** As you carry a dumbbell, do the following:
  1. Move it back and forth from hand to hand. Pass it from one hand to the other at different levels—waist level, shoulder level, up even with your head. Always strive to make your motions as smooth and controlled as you can.
  2. Holding your arm straight down by your side with the dumbbell in your hand, rotate your hand in toward your body and outward away from your body repetitively. Change hands and repeat.
  3. Holding the dumbbell in front of you at about waist or chest height, make small circles in the air with the hand holding the dumbell, first clockwise, then counterclockwise. Repeat with the other hand.

Informal Strength Training: On strength training days (Monday and Thursday), in addition to the above exercises, carry an exercise device with you constantly (such as a small rubber ball, gripper, or a light dumbbell), and work with it whenever you think about it and have time.

②   **Fine Muscle Control** concerns your ability to handle and move objects normally with your hands. Not only do you need strong hand muscles that you can use to grasp and move objects into the right position at the right time, you need to be able to use smaller objects as designed and be able to transfer them from hand to hand. You also need to be able to compensate for the weight and size of an object in your hand as you control it. You also should be able to use very precise movements for especially delicate tasks, such as picking up things between your thumb and forefinger, screwing in a tiny eyeglasses screw, or threading beads.

You should work on fine muscle control skills for one hour on fine muscle control days (Tuesday and Friday).

a.   **Picking Up Coins.** In a seated position, pick up coins one by one from a pile and put them into a stack. Once you have them stacked, practice moving them one by one from the first stack to a new stack. Then practice picking them up from a stack and putting them into a slot in a piggy bank or a slot cut into the top of a box.

b.   **Stacking, Moving and Sorting Coins.** Gather a bunch of coins of various types—pennies, nickels, dimes, quarters (at least 40).

    1.   Using your *right hand only*, take the coins out of the heap one by one and stack them by type of coin, making a stack for each type of coin. You'll have a penny stack, a dime stack, a nickel stack, and a quarter stack.

        Jumble up the coins again, then using your *left hand only*, pick up the coins and stack them by type in the same way. Keep the stacks of coins once you have finished this step.

    2.   For this next phase of the exercise, you need to be able to read the dates on the coins. If your vision doesn't permit this, skip this step. With one hand, pick up a coin from one of the stacks created in step 1. Transfer it to your other hand and note its date. Then place it flat on the table, starting a row for each different type of coin. Place the coins into rows in exact date order, with the earliest dates to the left and the latest dates to the right. You will wind up with a separate row each of pennies, nickels, dimes and quarters, each sorted into date order. This develops both your ability to grasp and move objects and your hand-eye coordination.

c.   **Stringing Beads.** Another thing you can do to improve your ability to handle small objects is to work with a bead stringing kit. Such kits come with beads of various sizes and colors, along with strings onto which the beads can be strung. Practice making necklaces and bracelets with colored beads to your liking.

d. **Origami Paper Folding.** As an alternative to bead stringing, you can take up origami, the Japanese art of paper folding. Get an origami kit containing both instructions and paper (or you can get a book on origami and follow its instructions as to what type of paper to get). Not only should most people find it interesting to work with paper to create folded pieces of art, your creations will undoubtedly get better as you progress, creating a visible record of your improvement.

e. **Kirigami Paper Cutting.** To increase your ability to work with scissors, you can take up kirigami, the Japanese art of paper cutting. As with origami, instruction kits and books are available. In kirigami, you work with scissors and paper to create some amazing effects—and hardly notice at the same time how much your hand skills are improving. See "Recommended Books and Other Resources" at the end of this book for books and kits for origami and kirigami.

❸ **Hand-Eye Coordination and Perceptual Skills.** That's a fancy way of saying your ability to watch something and move your hands correctly in response to what you see, or at the same time as you are watching it. A good example of this would be playing a game of ping-pong, in which you have to watch an object coming toward you and be able to hit it back to the other person at the right time, when it comes within reach. Before you attempt ping-pong, however, which is very quick and challenging, try the following simpler skills. You should spend one hour working on these hand-eye coordination and perceptual skills exercises.

a. **Typing** requires good hand-eye coordination. Work your hand-eye coordination by picking a written passage from a newspaper, magazine or book and typing it into a computer. Then give your work to someone who can read it back to you to show you what you have done and to let you know if you correctly copied the original passage. But don't worry too much about mistakes, because the most important part of these drills is the practice you are giving yourself. Lots of practice is what will help you to improve.

b. **Handwriting** requires good hand-eye coordination as well as fine muscle control. Select a written passage from a newspaper, magazine or book and practice writing it out in longhand. Then give your work to someone who can read it back to you to show you what you have done and to let you know if you correctly copied the original passage. But again, don't worry too much about the mistakes, because the most important part of these drills is the practice you are giving yourself. Lots of practice is what will help you to improve.

c. **Working a Jigsaw Puzzle.** Get a jigsaw puzzle to assemble whose number and shape of pieces present a good challenge for you. When you start, set goals for yourself—like "I am going to complete the border or the clouds in the sky today." Working the puzzle will help improve your ability to pick out an item based on its color and shape and use your hands to move it as desired.

d. **Playing a Video Game.** Invest the money in a handheld video game console and a couple of games. Carry the console with you and play games from time to time. You will learn to move your fingers based on what is shown on the console's screen. As an added plus, there are a number of good "brain expanding" games and foreign language teaching games available in video game format, enabling you to both expand your hand-eye coordination and develop other skills.

e. **Knitting, Crocheting, Tying Macramé, or Working Needlepoint.** While these skills will mostly interest women, these creative tasks are excellent for recovering anyone's hand-eye coordination and dexterity. (And by the way, needle skills aren't only for women—Daveda knows an excellent doctor who is expert at needlepoint—his beautiful needlepoint tapestries and artwork are hung all over his clinic's walls!)

When all your typing, writing, puzzle-working, game-playing (and needlework) skills are down pat … you're ready to play PING-PONG!

④ Positioning and Exertion-of-Force Control for Hand Muscles. Not only do you need your hands to be strong, you also need to be able to put them in the right place to do things and to exert the proper force on objects. Enabling you to do that is the purpose of this positioning and exertion-of-force control training.

The last three exercises below (b, c and d) require you to be able to walk without support, with both hands free. If you cannot do this, come back to these exercises after you have completed one of the walking recovery plans to increase your ability to walk.

a. **Toss Small Items.** Assume a seated position at a table or on the floor with a container such as a wastebasket about 5 feet away from you. Have a handful of small objects (like pennies or marbles) immediately in front of you. One by one, pick up the small objects and attempt to toss them into the container. See how many you can get into the container. Vary the kinds of objects you use and the distance between you and the container to increase (or decrease, if you want!) the challenge.

b. **Walking Ball Bounce.** To improve your ability to put your hands (and body) into place to accomplish a task, walk around a track with a small ball—like a tennis ball—in one of your hands. As you walk, bounce the ball in front of you and catch it with the other hand as you walk. After 15 minutes, change hands so you're throwing and catching with the opposite hands. Change every 15 minutes. Keep throwing the ball down with one hand so it bounces, and catching it with the other. Do this for an hour at a time. If you desire, you can listen to music, or work on your talking, while doing this.

c. **Standing Hand Ball.** As an alternative exercise, stand about 10 feet away from a wall, holding a tennis ball. Throw the tennis ball at the wall, causing it to bounce off the wall and return to you. Catch the tennis ball before it bounces. Repeat. For variation, work on hitting various different spots on the wall with the tennis ball. If you fail to catch the tennis ball, retrieve it, return to a spot facing the wall, and begin again. This should be done for an hour at a time when you do it.

d. **Shooting Baskets.** You can improve your hand positioning and exertion-of-force skills on a larger scale by shooting baskets:

1. Begin with a small basketball hoop and sponge rubber ball set designed to be used indoors, and practice shooting baskets. Start with the basket close enough to you for you to be able to get the objects into the basket fairly often, and increase the distance to the basket as your ability improves.

2. Using a lightweight large ball (like a volleyball), practice shooting baskets on a basketball court. As you improve you can increase the distance to the basket, until you are able to practice shooting baskets from the free-throw line.

You should also realize that your hand positioning and exertion-of-force control will naturally improve as you work not only on strength training for hand muscles, but also as you work on strengthening the other parts of your body using the walking recovery plans, yoga and core training.

Daily Worksheet Entry. Examples are:

Typing, handwriting, jigsaw puzzle – 1 hr.
Positioning and exertion-of-force control – 1 hr.

Recovery Plan 7

Ability to Speak Well

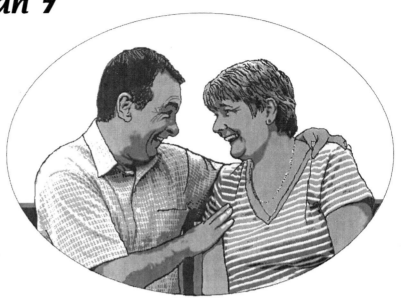

Date Begun:	Date Finished:	Repeat Dates:	Start:	Finish:
Goal:	To speak easily, clearly and naturally so that others instantly understand what you are saying.			
My Personal Goals for this Plan:				
Who Plan is For:	Anyone who is capable of making sounds; anyone who wants to recover their ability to speak clearly and naturally and be easily able to make himself or herself understood.			
Location:	At home or at a speech therapist's office.			

People to Hire:	A speech therapist to work with you on exercises that require that you speak properly, and who can give you helpful lists, forms and booklets. As an alternative, you might be able to find a speech therapy student who will be happy to work with you for a lower hourly fee or for the experience.
Special Requirements, Information or Features:	This stroke recovery plan is designed for a stroke survivor who is interested in getting the assistance of a speech therapist to help them recover their speaking ability. The therapist can tailor the exercises for you, make sure you do everything safely, and give you immediate feedback on how you are doing. **Swallowing.** Speech therapists are also trained to help people with swallowing problems. If you need swallowing assistance, request that your therapist also work with you on swallowing while you are together.
Components Trained:	**Articulation** (ability to make speech sounds correctly); **intonation** (varying your pitch); **rate** (varying your speed); **intensity** (varying your loudness).
Exercises Performed:	Sound-forming exercises to improve articulation; reading paragraphs aloud with proper emphasis to improve intonation; reading passages aloud to improve rate of speaking; speaking with the appropriate intensity (loudness or volume) to people different distances away to improve your control of intensity.
Equipment or Supplies to Buy:	Optional: a sound recorder (digital or tape) that you can speak into. Recording your exercises will help you evaluate your articulation, intonation, rate, and intensity.
Facility Equipment/ Supplies Used:	Lists, forms and booklets given to you by the speech therapist.

13-Week Training Plan:

Each week follow the schedule below. When a number appears after an exercise, refer to the explanation below this exercise schedule for instructions.

Weeks	Mon	Tue	Wed	Thu	Fri	Sat	Sun
1 – 13	Articulation Work❶ Intonation Work❷ Rate (speed) Work❸ Intensity (volume) Work❹ (Time: as directed by speech therapist)	Formal Articulation and Intonation Work on your own❺ (1 hr) Informal Articulation and Intonation Work on your own❻ (1 hr)	Rate and Intensity Work on your own❼ (1 hr 15 mins)	Articulation Work Intonation Work Rate Work Intensity Work	Formal Articulation and Intonation Work on your own (1 hr) Informal Articulation and Intonation Work on your own (1 hr)	Rate and Intensity Work on your own (1 hr 15 mins)	Off

Articulation, Intonation, Rate and Intensity Work. This plan asks you to meet with a speech therapist twice a week to work on your articulation, intonation, rate and intensity. (If Monday and Thursday are not convenient for you or the therapist, you may change those days and rearrange the other days.) Your therapist may also give you additional exercises for improving your speech.

Articulation. Articulation means being able to form and make the sounds of speech properly. In your sessions, the therapist will likely provide you with booklets of mouth, tongue and breath exercises and lists of sounds that you can make—all of which are designed to improve your articulation.

Intonation involves raising and lowering pitch (how low or high your voice sounds as you speak) to convey different meanings and emotions. To intonate correctly you need to be able to vary the pitch of your voice. The speech therapist has a number of ways to help you improve your pitch. You may, for example, be asked to read a paragraph while suiting your intonation to what you are saying.

Rate of Speech. The speech therapist can listen to you as you read lists of sounds, multi-syllable words, and text passages and make sure you speak at a proper speed. Most likely, you will find certain sounds hard to make. When you try to make those sounds, you may slow down or stop, causing you to have an unnatural and uneven rate of speaking. The speech therapist knows how to get you to speak sounds you find difficult more quickly so you get practice in making those sounds at the correct rate.

Intensity (Loudness). Your speech therapist may ask you to read a passage to people, each time from a different distance, to help you to speak at a proper volume.

 Articulation and Intonation Work On Your Own.

a.   **Formal Articulation and Intonation work.** On the two days a week listed in your schedule, perform the articulation and passage-reading exercises taught to you by your speech therapist. Use copies of material you get from the speech therapist (lists of exercises and selected written passages). Record yourself talking. From time to time, listen to your recordings, noting any sounds that don't sound quite right and passages that don't have quite the intonation desired. Tape yourself again, endeavoring to "improve" your rough spots. Repeat this process for an hour.

b.   **Informal Articulation and Intonation work.** On days on which you do formal articulation and intonation work on your own, you should do an additional hour of "informal" articulation and intonation work:

(1) One good idea is to sing along with recorded music. Such work will improve your ability to articulate and intonate. Don't worry if you are off-key or can't get the melody or words just right—just sing anyway!

           Taking Charge of Your Stroke Recovery

(2) Another excellent idea is to take a conversational or spoken foreign language course such as those available on CD and DVD. (4) You will learn how to make different sounds and to speak with different pitches. Just as you can sing along with recorded music, you can work with a foreign-language self-instruction recording or computer software.

Total time will be 2 hours—one hour on formal articulation and intonation, and the second hour on informal work.

Clarity Tips

During Roger's rehabilitation, he learned there are six things you can do to make your speech clearer:

1. Take a deep breath before you talk.

2. Begin speaking as soon as you breathe out.

3. Open your mouth wide.

4. Exaggerate the movements of your mouth.

5. Speak slowly.

6. Stress each word and syllable.

❼ Formal Rate and Intensity (Volume) Work On Your Own.

a. Do exercises given to you by your speech therapist. Record yourself speaking or reading, listen to the tape and evaluate how you did. Repeat the process, endeavoring to speak smoothly at a desirable speed and with appropriate volume (loudness).

b. Many experts believe your ability to vary the intensity of sounds can be increased with breath-control exercises. Specialists in breath-control maintain

---

(4) RosettaStone™ offers excellent foreign language courses which teach you to speak through pictures and sounds, using software you play on your computer. Search for this company on the Internet; they often also set up kiosks in shopping malls. A list of mall locations is available on their website at www.rosettastone.com, or call the 800 number listed on their website.

---

that few people breathe in a free, natural and harmonious way, but for the most part, they breathe too fast with constricted breath. This limits our ability to communicate well. Many other health practitioners believe there are numerous other health, healing, and fitness benefits of good breathing and that there is a direct relationship between lung function and overall health.

To directly work on your intensity, practice deliberately slowing down your inhalations, then lengthening your exhalations. Then practice deepening your breathing: take deeper, slower breaths, breathing from your lower abdomen rather than just your chest so that you are drawing your breath with your diaphragm. Work on your breathing for at least 15 minutes.

You should spend an hour and 15 minutes doing formal rate and intensity work on your own.

Daily Worksheet Entry. Examples are:

> **Articulation and intonation work, formal – 1 hr.**
> **Articulation and intonation work, informal – 1 hr.**
> **Rate and intensity work – 1 hr. 15 min.**

Recovery Plan 8

Thinking Skills

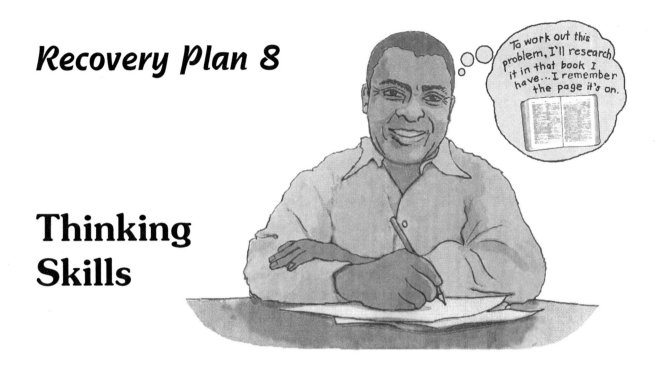

To work out this problem, I'll research it in that book I have...I remember the page it's on.

Date Begun:	Date Finished:	Repeat Dates:	Start:	Finish:
Goal:	To think more clearly			
My Personal Goals for this Plan:				
Who Plan is For:	Anyone			
Location:	At home			
People to Hire:	None			

Special Requirements, Information or Features:	This stroke recovery plan is designed for a stroke survivor who wants to be able to think and comprehend better. Being successful in life depends on these abilities: • to recall (call back into the mind something previously known or experienced), • to compare (observe and consider the similarities, differences, and other attributes of two or more things, one against the other or others), • to classify (arrange things into groups according to their features or characteristics), • to infer (arrive at an opinion or conclusion through observation or by reasoning), • to generalize (use particular facts or instances to form a general statement or principle), • to evaluate (consider and judge as to the value, quality, usefulness or importance of something). It has been scientifically demonstrated that such skills can be consciously learned and improved.
Components Trained:	Absorption (of knowledge), application (ability to use information), interaction (ability to convey information to others), association (ability to link recent experiences to earlier experiences, finding similarities, differences, and interrelationships).
Exercises Performed:	Reading of both factual material (such as a newspaper or magazine) and instructional material (such as plastic model assembly instructions). Various games, drills and exercises to improve thinking skills.
Equipment or Supplies Used:	A newspaper or magazine, blank writing paper, and a writing instrument for absorption, interaction and association work. For application work, you also need a plastic model for assembly, or an origami or kirigami instruction book; a puzzle book (mathematical puzzles, logic puzzles, or word puzzles) or a book of simple math problems.

13-Week Training:

Each week follow the schedule below. When a number appears after an exercise, refer to the explanation below this exercise schedule for instructions.

Weeks	Mon	Tue	Wed	Thu	Fri	Sat	Sun
1 – 13	Absorption Work❶ (1 hr)	Application Work❷ (1 hr) Association Work❸ (1 hr)	Interaction Work❹ (1 hr)	Absorption Work (1 hr)	Application Work (1 hr) Association Work (1 hr)	Interaction Work (1 hr)	Off

❶ **Absorption of Knowledge.** To increase your absorption, try to stay more open to information that comes your way—whether through reading, looking, listening, or conversation. Once you find information that is of interest to you, make sure you really understand it so you can make it part of your "knowledge base"—your mental store of information—and have it at your command.

One good way to ensure understanding, as well as to keep your mind "stretching," is to use the dictionary more frequently. When you come across a word you don't understand or aren't sure about, look it up in a good dictionary and use it in sentences until you feel comfortable with it. ⑤ Learning new words and using them when speaking and writing exercises your mind in a very beneficial way.

To develop your absorption-of-knowledge skill, do one or both of the following exercises:

---

⑤   If you don't have a dictionary you like, we can recommend three exceptional ones. An adult dictionary that contains a wide selection of words, yet which has extremely clear, easy definitions and lots of sample sentences is the *Macmillan English Dictionary for Advanced Learners of American English.* Another unique dictionary that uses very clear "action" definitions in complete sentences is The *Collins Cobuild English Dictionary for Advanced Learners.* It too makes learning a word very simple. Both dictionaries use plenty of example sentences and phrases so you can see how a word is actually used in speech. Third, if you'd like a large authoritative dictionary with very complete, advanced definitions, try *The New Oxford American Dictionary,* published by Oxford University Press. See "Recommended Books and Other Resources" in the back of this book for full publication information for these dictionaries.

Exercise #1: Remembering Information – this forces you to recall possibly useful items

a.   Go through a newspaper or magazine, putting a star by each piece of information you find that could be of some use to you.

b.   When you are done going through the newspaper or magazine, put it aside and make a list of all the things that you can remember checking. When this is done, compare what you listed with the publication where you placed stars.

c.   Referring to your list and the newspaper, make a second list of things that you forgot to put on your first list. Now put your lists aside.

d.   Now let's try this again! Look through the publication again to see what you marked. Put it aside, then make a new list of all the items you recall putting a star by. Check that list against the newspaper or magazine to see how you did and what you missed.

e.   Now, without referring to the publication, make a new list of items you forgot to put on your second list. When this is done, compare what you listed with the newspaper.

Exercise #2: Answering Questions – this forces you to extract information from material you read

a.   Read an article in a newspaper or magazine. Put it aside.

b.   Ask yourself: **Who** was involved in the matter discussed in the article? Speak your answer aloud, either to a caregiver, or *as if* a caregiver was with you.

c.   Ask yourself another question: **What** happened? Speak your answer aloud.

d.   And another: **When** did it happen? Speak your answer aloud.

e.   And another: **Where** did it happen? Speak your answer aloud.

f.   Yet another: **Why** did it happen? Speak your answer aloud.

g.   Ask yourself: **How** did it happen? Speak your answer aloud.

It is a good policy to always consider **WHO**, **WHAT**, **WHEN**, **WHERE**, **WHY**, and **HOW**, when you read things.

You should spend an hour at a time doing absorption-of-knowledge exercises.

 Application of Knowledge. To increase your application of knowledge—which is your ability to use information—you can do many things. Pick one of the exercises below during each application session and devote an hour to it.

Exercise #1: Working puzzles/building items

a.   Get a book of simple mathematics problems and work them. Alternatively, if you aren't good with math, you can get a book of non-math logical and word problems and work them. You can get a puzzle book (mathematical or logical puzzles, word and other kinds of puzzles) and work as many as you can. ⑥

b.   Get a plastic or wood assembly model of almost anything and use the instructions that came with it to build it. Make sure you use nontoxic products! As an alternative, you can get a book of instructions for creating Japanese origami figures (different animals and objects created through intricate folding of paper) and follow the instructions.

In the process of following directions to assemble a model or create origami figures, you will practice connecting or relating "real" items to "concepts."

Exercise #2: Playing the "Use For" game

a.   Pick an item at random: A book on a table. A glass in a cupboard. A kitchen knife. Anything.

---

⑥ There are many excellent books containing games and challenges designed to help anyone improve their thinking abilities, should you wish to go beyond the exercises provided here. An example is *Dental Floss for the Mind: A Complete Program for Boosting Your Brain Power,* by Michael Noir and Bernard Croisile (New York: McGraw-Hill, 2005). A search in a large bookstore such as Barnes & Noble or Borders Books & Music, or on www.Amazon.com on the Internet, will turn up other puzzle and thinking books that can provide fun and variety as you improve your thinking abilities.

---

b.　Come up with 10 original uses for the item. For example, if you picked a kitchen knife, you could say, it could be used to measure something (like a table is 8 kitchen knife-lengths long), it could be used to take the lid off a can, it could be used to make a hole in a wall, it could be used to dig a hole in dirt to plant a flower, it could be used as a pointer, etc.

c.　Share your ideas about the "new uses" for the item with a caregiver. Ask the caregiver if he or she can think of any different "new uses."

You should spend an hour at a time doing application-of-knowledge exercises.

❸　**Association.** This is your ability to link recent experiences to earlier ones. In doing this exercise, use your experience and existing knowledge to evaluate the item or event and come up with ways to improve it.

Exercise #1: Playing the "Improvement" game

a.　Pick an item. Come up with 10 ways you can think of to improve it. If you picked a book, for example, you could say that it would be improved if it was bound better, if it cost less, if it had clearer type, if it included more pictures, if it had a better table of contents, etc.

b.　Share your thoughts on improvements with a caregiver. Ask the caregiver what he or she thinks could be done to improve the item.

c.　As a variation, think of a past event of some kind—a convention, a party, a sporting event or charity function—any event you can recall attending, or that you have knowledge about. Come up with 10 ways it could be improved.

d.　Share your thoughts on these improvements with a caregiver. Ask the caregiver for his or her own ideas on improving the event.

Exercise#2: Playing the "What If" game

a.　Imagine a person who does a certain kind of job (like a plumber), or imagine an event. Now imagine if all plumbers were like that plumber, or if all events were like that event. Think, based on your past experiences, what the probable associated facts and their consequences would be. For instance, if the plumber happened to be particularly helpful, what if everyone were that helpful? If the plumber was not helpful at all, what if everyone were like that?

b. Discuss your "what ifs" with a caregiver.

You should spend an hour at a time working on Association.

❹ Interaction.

Exercise #1: Interaction with a caregiver

a. To increase your ability to interact with people, read a passage in the newspaper about some people doing something.

b. Write two separate short speeches about what you read. In both of your speeches, try to convince the "audience" to do what the people in the article did. (1) The first should be a speech aimed at someone who, with very little urging, would do exactly what the people in the article did. (2) The second should be a speech aimed at someone who thinks that what the people in the article did was wrong.

c. Deliver your two speeches to a caregiver, reading from your paper but using feeling and your powers of persuasion as you do so. Listen carefully to any comments or suggestions your caregiver may make about the speeches.

d. Modify the two speeches based upon what your caregiver said.

Exercise #2: Interaction with nonacquaintances

Do the following steps on different days, in the various locations suggested. Try to repeat at least one of these exercises each week until you feel very comfortable speaking to people you don't know.

a. Take a trip to a supermarket or another type of store likely to have a lot of shoppers or browsers. (You may shop if you wish.) Strike up a conversation with one of the shoppers you encounter in the store. You can discuss an item in the store, the selection, or any other subject that occurs to you. Keep the conversation going for at least two minutes.

b. Strike up a new conversation with another shopper in the same or in a different store. Keep the conversation going for at least four minutes.

c. Visit a park, shopping mall or other public area in your town. Strike up a conversation with someone you see there. Try to keep the conversation going at least five minutes.

Exercise #3: Interaction with groups of people (optional)

a.   Work on a speech about a topic of special interest to you—like what you did before having a stroke. Write out the speech or make notes on what you want to say.

b.   Another idea for a topic that could be especially interesting to you and others is what problems stroke caused you, what you are doing to recover from stroke, and what your recovery experiences have been to date.

c.   If you can, prepare a computer slideshow forming a background to your speech, using your notes or written speech as a guide.

d.   Contact local schools, groups, churches and the like, asking for an opportunity to deliver your speech.

e.   When an opportunity to present the speech arises, TAKE IT!

You should spend an hour at a time working on interaction exercises.

Daily Worksheet Entry. Examples are:

Absorption work – 1 hr.
Application work – 1 hr.
Association work – 1 hr.
Interaction work – 1 hr.

Recovery Plan 9

Vision and Ability to Use Your Eyes Better

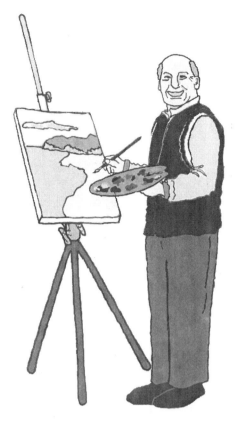

Date Begun:	Date Finished:	Repeat Dates:	Start:	Finish:
Goal:	To improve my use of my eyes to see and to increase my range of vision			
My Personal Goals for this Plan:				
Who Plan is For:	Anyone			
Location:	At home and in the yard; on a basketball court if available			
People to Hire:	None. This stroke recovery plan is designed for a stroke survivor working alone.			

Special Information and Requirements:	The sense of vision is made up of visual acuity (sharpness and ability of your eyes to detect details); eye function (if the eyes work properly and if there are any problems with the optic nerve); eye motility (if your eyes are positioned properly and move properly); and visual field (to what extent your eyes can see peripherally—to the sides).

This plan may not improve the visual difficulties that stem from physical or functional problems, nor the vision problems normally handled by corrective eyeglasses or contact lenses. However, any stroke survivor facing vision challenges should know that the medical profession offers many options for them. There are low vision specialists who may prescribe certain exercises to help improve vision. Mechanical devices, like prisms and contact lenses, may help. There are also a number of drugs that can improve vision. Finally, surgery may be prescribed—for example, eye muscle surgery to correct double vision that occurred as a result of the stroke. This surgery can be extremely helpful.

Make sure your eyes have been checked by an ophthalmologist or other eye specialist since your stroke and that you have up-to-date corrective lenses, if you need them, before you begin this plan.

The exercises in this plan can help you to improve your hand-eye coordination, your visual reaction time (ability to understand what you are seeing and respond promptly to it), your ability to focus, and your ability to see better with your peripheral (side) vision. The exercises should also help your visual acuity and visual field, unless you have any physical or functional problems that could stand in the way. |
| **Components Trained:** | Hand-eye coordination; visual reaction time; focusing; peripheral vision. |
| **Exercises Performed:** | Various exercises as detailed in the instructions. |

Equipment or Supplies Used:	• straight drinking straws
	• uncooked spaghetti strands
	• a basketball (or lighter-weight large ball like a volleyball for less athletic individuals) and a mounted basketball hoop
	• a bouncy rubber ball about baseball size to use playing catch and also to bounce off a wall
	• a book
	• a chair
	• picture puzzle books in which you compare pictures to spot the differences

13-Week Training Plan:

Each week follow the schedule below. When a number appears after an exercise, refer to the explanation below this exercise schedule for instructions.

Weeks	Mon	Tue	Wed	Thu	Fri	Sat	Sun
1 - 13	Hand-Eye Coordination❶ (1 hr) Reaction Time❷ (1 hr)	Near/Far Focusing❸ (10 mins, 6 times a day) Peripheral Vision❹ (10 mins, 6 times a day)	Off	Hand-Eye Coordination (1 hr) Reaction Time (1 hr)	Near/Far Focusing (10 mins, 6 times a day) Peripheral Vision (10 mins, 6 times a day) General Visual Acuity❺ (30 mins.)	Off	Off

❶ Hand-Eye Coordination.

a. A great exercise to enhance your hand-eye coordination is to thread the spaghetti. You need a drinking straw and a firm, uncooked piece of spaghetti to perform this exercise. With one hand, hold the straw about one or two feet in front of your face, at any angle. Insert the spaghetti into the hole at one end of the straw, then take it out the same side. Insert the spaghetti into the other end hole, then take it out. Alternate in each end of the straw. Do not let the spaghetti go so far into the straw that you can't take it back out the hole you inserted it in, and do not let the spaghetti fall back in. Vary the position of the straw and perform the exercise again.

b. If you are able to stand unsupported, you can perform a similar exercise on a basketball court. Use a lighter ball like a volleyball if your strength is limited. Practice shooting baskets from the free throw line. Between attempts, retrieve the basketball and return to the free-throw line and shoot again, attempting to make a basket. It is good to set a goal for yourself—like 10 successful free throws, then 20 or 25 when that becomes easy. Continue shooting until you reach your goal.

You should spend an hour a session doing hand-eye coordination work.

❷ Visual Reaction Time. A great exercise to improve your ability to respond appropriately to a moving object you see is to practice tossing a ball back and forth with a partner (increase the distance between you and your partner as your ability to catch the ball improves). If you can't find a partner, you can practice throwing a rubber ball against a wall and catching it on the rebound.

You should spend an hour a session doing reaction time work.

❸ Near and Far Focusing. A good way to improve your near and far focusing is to sit in a chair or on a bench, holding a book. First, focus on the book. Then focus on something about 10 feet away, preferably with something written on it. Then focus on something about 25 feet away. Then focus on something very far away, like an airplane moving across the sky. Repeat. When possible, as when looking at the book or at something about 10 feet away with something written on it, endeavor to read what you are looking at. Try to look at the various items quickly, but not so quickly that you can't focus on them well enough to read.

You should do near/far focusing work six times a day every day it is scheduled, for 10 minutes each time.

④ **Peripheral Vision.** A good way to improve your peripheral vision is to stand about 5 feet from a corner, where the two walls leading into the corner have objects on and against them. Staring at the corner, practice "seeing" the items on the walls with your peripheral vision. Practice seeing items farther and farther from the corner. Also, practice this standing at different distances from the corner.

You should do peripheral vision work six times a day, every day it is scheduled, 10 minutes each time.

⑤ **General Visual Acuity.** Get some picture puzzle books with visual exercises that have you compare pictures to spot the differences between then. This trains your visual acuity, ability to focus and to differentiate images. You should do 30 minutes of general visual acuity work on the scheduled day.

Daily Worksheet Entry. Examples are:

> **Hand-eye coordination – 1 hr.**
> **Reaction time – 1 hr.**
> **Near/far focusing – 10 min., 6 times/day**
> **Peripheral vision – 10 min., 6 times/day**
> **Gen. visual acuity – 30 min.**

Recovery Plan 10

Ability to Eat, Drink and Swallow Normally

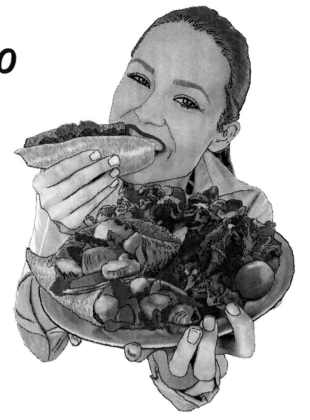

Date Begun:	Date Finished:	Repeat Dates:	Start:	Finish:
Goal:	To swallow better and have no difficulty whatever with eating, drinking and swallowing.			
My Personal Goals for this Plan:				
Who Plan is For:	Anyone.			
Location:	At home.			
People to Hire:	A speech therapist (optional but recommended).			

Special Information or Requirements:	This stroke recovery plan is designed for an average person working at home, with another person present.
	Having trouble swallowing can be devastating. If a stroke survivor has trouble swallowing, there will undoubtedly be types of food and drink he or she needs to avoid because they cause choking and coughing. There is a risk that such food and drink will go into the lungs, threatening the stroke survivor's life. In the worst cases, a stroke survivor cannot eat or drink at all, and must get nutrition though a tube threaded down their nose or surgically implanted directly into their stomach. To have a normal life, the stroke survivor needs to be able to recover the ability to eat, drink and swallow anything normally.
	If you are facing swallowing challenges, you should know that the medical profession offers many options for you. Speech therapists are trained to deal with swallowing problems and they have a multitude of different devices and equipment that can be used to improve swallowing. We recommend that if you have swallowing difficulties, you explore everything a speech therapist has to offer. However, if you cannot afford to hire a speech therapist, you can still do this plan and improve your swallowing.
	Swallowing can be viewed as made up of three phases: an oral phase, a throat phase, and an esophageal phase.
	(1) The **oral phase** involves the jaws, lips, tongue, teeth, cheeks and palate (roof of the mouth). This involves breaking down the food to prepare it for swallowing and delivering it to the back of the mouth when it is ready to swallow.
	(2) During the **throat phase**, a swallow-ready substance moves from the mouth, through the throat and into the esophagus. It is during this phase that food may inadvertently enter the airway. The throat phase involves multiple structures. Muscles at the base of the tongue, the soft palate (muscle at the

	back part of the roof of the mouth), the flap that covers the airway, the pharynx (throat), the larynx (voice box), and the muscle at the top of the esophagus all need to move quickly in concert.
	(3) The **esophageal phase** involves movement of food from the esophagus ("food pipe") into the stomach though a wavelike series of muscle actions. Food or liquid moving back up into the esophagus from the stomach (reflux) can be a problem.
	If you have a swallowing problem, it is critical that you swallow safely. **Make sure that you always have someone around you when you eat or drink and when you swallow anything**. If a problem develops that you cannot deal with, the person watching you can act immediately to help you.
	(If your weight drops as a likely result of your not getting enough food and drink, please let your doctor know. There is a place to record your weight each day at the top of the Daily Worksheets in this workbook.)
Components Trained:	The functions involved with each of the three swallowing phases mentioned above.
Items Needed:	Food and drink of varying consistencies.
Equipment or Supplies to Buy:	Thickener (to increase the consistency of foods and drinks you find too "thin"). ⑦ A straw. A cotton ball.

---

⑦ Food thickeners designed specifically to assist people with swallowing difficulties are available in medical supply stores and at commercial medical supply websites such as www.EasierLiving.com.

13-Week Training Plan:

Each week follow the exercise schedule below. When a number appears after an exercise, refer to the numbered explanation below this schedule for instructions.

Weeks	Mon	Tue	Wed	Thu	Fri	Sat	Sun
1 - 13	Oral Phase Work❶ (10-15 mins, before each meal)	Throat Phase Work❷ (10-15 mins, before each meal)	Food Pipe Work❸ (10-15 mins, before each meal)	Oral Phase Work (10-15 mins, before each meal)	Throat Phase Work (10-15 mins, before each meal)	Food Pipe Work (10-15 mins, before each meal)	Off❹

Important General Eating and Drinking Instructions

1. In all cases, when you eat, sit up tall and remain in that position for 30 minutes after the meal is over.

2. Take small bites of food and sips of liquid, one at a time.

3. Make sure that all your food and drink has a consistency you can handle (such as honey-like, or nectar-like). You can add thickener to food and drink to make it easier to deal with.

4. From time to time, swallow or sip something that is "difficult" for you to deal with (with a caregiver watching you so they can take immediately action to help you if necessary). If you swallow something difficult, it makes sense to next swallow something easy. Alternate hard and easy swallows (just like many people alternate swallowing food and liquid).

5. As you are able, you can increase the size of bites to maximize your swallowing challenges and improvement.

6. If you start to cough or clear your throat, swallow immediately. If you continue to cough, **CLEAR IT ALL OUT** of your mouth and throat and swallow.

Tip for Improving Swallowing. It is a good idea to keep Lemon Chill® brand soft frozen lemonade in your freezer. This is a refreshing, naturally flavored product that is like a soft-frozen sherbet or ice, and eaten with a spoon. If eating it doesn't cause any problems for you, you can have it from time to time for dessert and snacks. People have found that lemon flavoring stimulates throat muscles. Consuming lemon flavored items can help you swallow better. (If this brand isn't available in your area, try to find another naturally flavored, soft frozen lemon product in place of it.)

Instructions for Swallowing Exercises

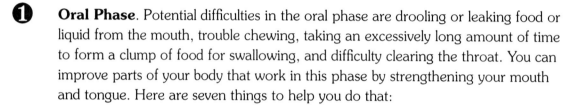 **Oral Phase**. Potential difficulties in the oral phase are drooling or leaking food or liquid from the mouth, trouble chewing, taking an excessively long amount of time to form a clump of food for swallowing, and difficulty clearing the throat. You can improve parts of your body that work in this phase by strengthening your mouth and tongue. Here are seven things to help you do that:

a.   Pucker your lips like you are going to kiss someone. Focus on making your lips as round as possible. Relax your face. Repeat.

b.   Smile as widely and as evenly as you can. Relax your face. Repeat.

c.   Pucker. Smile. Relax your face. Repeat.

d.   Puff out your cheeks with air, not letting air escape from your lips. Relax your face. Repeat.

e.   Move your tongue back and forth, from side to side, touching each corner of your mouth.

f.   With your mouth open wide, first touch your top lip with your tongue, then touch your bottom lip with your tongue.

g.   With your tongue, circle your lips in a clockwise direction. Then circle your lips in a counterclockwise direction with your tongue. Imagine there is something on your lips that you are cleaning off with your tongue.

You should do the above oral phase work for ten or fifteen minutes before you eat each time, on days on which it is scheduled.

❷ **Throat Phase.** Difficulties in this stage are choking and coughing when items go down the "wrong pipe," problems if food or liquid enters the lungs, and the sensation of food "sticking in the throat." You can improve the parts of your body that work in this phase by moving your Adam's apple. (Everyone has one, even if it doesn't show!) Here are two exercises you can do for this:

a. Without anything in your mouth, swallow, noticing the "feeling" of your Adam's apple moving. Swallow again, holding your Adam's apple at its highest position with your throat muscles for three seconds before letting it drop. This work on controlling the movement of your Adam's apple will help improve your ability to swallow. (Ladies, don't worry that your Adam's apple might grow more prominent by doing these exercises—that isn't possible since it is made of cartilage and its size doesn't change once it's formed!)

b. Say a vowel sound like "eee" in as low a voice as possible, then say the same sound in as high a voice as possible. While doing this, place a finger on your throat and "feel" your Adam's apple move. You are interested in making your Adam's apple move as much as possible.

On days that throat phase work is scheduled, you should practice it for ten or fifteen minutes, before you eat.

❸ **Esophageal (Food Pipe) Phase.** Reflux is the most common problem in this phase. The best exercise to solve food pipe problems is to eat foods that are slightly difficult for you. Here are the most common types of foods that are difficult to eat and which you should practice eating:

a. Softer foods (with more liquid in them) are harder to eat than harder foods.

b. Dry and flaky foods (like crackers or flaky pastry) are harder to eat than foods that don't fall apart in the mouth.

c. Food that is difficult to chew (like certain meats and raw fruits and vegetables) is harder to eat than easily chewed food.

d. Sticky and gummy food (like peanut butter) is harder to eat than food that is unlikely to stick in the mouth or throat and can thus more easily be prepared by the mouth for swallowing.

You can also improve the parts of your body that work in this phase by doing the following things:

a.   While sitting down in a chair, push down on the arms and hold your breath for as long as possible. You are endeavoring to increase your breath control.

b.   Place a cotton ball on a table in front of you. Take a straw in your hand. With one end of the straw in your mouth, suck in, picking up the cotton ball with the other end of the straw. Endeavor to hold the cotton ball on the other end of the straw by sucking on the straw for as long as you can. This exercise works to increase your breath control and capacity.

You should do food pipe work for ten or fifteen minutes before you eat on days on which it is scheduled.

 On your day off, eat and drink normally, making sure someone is always with you. Take note of the current status of your swallowing skill so you can fill it in on your Daily and Weekly Worksheets.

Daily Worksheet Entry. Examples are:

> **Oral phase work – 10 min., before meals**
> **Throat phase work – 10 min., before meals**
> **Food pipe work – 15 min., before meals**

Recovery Plan 11

Alleviation of Single-Sided Weakness

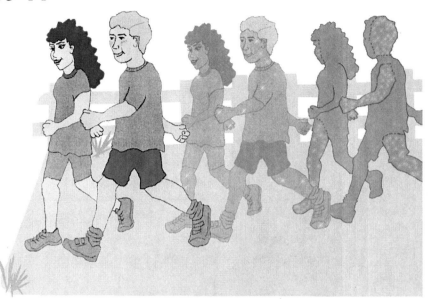

Date Begun:	Date Finished:	Repeat Dates:	Start:	Finish:
Goal:	To eliminate all single-sided weakness in my body and regain normal strength, feeling and function in those areas.			
My Personal Goals for this Plan:				
Who Plan is For:	Any stroke survivor with single-sided weakness of the face, hand, arm or leg (but not actual paralysis).			
Location:	Your home; a health club or gym for resistance training and access to a treadmill; an athletic track (or quiet street with sidewalks); a handball court or other location with a large wall to bounce a ball against; a yoga facility for yoga (or a group yoga class held at your health club).			

People to Hire:	Depending on which single-sided weakness you are working to correct, you may need to hire: (1) a personal trainer (for two sessions a week at a gym or health club). This person should be capable of and interested in working with a stroke survivor and able to design an appropriate workout for people of varying physical abilities; (2) A certified yoga instructor (for one session a week), or alternatively, take a group yoga class at your health club. The yoga instructor should be capable of and interested in working with a stroke survivor.
Special Requirements, Information or Features:	The arm and leg single-sided weakness plans require you to travel regularly to a gym or health club (and a yoga facility if there are no classes at your health club) and work with instructors there.
Components Trained:	One-sided weakness of the face, arms, hand or leg: facial muscle strengthening; hand, arm and leg strength training; hand positioning control; hand-eye coordination; cardio walking; resistance training; balance.
Exercises Performed:	Resistance training exercises for strength; yoga for flexibility and balance; cardio walking for endurance.
Equipment or Supplies to Buy:	Various household objects as described in the hand, arm and leg sections of this plan. A heart-rate monitor if required by your doctor (if your health club's cardio equipment does not incorporate heart-rate monitors).
Facility Equipment/ Supplies Used:	Machine weights, free weights, weighted balls, mats, tilt boards, etc., at a health club or gym where you meet with the personal trainer; yoga props at a yoga studio where you meet with the yoga instructor; a treadmill at the health club or gym.

Single-sided weakness expresses itself as a "tingling" or "numbness" on one side of the body or in certain areas or limbs, coupled with general weakness of the affected side. It may affect one side of the face, one arm and hand, one side of the trunk, or one leg. It occurs commonly in cases of stroke. If you have total paralysis, or paralysis of any limbs, you are going to need to get help from physicians and therapists so you can move again. Once you can move, you can take charge of your treatment with these plans and deal with any residual single-sided weakness.

Working to *lessen or relieve* single-sided weakness is not quite the same as working to *increase or regain* a physical function or skill, but there isn't too much difference in approaches between their recovery plans. The main practical difference in working to rehabilitate single-sided weaknesses is in measuring results. If you use one of the other recovery plans to regain a function or skill, you can decide whether or not you have regained that function to your satisfaction. But if you are using the plan to overcome a deficiency such as single-sided weakness, you need to ask yourself whether or not the deficiency has been diminished to your satisfaction, or eradicated.

With facial weakness, for example, you can ask whether food that you are not aware of is collecting on your face when you eat, alerting other people (but not you) that there is a "problem." With single-sided arm or leg weakness, you can note how much of the time you feel *reduced* or *no* numbness or tingling in the affected limb—or you can take note of how much time goes by without your even thinking about this problem. You might also notice *increasing* strength in your weaker hand, arm or leg, depending on which weakness you've been working to reduce.

With that difference, then, here is a plan to overcome single-sided weakness.

FOR CASES OF SINGLE-SIDED WEAKNESS AFFECTING YOUR FACE

Perhaps you wish you could eat or speak better. Perhaps you wish you could express emotions with your face better. If you think that having better control and strength of your facial muscles could solve your problems, you should do the following exercises, which also enhance swallowing, as follows:

Weeks	Mon	Tue	Wed	Thu	Fri	Sat	Sun
1 - 13	Facial Muscle Work❶ (30 mins)	Facial Muscle Work (30 mins)	Facial Muscle Work (30 mins)	Facial Muscle Work (30 mins)	Facial Muscle Work (30 mins)	Facial Muscle Work (30 mins)	Off

❶ **Facial Muscle Work.** For facial muscle work, perform the following exercises for at least a half hour on days on which it is scheduled:

a. Pucker your lips like you are going to kiss someone. Focus on making your lips as round as possible. Relax your face. Repeat.

b. Smile as widely and as evenly as you can. Relax your face. Repeat.

c. Pucker. Smile. Relax your face. Repeat.

d. Puff out your checks with air, while preventing air from escaping through your lips. Relax your face. Repeat.

e. Move your tongue back and forth, from side to side, touching each corner of your mouth.

f. With your mouth open wide, first touch your top lip with your tongue, and then touch your bottom lip with your tongue.

g. With your tongue, circle your lips in a clockwise direction. Then circle your lips in a counterclockwise direction with your tongue. Imagine there is something on your lips that you are cleaning off with your tongue.

h. Without any food or drink in your mouth, swallow, noticing the "feeling" of your Adam's apple moving. Swallow again, holding your Adam's apple at its highest position with your throat muscles for three seconds before letting it drop. This work on controlling the movement of your Adam's apple will help improve your facial muscle strength. (Ladies, don't worry that your Adam's apple might grow more prominent by doing these exercises—that isn't possible since it is made of cartilage and its size doesn't change once it's formed!)

i. Say a vowel sound like "eee" in as low a voice as possible, then say the same sound in as high a voice as possible. While doing this, place a finger on your throat and "feel" your Adam's apple move. You are interested in making your Adam's apple move as much as possible.

j.   While sitting down in a chair, push down on the arms and hold your breath for as long as possible. You are endeavoring to increase your breath control.

k.   Place a cotton ball on a table in front of you. Take a straw in your hand. With one end of the straw in your mouth, suck in, picking up the cotton ball with the other end of the straw. Endeavor to hold the cotton ball on the other end of the straw by sucking on the straw for as long as you can. This exercise works to increase your breath control and capacity.

FOR CASES OF SINGLE-SIDED WEAKNESS AFFECTING YOUR ARMS OR HANDS

Having a weak arm can cause many problems. One of your hands and arms is normally dominant; if the dominant side of your body is weakened, you could have many hand control problems with fine movements. Having a tingling or numb arm can make it hard for you to rest, increasing your fatigue and making you do things less well. It is hard to drive if both your hands and arms don't work well. To reduce the effects of single-sided weakness affecting an arm and/or hand, you can do the hand control exercises, as follows:

13-Week Training Plan:

Each week follow the exercise schedule below. When a number appears after an exercise, refer to the corresponding explanation below the schedule for instructions.

Weeks	Mon	Tue	Wed	Thu	Fri	Sat	Sun
1 - 13	Strength Training❶ (1 hr) Fine Muscle Control❷ (1 hr)	Hand-Eye Coordination❸ (1 hr) Positioning and Exertion-of-Force Control❹ (1 hr)	Off	Strength Training (1 hr) Fine Muscle Control (1 hr)	Hand-Eye Coordination (1 hr) Positioning and Exertion-of-Force Control (1 hr)	Off	Off

❶ **Strength Training for Hand Muscles.** Do the following exercises for periods of 10 minutes each, for a total of one hour of concentrated hand-strength training.

- **Small, Soft Rubber Ball:** squeeze a small, soft rubber ball repetitively, first with one hand, and then the other. This will increase the strength of your hand muscles and your grip.

- **Gripper:** Open and close the gripper repetitively with one hand, then the other, to increase the strength of your grip. See information about grippers in the plan chart above. It is possible that even a sport gripper may be too stiff for some people to close initially, so if this is the case, do the above exercise of squeezing a small soft rubber ball until you are strong enough to begin using the gripper.

- **Soft Rubber Handball (Small) or Tennis Ball:** With your hands close together, change the ball from hand to hand. When you can do that smoothly, toss it from one hand to the other. Widen the distance between your hands every few days as you become more proficient. Also vary the distance between your hands as you toss it from one hand to the other.

- **Small Dumbbell:** As you carry a dumbbell, (a) move it back and forth from hand to hand, and from side to side. Pass it from one hand to the other at different levels—waist level, shoulder level, up even with your head. Always strive to make your motions as smooth and controlled as you can. (b) Holding your arm straight down by your side with the dumbbell in your hand, rotate your hand in toward your body and outward away from your body repetitively. Change hands and repeat. (c) Holding the dumbbell in front of you at about waist or chest height, make small circles in the air with the hand holding the dumbbell, first clockwise, then counterclockwise. Repeat with the other hand.

Informal Strength Training: On strength training days (Monday and Thursday), in addition to the above exercises, carry an exercise device with you constantly (such as a small rubber ball, gripper, or a light dumbbell), and work with it whenever you think about it and have time.

❷ **Fine Muscle Control** concerns your ability to handle and move objects normally with your hands. Not only do you need strong hand muscles that you can use to grasp and move objects into the right position at the right time, you need to be able to use smaller objects as designed and be able to transfer them from hand to hand.

You also need to be able to compensate for the weight and size of an object in your hand as you control it. You also should be able to use very precise movements for especially delicate tasks, such as picking up things between your thumb and forefinger, screwing in a tiny eyeglasses screw, or threading beads.

You should work on fine muscle control skills for one hour on fine muscle control days (Tuesday and Friday).

a. **Picking up Coins.** In a seated position, pick up coins one by one from a pile and put them into a stack. Once you have them stacked, practice moving them one by one from the first stack to a new stack. Then practice picking them up from a stack and putting them into a slot in a piggy bank or a slot cut into the top of a box.

b. **Stacking, Moving and Sorting Coins.** Gather a bunch of coins of various types—pennies, nickels, dimes, quarters (at least 40).

1. Using your *right hand only*, take the coins out of the heap one by one and stack them by type of coin, making a stack for each type of coin. You'll have a penny stack, a dime stack, a nickel stack, and a quarter stack.

    Jumble up the coins again, then using your *left hand only*, pick up the coins and stack them by type in the same way. Keep the stacks of coins once you have finished this step.

2. For this next phase of the exercise, you need to be able to read the dates on the coins. If your vision doesn't permit this, skip this step. With one hand, pick up a coin from one of the stacks created in step 1. Transfer it to your other hand and note its date. Then place it flat on the table, starting a row for each different type of coin. Place the coins into rows in exact date order, with the earliest dates to the left and the latest dates to the right. You will wind up with a separate row each of pennies, nickels, dimes and quarters, each sorted into date order. This develops both your ability to grasp and move objects and your hand-eye coordination.

c. **Stringing Beads.** Another thing you can do to improve your ability to handle small objects is to work with a bead stringing kit. Such kits come with beads of various sizes and colors, along with strings onto which the beads can be strung. Practice making necklaces and bracelets with colored beads to your liking.

d.   **Origami Paper Folding.** An alternative to bead stringing, you can take up origami, the Japanese art of paper folding. Get an origami kit containing both instructions and paper (or you can get a book on origami and follow its instructions as to what type of paper to get). Not only should most people find it interesting to work with paper to create folded pieces of art, your creations will undoubtedly get better as you progress, creating a visible record of your improvement.

e.   **Kirigami Paper Cutting.** To increase your ability to work with scissors, you can take up kirigami, the Japanese art of paper cutting. In kirigami, you work with scissors and paper to create some amazing effects—and hardly notice at the same time how much your hands are improving. As with origami, instruction kits and books are available (see "Recommended Books and Other Resources" at end of this book).

❸ **Hand-Eye Coordination and Perceptual Skills.** That's a fancy way of saying your ability to watch something and move your hands correctly in response to what you see, or at the same time as you are watching it. A good example of this would be playing a game of ping-pong, in which you have to watch an object coming toward you and be able to hit it back to the other person at the right time, when it comes within reach. Before you attempt ping-pong, however, which is very quick and challenging, try the following simpler skills. You should spend one hour working on these hand-eye coordination and perceptual skills exercises.

a.   **Typing** requires good hand-eye coordination. Work your hand-eye coordination by picking a written passage from a newspaper, magazine or book and typing it into a computer. Then give your work to someone who can read it back to you to show you what you have done and to let you know if you correctly copied the original passage. But don't worry too much about mistakes, because the most important part of these drills is the practice you are giving yourself. Lots of practice is what will help you to improve.

b.   **Handwriting** requires good hand-eye coordination as well as fine muscle control. Select a written passage from a newspaper, magazine or book and practice writing it out in longhand. Then give your work to someone who can read it back to you to show you what you have done and to let you know if you correctly copied the original passage. But again, don't worry too much about the mistakes, because the most important part of these drills is the practice you are giving yourself. Lots of practice is what will help you to improve.

c. **Working a Jigsaw Puzzle.** Get a jigsaw puzzle to assemble whose number and shape of pieces present a good challenge for you. Set goals for yourself—like "I am going to complete the border or the clouds in the sky today." Working on the puzzle will help improve your ability to pick out an item based on its color and shape, and to use your hands to move it as desired.

d. **Playing a Video Game.** Invest the money in a handheld video game console and a couple of games. Carry the console with you and play games from time to time. You will learn to move your fingers based on what is shown on the console's screen. As an added plus, there are a number of good "brain expanding" games and foreign language teaching games available in video game format, enabling you to both expand your hand-eye coordination and develop other skills.

e. **Knitting, Crocheting, Tying Macramé, or Working Needlepoint.** While these skills will mostly interest women, these creative tasks are excellent for recovering anyone's hand-eye coordination and dexterity. (By the way, needle skills aren't only for women—Daveda knows an excellent doctor who is expert at needlepoint—his beautiful needlepoint tapestries and artwork are hung all over his clinic's walls!)

When all your typing, writing, puzzle-working, game-playing (and needlework) skills are down pat ... you're ready to play PING-PONG!

④ Positioning and Exertion-of-Force Control for Hand Muscles. Not only do you need your hands to be strong, you also need to be able to put them in the right place to do things and to exert the proper force on objects. Enabling you to do that is the purpose of this positioning and exertion-of-force control training.

The last three exercises below (b, c and d) require you to be able to walk without support, with both hands free. If you cannot do this, come back to these exercises after you have completed one of the walking recovery plans to increase your ability to walk.

a. **Toss Small Items.** Assume a seated position at a table or on the floor with a container such as a wastebasket about 5 feet away from you. Have a handful of small objects (like pennies or marbles) immediately in front of you. One by one, pick up the small objects and attempt to toss them into the container. See how many you can get into the container. Vary the kinds of objects you use and the distance between you and the container to increase (or decrease, if you want!) the challenge.

b.   **Walking Ball Bounce.** To improve your ability to put your hands (and body) into place to accomplish a task, walk around a track with a small ball—like a tennis ball—in one of your hands. As you walk, bounce the ball in front of you and catch it with the other hand. Keep throwing the ball down with one hand so it bounces and catching it with the other. After 15 minutes, change hands so you're throwing and catching with the opposite hands. Change every 15 minutes. When you do this, do it for an hour at a time. If you desire, you can listen to music, or work on your talking, while doing this.

c.   **Standing Hand Ball.** As an alternative exercise, stand about 10 feet away from a wall, holding a tennis ball. Throw the tennis ball at the wall, causing it to bounce off the wall and return to you. Catch the tennis ball before it bounces. Repeat. For variation, work on hitting various different spots on the wall with the tennis ball. If you fail to catch the tennis ball, retrieve it, return to a spot facing the wall, and begin again. This should be done for an hour at a time when you do it.

d.   **Shooting Baskets.** On a larger scale, you can improve your hand positioning and exertion-of-force skills by shooting baskets:

    1. Begin with a small basketball hoop and sponge rubber ball set designed to be used indoors, and practice shooting baskets. Start with the basket close enough to you for you to be able to get the objects into the basket fairly often, and increase the distance to the basket as your ability improves.

    2. Using a lightweight large ball (like a volleyball), practice shooting baskets on a basketball court. As you improve you can increase the distance to the basket, until you are able to practice shooting baskets from the free-throw line.

You should also realize that your hand positioning and exertion-of-force control will naturally improve as you work not only on strength training for hand muscles above, but also as you work on strengthening the other parts of your body using the walking recovery plans, yoga and core training.

FOR CASES OF SINGLE-SIDED WEAKNESS AFFECTING YOUR LEGS

Just as a tingling or numb arm can bother you and keep you awake, a tingling or numb leg can do the same. It can also fail you when you are walking, causing you to fall. To reduce the effects of single-sided weakness affecting a leg, you can adopt a walking program, as follows:

13-Week Training Plan:

Each week follow the workout schedule below. When a number appears after an exercise in the schedule, refer to the explanation below this exercise schedule for instructions.

Weeks	Mon	Tue	Wed	Thu	Fri	Sat	Sun
Weeks 1 - 13	Resistance Training❶ (1 hr) Cardio Walking❷ (1 hr)	Cardio Walking (1 hr)	Off	Resistance Training (1 hr) Cardio Walking (1 hr)	Cardio Walking (1 hr)	Yoga❸ (1 hr)	Off

Instructions

 Resistance Training (muscle resistance) is done under the guidance and supervision of a personal trainer, who will help you determine which fixed-weight machines to use, how much weight to begin with and how many repetitions of each movement to make (called "reps"), depending upon your present strength and mobility. Specific resistance training exercise workouts are presented in Recovery Plan 2 that your personal trainer can use in designing your exercise plan if he or she wishes.

Each resistance training session lasts about an hour. On days with both resistance training and cardio walking, try to perform resistance training *before* cardio walking. Your personal trainer should make sure you warm up appropriately during each exercise session. This is important so as to *avoid injury*.

This walking plan features upper and lower body resistance training. You need both upper and lower body strength to walk well and especially to completely remedy any single-sided weakness. A strong upper body keeps you balanced and allows you to support yourself when walking or when you need to grab hold of something to regain balance, or support yourself to keep from falling. It likewise enables you to smoothly carry loads, which may be heavy or of odd size or shape, so their weight is unevenly distributed.

Core Training. Your personal trainer will also likely understand the importance of "core training"—exercises that strengthen and stabilize the spine and pelvis. Many fitness specialists think that having a well-trained core is the KEY to being able to walk well. Strong core muscles also provide support and stability to the spine's network of nerves, in that the spine is less subject to misalignment and resulting impingement on the nerves. Your personal trainer should guide you through appropriate core training exercises. However, if your trainer doesn't mention it, be sure to ask that core training be included in your workout. (Core exercises are included in Recovery Plan 2 on pages 62-64 that you can adopt for use in this plan if you wish.)

Daily Worksheet Entry. A standard worksheet entry for the resistance training workouts could appear as follows (the first number is the weight used, the slashes show the number of repetitions in each of three sets). Change the exercise names or amounts based on your actual workouts. (And if it's easier for you while you're just getting going, ask your personal trainer to enter your weights and number of reps in your workbook for you as you work out).

> **Core Work – 10 minutes**
> **Lateral Raise – 25 – 8/8/8**
> **Pull down – 50 – 8/8/8**
> **Seated Squat – 80 – 8/8/8**
> **Triceps Overhead Press – 40 – 8/8/8**
> **Seated Biceps Incline Curl – 35 – 8/8/8**

Cardio Walking is done on a treadmill with the help of your personal trainer. The treadmill is somewhat like a walker—if you can use a walker, you can use a treadmill. Each cardio walking session should last as long as you can continue to walk on the treadmill with proper form, up to one hour maximum. If you are very weak or out of shape, start at 20 or 30 minutes and push yourself to increase your time every week, as you are able. Proper form would consist of moving straight forward, holding your body erect. Move smoothly, getting all the balance you need from the act of "walking." Keep one of your feet firmly planted on the ground (or treadmill platform) at all times, "vaulting" your body directly over your forward leg. (This means try not to rock side to side as you walk, as can happen if you keep your feet too far apart in an effort to balance yourself).

If your doctor has requested that you not exceed a certain maximum heart rate during cardio exercise, have your personal trainer show you how to monitor this using your heart rate monitor or the sensors on the cardio machines.

There are two variations you can perform on the treadmill:

a. **Walk at different speeds:** Begin with slower speeds until you gain sufficient strength and endurance to increase the speed. As soon as possible, begin varying and alternating your speeds from slower to faster, then slower again *within the same workout session,* so you are raising the demand on your muscles.

Note that walking at a *slower* speed, such as 0.5 miles per hour (or the slowest speed that the treadmill permits) is just as important for improving your ability to walk as the faster speeds. This is because it is more difficult to maintain your balance and proper form at slower speeds—it requires more muscle control. So even as you become able to walk faster, always include at least half your time walking at the slowest speed.

b. **Walk with different levels of support:** (1) holding on with both hands; (2) holding on with one hand; (3) only grasping or leaning against the treadmill handrail if you feel yourself losing your balance, but otherwise walking without support.

Your goal is to become able to walk without using any support at all (without holding the handrails or handlebars). Your increasing strength will begin to alleviate any single-sided weakness in your trunk and legs.

Daily Worksheet Entry. A standard worksheet entry for this could be:

> **Treadmill –**
>> **Distance – 2 miles**
>> **Time –1 hour**
>> **Speed – 1.6–2.4 mph** (entered into the treadmill).
>> **Time walked without support – 1 min. 15 seconds**
>> (time measured by the treadmill)

❸ **Yoga** is done under the guidance and supervision of a certified yoga instructor in your health club or at a yoga facility. Each yoga session should last about an hour. **Daily Worksheet Entry.** A standard worksheet entry for this is:

> **Yoga as directed by my yoga instructor**
> (or name the individual postures you assumed)

Recovery Plan 12

Improvement of Nutrition

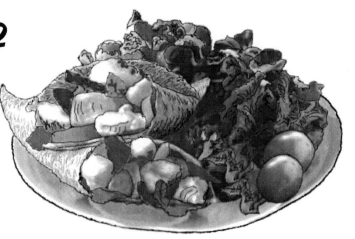

We suggest that all stroke survivors do this plan at the same time as your other recovery plans. We also suggest that you continue with this plan even after you finish all your other recovery plans. It might be a good idea to have a nutritionist review your nutrition regimen from time to time to make sure it meets your needs. You can then add or subtract nutrients according to your nutritionist's recommendations.

Date Begun:	
Goal:	(1) To get every nutrient needed to support brain healing and function; (2) to increase your overall body health to support your strength training and your return to optimum physical functioning.
My Personal Goals for this Plan:	
Who Plan is For:	Anyone.
Locations:	Health food store, doctor's office to approve nutritional supplements and check for conflicts with medicines.

People to Hire:	None.
Special Requirements, Information or Features:	It makes no sense to exercise to recover, while making recovery harder by not giving your brain what it *needs* to recover! Scientists believe that a shoreline diet caused our ancestors' brains to eventually double in size and help them take on great new skills (like using tools and communicating).[viii] The nutrition plan recommended here provides for similar nutrients. We feel taking these nutrients is bound to help you recover from stroke.
Supplies to Purchase:	Nutritional supplements and nutrient-rich foods as listed in the Detailed Stroke Recovery Nutrient Information & Selection Table.

Instructions for Following the Nutrition Plan

| 1. | Based on the information in the **Supplement Quick Selection List** and the **Detailed Stroke Recovery Nutrient Information & Selection Table** starting on page 153, decide what nutrients you want to take. In the Detailed Selection Table, put a check in the "I Want This" box next to each nutrient. Take note of the sources of each nutrient listed in the right-hand column. Some are foods and some are available mainly in nutritional supplements such as capsules, tablets, liquids, etc.

The **Supplement Quick Selection List** helps you quickly search for supplements that provide specific benefits people often inquire about, but doesn't cover all the nutrients discussed in the Detailed Selection Table. Be sure to go through the longer table so you don't miss any important nutrients. |
|---|---|
| 2. | Take the checked list to your doctor and get his or her approval for you to take the selected nutrients and amounts* and make sure there is no conflict with any medications you are taking. When you have your doctor's approval, put a check in the "Doctor Approval" box next to that nutrient in the table.

* Amounts recommended are based on selected sources researched by the authors and are not intended to constitute or substitute for the advice of professional healthcare and nutritional providers. |

3.	Each day it might help to plan what you will eat to include the foods and supplements that contain the nutrients you want to take. Be sure to record on your Daily Worksheets the nutrient-rich foods and the supplements you consume daily.
4.	Every week, review the previous week's entries. Ensure that you are getting all the nutrients you desire, either in your foods or in supplements.
5.	If you are concerned that you are not getting enough of a certain nutrient from the foods you eat, take the nutrient in the form of a supplement.
6.	If you are ever in doubt about what to eat—for example, if this workbook is not handy—eat and drink items that you would likely find on a shoreline—fatty fish, iodine-rich foods, fruits, vegetables, whole grains— and avoid starches and refined carbohydrates. Meat, poultry and eggs are also good sources of protein.

More Information on Eating Healthily

Organic Foods and Avoidance of Toxins

Common sense suggests that it would be a good idea to reduce the number of non-food, non-nutritional and potentially harmful chemicals entering our bodies. Organic foods (those raised without use of chemical fertilizers, pesticides or other contaminants) can enhance health. Many studies have been done showing that toxic metals such as mercury and industrial chemicals such as PCBs are found widely in our food and water sources and accumulate in animal and human tissues. As another example, aluminum and Teflon® from cookware are also said by some scientists to be harmful when absorbed by the body and may contribute to the development of dementia.

The accumulation of toxins in the body has been shown to cause many health problems, including disrupting the action of hormones that act as chemical messengers to and from the brain as they regulate vital functions throughout the entire body. Certified organic foods, both vegetables and fish, meat and poultry, fruit and juices, contain fewer, or no, toxic chemicals and have more health-giving nutrients. We suggest you consider purchasing organic foods. At the store, read the labels to find out what percentage of any item is actually organic. And don't forget to wash your fresh produce before eating it!

Cooking Oils and Fats

We also suggest that you consider reducing or eliminating from your diet the *refined and cooked* vegetable oils found on most grocery-store shelves, as well as margarine and other "spreads" that contain hydrogenated oils and trans fats. The latest research shows that these processed, heated oils are extremely damaging to your arteries and overall health.

You can replace processed oils with uncooked, expeller-pressed seed, nut and vegetable oils available at health food stores and in increasing numbers of supermarkets. Such unrefined oils and fats, produced through mechanical extraction instead of heat or chemical extraction, have their innate healthful properties intact. Unrefined coconut oil comes naturally in a semi-solid form like shortening and has been vindicated as an extremely healthful oil, possessing antiviral, antibacterial and antiprotozoal properties. Some unrefined oils are helpfully labeled "high heat," which means they are suitable for cooking and won't become harmful to health when used for that purpose.

Additionally, the most recent science is showing that traditionally used saturated fats such as the following are healthful rather than harmful, especially if they are cooked or heated as little as possible:

- Butter
- Beef and lamb tallow
- Lard
- Chicken, goose and duck fat
- Coconut, palm and sesame oils
- Cold pressed olive oil
- Cold pressed flax oil
- Marine oils[ix]

Significant questions still exist about the safety of canola oil for human consumption despite its prevalence in commercial foods. In the article, "The Great Con-ola," authors Sally Fallon and Mary G. Enig, Ph.D., point out that studies with animals have shown canola oil to have harmful effects on the cardiovascular system. They also write,

> "Like rapeseed oil, its predecessor, canola oil . . . causes vitamin E deficiency . . . and shortened life-span in stroke-prone rats when it was the only oil in the animals' diet."[x]

Supplement Quick Selection List

TO INCREASE YOUR ENERGY LEVEL, consider:

Ginseng	Magnesium	Minerals
Royal Jelly	ALC	B Vitamins

TO HAVE A "YOUNGER" BRAIN—MORE LIKELY FOR IT TO AGE WELL, consider:

Vitamin E	Co-Q10	Minerals
Vitamin C	ALC	

TO INCREASE BLOOD FLOW IN THE BRAIN, AMPLIFYING POSITIVE EFFECTS, consider:

EFAs (LA & ALA)	Gingko Biloba
Gotu Kola	Vinpocetine

FOR A "SHARPER" MIND, consider:

B Vitamins	NAC	Folic Acid
Co-Q10	Gingko Biloba	

TO ENHANCE MEMORY, consider:

Rosemary	PS	Lipoic Acid
Minerals	Gingko Biloba	Folic Acid

TO IMPROVE LEARNING, consider:

Calcium	Co-Q10

FOR A BETTER MOOD, consider:

Kava Kava	Vitamin D

TO REDUCE INFLAMMATION AND PAIN, consider:

EFAs (LA & ALA)
Vitamin E capsules (mixed tocopherols)
OPC-3 (powerful antioxidant)
Serratia peptidase enzyme[xi]
Ganoderma Lucidum (medicinal mushroom extract)

DETAILED STROKE RECOVERY NUTRIENT INFORMATION AND SELECTION TABLE				
Nutrient/ Suggested Daily Dose	Comments About This Nutrient	Sources	I Want This	Doctor Approval
Essential fatty acids (LA, ALA, EPA, and DHA)— 1000 mg;	About 60% of your brain is formed of essential fatty acids (EFAs)—good fats that cannot be made by your body so must be consumed from foods or supplements. EFAs make your brain cell membranes flexible and better able to communicate with other brain cells—so you can think quicker and better! If there are not enough essential fatty acids on hand to make new brain cells, and to repair old ones, the brain uses bad fats (like trans-fats), which make relatively rigid brain cell membranes. Brain cells with bad-fat-constructed (rigid) membranes don't communicate as well as brain cells with essential fatty acid-constructed (flexible) membranes. For this reason, you sometimes hear the saying: "sluggish fat produces a sluggish brain, and good fat produces a great brain." The two most important EFAs, "parent" omega-6 (linoleic acid, or LA) and "parent" omega-3 (alpha-linolenic acid, or ALA), work together, providing numerous health benefits to all cells including superior cellular oxygenation and powerful anti-inflammatory effects. New developments show that the greatest benefits result when they are taken together in proportions of from 1:1 (one part omega-6 LA to	Fatty fish (like salmon, tuna and sardines) is an excellent source of these fats. However, most people do not eat enough fatty fish to obtain sufficient essential fatty acids in their diets, making taking supplements advisable. LA and ALA oils (omega-6 and omega-3) should be from raw, unprocessed and organic sources such as seed and nut oils. (Cooking and refining remove the health-giving properties.)		

DETAILED STROKE RECOVERY NUTRIENT INFORMATION AND SELECTION TABLE				
Nutrient/ Suggested Daily Dose	Comments About This Nutrient	Sources	I Want This	Doctor Approval
	one part omega-3 ALA) to 2:1 (two parts omega-6 LA to one part omega-3 ALA). You should not take omega-3 EFAs to the exclusion of omega-6, despite what has been promoted so widely.[xii]			
Vitamin E— 400 IU	Many researchers believe Vitamin E is a "smart pill." Researchers at the Chicago Health and Aging Project have reported that people who consume high levels of vitamin E are eight to ten years smarter than their counterparts who consume little vitamin E. Vitamin E has also been shown to be protective against different forms of cognitive decline and dementia. Thus, many people think that taking vitamin E supplements can enable you to gain a decade's worth of brainpower. Vitamin E offers antioxidant protective function and is often considered to be the most important brain antioxidant, because it is fat-soluble and the brain is composed of about 60% fat (an antioxidant is a substance that protects cell membranes by destroying free radicals, which cause oxidative damage). By helping to keep the brain cell membranes healthy, vitamin E helps keep the entire cell healthy as well. There are many other positive health benefits to vitamin E, including an over 52 percent reduction in the risk of	Because people drink so much coffee, it has become the number one source of antioxidants in the American diet—and nothing else even comes close—according to a report delivered to the American Chemical Society back in 2005. However, some people cannot tolerate coffee or caffeine, and some negative health effects have been observed (for example, caffeine triggers migraines in many people). Fruits and vegetables are good sources of antioxidants, or you can opt to take a vitamin E supplement.		

DETAILED STROKE RECOVERY NUTRIENT INFORMATION AND SELECTION TABLE

Nutrient/ Suggested Daily Dose	Comments About This Nutrient	Sources	I Want This	Doctor Approval
	stroke from taking a vitamin E supplement each day. (8)			
Vitamin C— 400 mg	Vitamin C has a similar structure to glucose, your brain's sugar fuel. Because it is much like glucose, vitamin C shows up in large concentrations in the brain. Not only does vitamin C offer its own antioxidant protection, it is reported to boost the effectiveness of vitamin E. Because vitamin C and vitamin E are known to work hand in hand, researchers often administer them together.	Fruits. Supplements.		
Ginseng— 400 mg	Studies reveal that ginseng allows people to work longer and harder at mental tasks (which may appeal to you!).	Supplements.		
Kava kava—30% extract— 300 mg	Kava kava (both the plant and the beverage made from it) is said to elevate mood and relieve stress.	Supplements.		
Royal jelly— 500 mg	Royal jelly, which is the sole food of the queen bee, is a rich source of B-vitamins and essential fatty acids.	Supplements.		

(8) Some researchers have found that taking Vitamin E supplements may increase the chance of a hemorrhagic stroke (from bleeding, which constitutes about 1 out of 5 strokes), because vitamin E tends to thin the blood. It is this same blood thinning quality, however, which has been shown to protect against ischemic strokes (from a blood clot) and reduce the incidence of heart attacks. Vitamin E's protective and beneficial effects to the entire body are substantial. Follow your doctor's guidance if you have concerns about hemorrhagic stroke.

DETAILED STROKE RECOVERY NUTRIENT INFORMATION AND SELECTION TABLE

Nutrient/ Suggested Daily Dose	Comments About This Nutrient	Sources	I Want This	Doctor Approval
Gotu kola— 400 mg	Gotu kola, from a creeping marsh plant that is used in India much like the Chinese use ginseng, is said to improve circulation to the brain, improving learning and memory. Although gotu kola is sometimes confused with kola nut (which contains a lot of caffeine), gotu kola contains no caffeine, and people who are interested in boosting their energy without consuming caffeine often use it.	Supplements.		
Rosemary (oil)—30 ml, one drop on each temple	Rosemary, the "dew of the sea," considered by ancient Egyptians, Hebrews, Greeks and Romans to be sacred, has been used for centuries to enhance memory.	Supplements.		
Minerals—as provided by a good mineral supplement. It is important that you ingest at least 150 mcg of iodine!	Minerals—including potassium, magnesium, calcium, iodine, iron, zinc, chromium, boron, manganese, and molybdenum— are reported to provide key ingredients for neuro-transmission—your brain's communication with your body. One mineral that has attracted a lot of attention in the area of brain science is iodine. Iodine is known to be commonly present in marine foods. Iodine forms thyroid hormones. Thyroid hormones play a basic role in biology—regulating the basal metabolic rate. The United States FDA recommends 150 micrograms of iodine per day for both men and women. The FDA considers iodine necessary for proper production of thyroid hormones.	Dairy foods, leafy green vegetables, nuts, tomatoes, bananas, table salt, meat, eggs, legumes (peas and beans) and enriched (iron-containing) grains. Much research holds that humans often benefit from mineral supplementation. Vitamins and minerals are interdependent, requiring the presence of others for full benefit; thus, taking a multivitamin without minerals is not nearly as effective as taking one with minerals. Natural sources of iodine include sea life, such as kelp and		

DETAILED STROKE RECOVERY NUTRIENT INFORMATION AND SELECTION TABLE

Nutrient/ Suggested Daily Dose	Comments About This Nutrient	Sources	I Want This	Doctor Approval
	In areas where there is little iodine in the diet—such as remote inland areas where no marine foods are eaten—iodine deficiency gives rise to a thyroid problem, which can cause extreme fatigue, mental slowing and depression. It is especially important that iodine be part of a recovering stroke survivor's diet.	certain seafoods, as well as plants grown in iodine-rich soil. Salt for human consumption is often enriched with iodine and is referred to as iodized salt.		
B1—50 mg **or** **Benfotiamine—** **200-400 mg** **B3—50 mg** **Folic acid—** **400 mcg**	Scientists say that B vitamins (and their relations) are critical for brain health because they lower the level of homocysteine—an amino acid found naturally in the body—that is reported to reduce blood flow to the brain and kill brain cells. Researchers have found a clear link between elevated homocysteine and decreased mental performance. Elevated homocysteine has been found to slow reaction times. Folic acid improves memory and mental ability. In a 3-year trial reported in *The Lancet* in January 2007, 818 people over age 50 who took 800 micrograms of folic acid daily (twice the current RDA), all demonstrated short-term memory, mental agility and verbal fluency that was improved over those who took a placebo.[xiii] Benfotiamine (a fat-soluble form of vitamin B-1) is extremely effective in alleviating and healing	Although B vitamins exist throughout our food supply—showing up in meat, fish, eggs, whole grains and fortified cereals—they are frequently lost before they are consumed. Microwave cooking and high heat destroy them. B vitamins are also water-soluble. They are often absorbed into cooking fluids and lost. Vitamin B1 is destroyed by alcohol; alcoholics are often deficient in this nutrient. Since animal products are a significant source of many B vitamins, vegetarians are at risk of running low on them. All in all, the best source for B-vitamins (and their relations) is a supplement.		

DETAILED STROKE RECOVERY NUTRIENT INFORMATION AND SELECTION TABLE

Nutrient/ Suggested Daily Dose	Comments About This Nutrient	Sources	I Want This	Doctor Approval
B12—500 mcg **or** **Methylcobalamin— 1 mg sublingually** **Choline—425 mg** **Tyrosine—500 mg** **Tryptophan— 500 mg**	painful nerve conditions such as the numbness, tingling and pain of neuropathy. Its proven healing benefit to nerves may make it helpful for stroke survivors. Benfotiamine users experience increased nerve conduction velocity, increased ability of the nerves to detect an electrical current and respond to electrical stimulation, and regulation of the heartbeat. Users have experienced a 50% reduction in diabetic nerve pain; it can prevent diabetic retinopathy. Because it is fat-soluble, it stays in the system (and brain) longer and is far more bioactive than common B-1, with far less toxicity and no adverse side effects shown. Choline is a chemical precursor or "building block" needed to produce the neurotransmitter acetylcholine, and research suggests that memory, intelligence and mood are mediated at least in part by acetylcholine metabolism in the brain. Methylcobalamin is the only form of vitamin B12 found in the brain and that is active in the central nervous system. It supports a healthy brain and spinal cord and may support cognitive function. It is essential for cell growth and replication. The liver can't convert cyanocobalamin (the usual supplement form of	Tryptophan is naturally occuring in various proteins such as nuts, seeds, red meat, tuna, turkey and shellfish. It also occurs in as bananas and soy. Supplements.		

DETAILED STROKE RECOVERY NUTRIENT INFORMATION AND SELECTION TABLE

Nutrient/ Suggested Daily Dose	Comments About This Nutrient	Sources	I Want This	Doctor Approval
	B12), into sufficient amounts of methylcobalamin to support proper nerve function. But methylcobalamin is neuroprotective, accelerates nerve cell growth, and promotes healthy homocysteine levels. Tyrosine reportedly improves mental alertness and quick response, eases anxiety and helps to relieve tension. Tryptophan makes you feel more relaxed. Tryptophan reportedly helps your thinking stay clearer and eases the effects of stress.			
Calcium— 1200 mg	Calcium has been found to boost the potential of nerve and muscle cells so they communicate better.	Milk, cheese and yogurt. Supplements.		
Magnesium— 400 mg	Magnesium is reported to increase cell energy and help produce neurotransmitters. It also has a calming effect, and helps muscles relax.	Pumpkin and squash seeds, nuts (brazil nuts, almonds and cashews) and bran cereal. Supplements.		
Co-Q10— 200 mg	Although Co-Q10 is common (sometimes called the "spark plug" that generates energy within each cell in your body), especially in your metabolically active brain, your body produces less and less Co-Q10 as you age. There is a strong belief in the scientific community that low levels of Co-Q10 cause mental decline as you age. Scientists argue that if you can't think, learn or remember things, it is because you don't have enough Co-Q10 to power your brain.	Beef, pork and eggs. There are plenty of vegetable sources of CoQ10, the richest currently known being spinach, broccoli, peanuts, wheat germ and whole grains—in that order—although the amount of Co-Q10 found in vegetables is significantly smaller than that found in meat.		

DETAILED STROKE RECOVERY NUTRIENT INFORMATION AND SELECTION TABLE				
Nutrient/ Suggested Daily Dose	**Comments About This Nutrient**	**Sources**	**I Want This**	**Doctor Approval**
Lipoic acid— 200 mg	Alpha Lipoic Acid, administered in concert with Acetyl-L-carnitine, has been found to enhance memory function without damaging brain cells. This is not a minor accomplishment, as drugs that are strong enough to alter brain chemistry often kill brain cells.	Lipoic acid is found in a variety of foods, notably kidney, heart and liver meats as well as spinach, broccoli and potatoes.		
NAC— 800 mg	N-Acetyl-Cysteine (NAC), taken orally, raises blood levels of glutathione. Glutathione production declines with age. Glutathione has been shown to boost immune system function. Some researchers report that glutathione is designed to protect the brain and nervous system. NAC has powerful antioxidant effects. In addition to protecting the body from oxidative damage resulting from metabolic and environmental toxins, NAC has shown positive effects on liver function, protecting the liver from heavy metals like lead and mercury. Acetyl-L-carnitine, which is the chemically active form of the amino acid carnitine, is naturally produced by the body and found in food. Carnatine plays important roles in generation of brain energy. People with Alzheimer's disease have been found to have markedly low levels of carnitine. Thus, often people with Alzheimer's disease are given Acetyl-L-carnitive	NAC is found in a variety of protein sources including ricotta cheese, cottage cheese, yogurt, pork, red meat, poultry, wheat germ, granola, oat flakes, garlic, onions, broccoli, and brussels sprouts. Meat, poultry, fish and dairy products are the richest sources of acetyl-L-carnitine.		

DETAILED STROKE RECOVERY NUTRIENT INFORMATION AND SELECTION TABLE

Nutrient/ Suggested Daily Dose	Comments About This Nutrient	Sources	I Want This	Doctor Approval
Acetyl-L-carnitine— 800 mg	supplements to counter the degenerative effects of that disease.			
Phosphatidylserine —200 mg	Phosphatidylserine (PS), a fatlike substance concentrated in brain cell membranes, is held by some people to improve the memory of memory-impaired people.	Supplements. Note that there is a cloud on phosphatidylserine (PS) supplements. Historically they were made with cows' brains. Today, because of concerns that cow brain supplements might spread diseases, PS supplements are made with soy. Some people think that the new soy-derived PS supplements are ineffective.		
Ginkgo biloba—360 mg	Many studies have found that ginkgo biloba improves blood flow to the brain and enhances mental function and memory. A study reported in the Journal of American Medical Association (JAMA) reported that about 30% of the people, including stroke survivors, who took a daily dose of ginkgo extract showed improvements on tests of reasoning, memory and behavior.	Exclusively in supplements. Many people think that taking ginkgo biloba supplements is a good idea. Ginkgo Biloba is safe; physicians in Europe have used it for decades to enhance brain function. Also, healers in China have used it for thousands of years.		
Vitamin D— 400 IU	Vitamin D reportedly helps you improve your mood. It has been shown to improve the mood of people who suffered from seasonal affective disorder (SAD)—that is, people who feel sad during periods when they are exposed to less sunlight.	Milk, a fortified rice or soy beverage, canned salmon and canned tuna.		

DETAILED STROKE RECOVERY NUTRIENT INFORMATION AND SELECTION TABLE				
Nutrient/ Suggested Daily Dose	Comments About This Nutrient	Sources	I Want This	Doctor Approval
	Sunlight is thought to trigger the production of seratonin, a chemical in the brain that controls mood. In addition to its mood-enhancing properties, vitamin D is a strong antioxidant, and it protects brain cells from free radical attacks, which some researchers think causes mental performance problems. Vitamin D has more recently been shown to have a strong protective effect against cancer.			
Vinpocetine—10 mg	Vinpocetine has been found to increase blood flow in areas of reduced blood flow.	Supplements. For more than two decades, vinpocetine has been used in Europe and in Japan to treat stroke survivors having reduced blood circulation. Vinpocetine became available over the counter in the United States in the late 1990's. Vinpocetine's ability to increase blood flow can cause a severe problem for people on some form of blood thinner (such as Coumadin or Plavix). Because vinpocentine can cause problems for people on blood thinners, and because physicians put many stroke survivors on blood thinners, vinpocetine is little used. Be sure to check with your doctor before taking it.		

Recovery Plan 13

Self-Selected

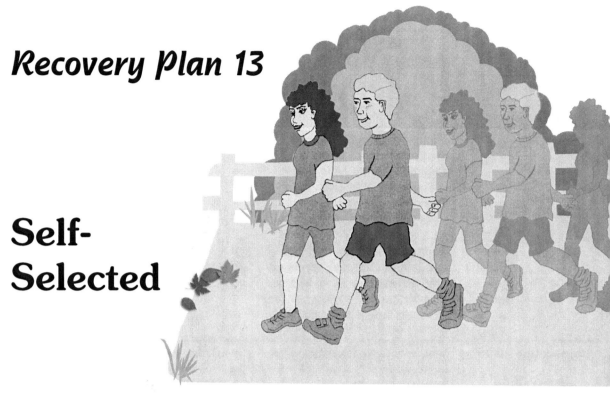

For Recovery/Development of _____

Date Begun:	Date Finished:	Repeat Dates:	Start:	Finish:
Personal Goals for this Plan:				
Location(s):				
People to Hire:				

Special Requirements, Information or Features:	
Components of Function to be Trained:	
List of Exercises to be Performed:	
Facility Equipment/ Supplies Needed:	
Equipment and Supplies to Buy:	

13-Week Training Plan:

Weeks	Mon	Tue	Wed	Thu	Fri	Sat	Sun
1 – 13							

Exercise Details	
Monday	**Description of Exercises:** **Special timing/duration of exercises:**
Tuesday	**Description of Exercises:** **Special timing/duration of exercises:**

Wednesday	**Description of Exercises:** **Special timing/duration of exercises:**
Thursday	**Description of Exercises:** **Special timing/duration of exercises:**
Friday	**Description of Exercises:** **Special timing/duration of exercises:**
Saturday	**Description of Exercises:** **Special timing/duration of exercises:**
Sunday	**Description of Exercises:** **Special timing/duration of exercises:**

Recovery Plan 14

Self-Selected

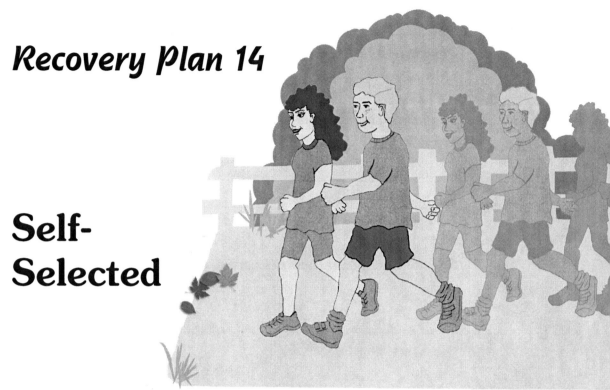

For Recovery/Development of _____

Date Begun:	Date Finished:	Repeat Dates:	Start:	Finish:
Personal Goals for this Plan:				
Location(s):				
People to Hire:				

Special Requirements, Information or Features:	
Components of Function to be Trained:	
List of Exercises to be Performed:	
Facility Equipment/ Supplies Needed:	
Equipment and Supplies to Buy:	

13-Week Training Plan:

Weeks	Mon	Tue	Wed	Thu	Fri	Sat	Sun
1 – 13							

Exercise Details		
Monday	**Description of Exercises:** **Special timing/duration of exercises:**	
Tuesday	**Description of Exercises:** **Special timing/duration of exercises:**	

Wednesday	Description of Exercises:
	Special timing/duration of exercises:
Thursday	Description of Exercises:
	Special timing/duration of exercises:
Friday	Description of Exercises:
	Special timing/duration of exercises:
Saturday	Description of Exercises:
	Special timing/duration of exercises:
Sunday	Description of Exercises:
	Special timing/duration of exercises:

Recovery Plan 15

As Instructed by a Healthcare Advisor

For Recovery/Development of _____

Date Begun:	Date Finished:	Repeat Dates:	Start:	Finish:
Personal Goals for this Plan:				
Location(s):				
People to Hire:				

Special Requirements, Information or Features:	
Components of Function to be Trained:	
List of Exercises to be Performed:	
Facility Equipment/ Supplies Needed:	
Equipment and Supplies to Buy:	

13-Week Training Plan:

Weeks	Mon	Tue	Wed	Thu	Fri	Sat	Sun
1 – 13							

Exercise Details	
Monday	**Description of Exercises:** **Special timing/duration of exercises:**
Tuesday	**Description of Exercises:** **Special timing/duration of exercises:**

Wednesday	**Description of Exercises:** **Special timing/duration of exercises:**
Thursday	**Description of Exercises:** **Special timing/duration of exercises:**
Friday	**Description of Exercises:** **Special timing/duration of exercises:**
Saturday	**Description of Exercises:** **Special timing/duration of exercises:**
Sunday	**Description of Exercises:** **Special timing/duration of exercises:**

Recovery Plan 16

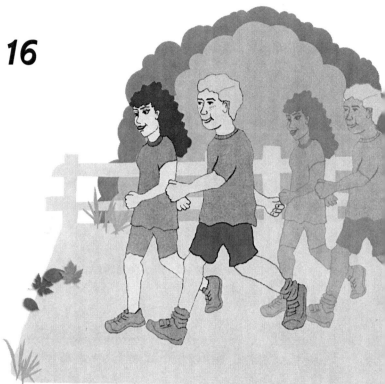

As Instructed by a Healthcare Advisor

For Recovery/Development of _____

Date Begun:	Date Finished:	Repeat Dates:	Start:	Finish:
Personal Goals for this Plan:				
Location(s):				
People to Hire:				

Special Requirements, Information or Features:	
Components of Function to be Trained:	
List of Exercises to be Performed:	
Facility Equipment/ Supplies Needed:	
Equipment and Supplies to Buy:	

13-Week Training Plan:

Weeks	Mon	Tue	Wed	Thu	Fri	Sat	Sun
1 – 13							

	Exercise Details
Monday	**Description of Exercises:** **Special timing/duration of exercises:**
Tuesday	**Description of Exercises:** **Special timing/duration of exercises:**

Wednesday	Description of Exercises:
	Special timing/duration of exercises:
Thursday	Description of Exercises:
	Special timing/duration of exercises:
Friday	Description of Exercises:
	Special timing/duration of exercises:
Saturday	Description of Exercises:
	Special timing/duration of exercises:
Sunday	Description of Exercises:
	Special timing/duration of exercises:

Part 3:

Worksheets To
Keep Track of Your
Recovery Progress

Start of Week Worksheet—Week No. 1

Date: Week Beginning Monday, _____, 20___

After you have had a stroke, you might realize there are many things you can't control. You can't control your age. You can't control having had a stroke, what type of stroke you had, where in your brain the stroke occurred or how the stroke affected you. You can't control the treatment you received. You can't control what you did before you had the stroke. However, you CAN CONTROL what you do after having the stroke. If you do the right things, you can recover from stroke. If you do what this workbook suggests, you can meet your goal—to recover completely and be better than you ever were before.

Roger Maxwell

Start of Week Statistics:

MEASUREMENTS—MEN:

Waist:_____   Chest:_____

Upper Leg: ____ Upper Arm:_____

MEASUREMENTS—WOMEN:

Waist:_____   Hips:_____

Upper Leg: ____ Upper Arm:____

WEIGHT: _____

BLOOD PRESSURE:

_____ over _____

Fill out the following information to guide you during the coming week.

Last week's successes and progress:_____

_____

_____

How well I am physically functioning right now: _____

_____

_____

Goals and expectations for this week:_____

_____

_____

Skills or exercises I want to especially focus on improving this week:_____

_____

_____

Shopping List: brain nutrient foods to add to diet this week:

_____   _____

_____   _____

If my weight or blood pressure are high, plan to reduce them (current/continuing):

_____

Daily Worksheet

Day of the Week:	Date:	Day No.	Max. Heart Rate:	A.M. Weight:	A.M. Blood Pressure: _____ OVER _____

Glasses of water drunk today (check):   ○   ○   ○   ○   ○   ○   ○   ○

WALKING Plan No. _____
Week No.:_____ **Day No.:**_____

RECOVERY PLAN: _____
Week No. _____ **Day No.:**_____

RECOVERY PLAN: _____
Week No. _____ **Day No.:**_____

CORE WORK:
Total Time _____

RESISTANCE TRAINING:
1) Machine/Exerc._____
   Weight_____ Reps ____/____/____
2) Machine/Exerc._____
   Weight_____ Reps ____/____/____
3) Machine/Exerc._____
   Weight_____ Reps ____/____/____
4) Machine/Exerc._____
   Weight_____ Reps ____/____/____
5) Machine/Exerc._____
   Weight_____ Reps ____/____/____
6) Machine/Exerc._____
   Weight_____ Reps ____/____/____
7) Machine/Exerc._____
   Weight_____ Reps ____/____/____
8) Machine/Exerc._____
   Weight_____ Reps ____/____/____
Resistance Tr. Total Time_____

CARDIO WALKING:
Treadmill: Distance _____
   Time _____ Speed _____
   Time walked without support _____
Elliptical: Distance _____Time _____
   Reversed direction every _____ minutes
   Time walked without support _____
Stepper: Distance _____Time _____
   Time walked without support _____
Track: Distance _____Time _____
   Speed or pace (if recorded) _____
   Time walked without support _____
   Fastest lap _____
   Fastest lap without support_____
Total Cardio Walking Time:_____
Max. Heart Rate Noted:_____

Exercises/Drills Done:
_____Time_____
_____Time_____
_____Time_____
_____Time_____
_____Time_____
_____Time_____
_____Time_____
_____Time_____
_____Time_____
_____Time_____
Total Time Spent_____

NUTRITION PLAN:
Nutrient-rich foods eaten | quantity:
BREAKFAST:
_____|_____
_____|_____
_____|_____
_____|_____
Drinks:_____
LUNCH:
_____|_____
_____|_____
_____|_____
_____|_____
_____|_____
Drinks:_____
Snacks:_____
DINNER:
_____|_____
_____|_____
_____|_____
_____|_____
_____|_____
_____|_____
_____|_____
Drinks:_____
Snacks:_____

Exercises/Drills Done:
_____Time_____
_____Time_____
_____Time_____
_____Time_____
_____Time_____
_____Time_____
_____Time_____
_____Time_____
_____Time_____
_____Time_____
Total Time Spent_____

SUPPLEMENTS TAKEN:
_____|_____
_____|_____
_____|_____
_____|_____
_____|_____
Supplements I Need to Buy:
_____|_____
_____|_____
MEDICINES TAKEN:
_____|_____
_____|_____
_____|_____
_____|_____
_____|_____

YOGA TRAINING:
Exercises:_____
_____
_____
_____
_____
_____
Total Yoga Time: _____
Notes:_____

RECOVERY BASICS:
☐ **Were physical exercise targets (time and total no. of reps) met?**
☐ **Did I focus well on exercises?**
☐ **Did I work intensively + aggressively?**
☐ **Did I push myself to increase difficulty?**

NOTES, SUCCESSES, BREAKTHROUGHS, PROGRESS!
_____
_____
_____
_____
_____

Daily Worksheet

Day of the Week:	Date:	Day No.	Max. Heart Rate:	A.M. Weight:	A.M. Blood Pressure: _____ OVER _____

Glasses of water drunk today (check): ○ ○ ○ ○ ○ ○ ○ ○

WALKING Plan No. _____

Week No.:_____ **Day No.:**_____

CORE WORK:

Total Time _____

RESISTANCE TRAINING:

1) Machine/Exerc._____

Weight_____ Reps _____/_____/_____

2) Machine/Exerc._____

Weight_____ Reps _____/_____/_____

3) Machine/Exerc._____

Weight_____ Reps _____/_____/_____

4) Machine/Exerc._____

Weight_____ Reps _____/_____/_____

5) Machine/Exerc._____

Weight_____ Reps _____/_____/_____

6) Machine/Exerc._____

Weight_____ Reps _____/_____/_____

7) Machine/Exerc._____

Weight_____ Reps _____/_____/_____

8) Machine/Exerc._____

Weight_____ Reps _____/_____/_____

Resistance Tr. Total Time_____

CARDIO WALKING:

Treadmill: Distance _____

Time _____ Speed _____

Time walked without support _____

Elliptical: Distance _____Time _____

Reversed direction every _____ minutes

Time walked without support _____

Stepper: Distance _____Time _____

Time walked without support _____

Track: Distance _____Time _____

Speed or pace (if recorded) _____

Time walked without support _____

Fastest lap _____

Fastest lap without support_____

Total Cardio Walking Time:_____

Max. Heart Rate Noted:_____

RECOVERY PLAN: _____

Week No. _____ **Day No.:**_____

Exercises/Drills Done:

_____Time_____

_____Time_____

_____Time_____

_____Time_____

_____Time_____

_____Time_____

_____Time_____

_____Time_____

_____Time_____

_____Time_____

Total Time Spent_____

NUTRITION PLAN:

Nutrient-rich foods eaten | quantity:

BREAKFAST:

_____ | _____

_____ | _____

_____ | _____

_____ | _____

Drinks:_____

LUNCH:

_____ | _____

_____ | _____

_____ | _____

_____ | _____

_____ | _____

Drinks:_____

Snacks:_____

DINNER:

_____ | _____

_____ | _____

_____ | _____

_____ | _____

_____ | _____

_____ | _____

Drinks:_____

Snacks:_____

RECOVERY PLAN: _____

Week No. _____ **Day No.:**_____

Exercises/Drills Done:

_____Time_____

_____Time_____

_____Time_____

_____Time_____

_____Time_____

_____Time_____

_____Time_____

_____Time_____

_____Time_____

_____Time_____

Total Time Spent_____

SUPPLEMENTS TAKEN:

_____ | _____

_____ | _____

_____ | _____

_____ | _____

_____ | _____

Supplements I Need to Buy:

_____ | _____

_____ | _____

MEDICINES TAKEN:

_____ | _____

_____ | _____

_____ | _____

_____ | _____

_____ | _____

YOGA TRAINING:

Exercises:_____

_____

_____

_____

_____

_____

_____

Total Yoga Time: _____

Notes:_____

RECOVERY BASICS:

☐ **Were physical exercise targets (time and total no. of reps) met?**

☐ **Did I focus well on exercises?**

☐ **Did I work intensively + aggressively?**

☐ **Did I push myself to increase difficulty?**

NOTES, SUCCESSES, BREAKTHROUGHS, PROGRESS!

_____

_____

_____

_____

_____

Daily Worksheet

Day of the Week:	Date:	Day No.	Max. Heart Rate:	A.M. Weight:	A.M. Blood Pressure: _____ OVER _____

Glasses of water drunk today (check): ○ ○ ○ ○ ○ ○ ○ ○

WALKING Plan No. _____

Week No.:_____ Day No.:_____

CORE WORK:

Total Time _____

RESISTANCE TRAINING:

1) Machine/Exerc._____

Weight_____ Reps _____/_____/_____

2) Machine/Exerc._____

Weight_____ Reps _____/_____/_____

3) Machine/Exerc._____

Weight_____ Reps _____/_____/_____

4) Machine/Exerc._____

Weight_____ Reps _____/_____/_____

5) Machine/Exerc._____

Weight_____ Reps _____/_____/_____

6) Machine/Exerc._____

Weight_____ Reps _____/_____/_____

7) Machine/Exerc._____

Weight_____ Reps _____/_____/_____

8) Machine/Exerc._____

Weight_____ Reps _____/_____/_____

Resistance Tr. Total Time_____

CARDIO WALKING:

Treadmill: Distance _____

Time _____ Speed _____

Time walked without support _____

Elliptical: Distance _____Time _____

Reversed direction every _____ minutes

Time walked without support _____

Stepper: Distance _____Time _____

Time walked without support _____

Track: Distance _____Time _____

Speed or pace (if recorded) _____

Time walked without support _____

Fastest lap _____

Fastest lap without support_____

Total Cardio Walking Time:_____

Max. Heart Rate Noted:_____

RECOVERY BASICS:

☐ **Were physical exercise targets (time and total no. of reps) met?**

☐ **Did I focus well on exercises?**

☐ **Did I work intensively + aggressively?**

☐ **Did I push myself to increase difficulty?**

RECOVERY PLAN: _____

Week No. _____ Day No.:_____

Exercises/Drills Done:

_____Time_____

_____Time_____

_____Time_____

_____Time_____

_____Time_____

_____Time_____

_____Time_____

_____Time_____

_____Time_____

_____Time_____

Total Time Spent_____

NUTRITION PLAN:

Nutrient-rich foods eaten ǀ quantity:

BREAKFAST:

_____ǀ_____

_____ǀ_____

_____ǀ_____

_____ǀ_____

Drinks:_____

LUNCH:

_____ǀ_____

_____ǀ_____

_____ǀ_____

_____ǀ_____

_____ǀ_____

Drinks:_____

Snacks:_____

DINNER:

_____ǀ_____

_____ǀ_____

_____ǀ_____

_____ǀ_____

_____ǀ_____

_____ǀ_____

Drinks:_____

Snacks:_____

RECOVERY PLAN: _____

Week No. _____ Day No.:_____

Exercises/Drills Done:

_____Time_____

_____Time_____

_____Time_____

_____Time_____

_____Time_____

_____Time_____

_____Time_____

_____Time_____

_____Time_____

Total Time Spent_____

SUPPLEMENTS TAKEN:

_____ǀ_____

_____ǀ_____

_____ǀ_____

_____ǀ_____

Supplements I Need to Buy:

_____ǀ_____

_____ǀ_____

MEDICINES TAKEN:

_____ǀ_____

_____ǀ_____

_____ǀ_____

_____ǀ_____

_____ǀ_____

YOGA TRAINING:

Exercises:_____

_____

_____

_____

_____

Total Yoga Time: _____

Notes:_____

NOTES, SUCCESSES, BREAKTHROUGHS, PROGRESS!

_____

_____

_____

_____

Daily Worksheet

Day of the Week:	Date:	Day No.	Max. Heart Rate:	A.M. Weight:	A.M. Blood Pressure: _____ OVER _____

Glasses of water drunk today (check): ○ ○ ○ ○ ○ ○ ○ ○

WALKING Plan No. _____

Week No.: _____ **Day No.:** _____

CORE WORK:
Total Time _____

RESISTANCE TRAINING:

1) Machine/Exerc. _____

   Weight _____ Reps ____ / ____ / ____

2) Machine/Exerc. _____

   Weight _____ Reps ____ / ____ / ____

3) Machine/Exerc. _____

   Weight _____ Reps ____ / ____ / ____

4) Machine/Exerc. _____

   Weight _____ Reps ____ / ____ / ____

5) Machine/Exerc. _____

   Weight _____ Reps ____ / ____ / ____

6) Machine/Exerc. _____

   Weight _____ Reps ____ / ____ / ____

7) Machine/Exerc. _____

   Weight _____ Reps ____ / ____ / ____

8) Machine/Exerc. _____

   Weight _____ Reps ____ / ____ / ____

Resistance Tr. Total Time _____

CARDIO WALKING:

Treadmill: Distance _____

   Time _____ Speed _____

   Time walked without support _____

Elliptical: Distance _____ Time _____

   Reversed direction every _____ minutes

   Time walked without support _____

Stepper: Distance _____ Time _____

   Time walked without support _____

Track: Distance _____ Time _____

   Speed or pace (if recorded) _____

   Time walked without support _____

   Fastest lap _____

   Fastest lap without support _____

Total Cardio Walking Time: _____

Max. Heart Rate Noted: _____

RECOVERY BASICS:
☐ Were physical exercise targets (time and total no. of reps) met?
☐ Did I focus well on exercises?
☐ Did I work intensively + aggressively?
☐ Did I push myself to increase difficulty?

RECOVERY PLAN: _____

Week No. _____ **Day No.:** _____

Exercises/Drills Done:

_____ Time _____

_____ Time _____

_____ Time _____

_____ Time _____

_____ Time _____

_____ Time _____

_____ Time _____

_____ Time _____

_____ Time _____

_____ Time _____

Total Time Spent _____

NUTRITION PLAN:

Nutrient-rich foods eaten | quantity:

BREAKFAST:

_____ | _____

_____ | _____

_____ | _____

_____ | _____

Drinks: _____

LUNCH:

_____ | _____

_____ | _____

_____ | _____

_____ | _____

_____ | _____

_____ | _____

Drinks: _____

Snacks: _____

DINNER:

_____ | _____

_____ | _____

_____ | _____

_____ | _____

_____ | _____

_____ | _____

Drinks: _____

Snacks: _____

RECOVERY PLAN: _____

Week No. _____ **Day No.:** _____

Exercises/Drills Done:

_____ Time _____

_____ Time _____

_____ Time _____

_____ Time _____

_____ Time _____

_____ Time _____

_____ Time _____

_____ Time _____

_____ Time _____

_____ Time _____

Total Time Spent _____

SUPPLEMENTS TAKEN:

_____ | _____

_____ | _____

_____ | _____

_____ | _____

_____ | _____

Supplements I Need to Buy:

_____ | _____

_____ | _____

MEDICINES TAKEN:

_____ | _____

_____ | _____

_____ | _____

_____ | _____

_____ | _____

_____ | _____

YOGA TRAINING:

Exercises: _____

_____

_____

_____

_____

_____

Total Yoga Time: _____

Notes: _____

NOTES, SUCCESSES, BREAKTHROUGHS, PROGRESS!

_____

_____

_____

_____

_____

_____

Daily Worksheet

Day of the Week:	Date:	Day No.	Max. Heart Rate:	A.M. Weight:	A.M. Blood Pressure: _____ OVER _____

Glasses of water drunk today (check): ○ ○ ○ ○ ○ ○ ○ ○

WALKING Plan No. _____

Week No.:_____ Day No.:_____

CORE WORK:
Total Time _____

RESISTANCE TRAINING:
1) Machine/Exerc._____
  Weight_____ Reps _____/_____/_____
2) Machine/Exerc._____
  Weight_____ Reps _____/_____/_____
3) Machine/Exerc._____
  Weight_____ Reps _____/_____/_____
4) Machine/Exerc._____
  Weight_____ Reps _____/_____/_____
5) Machine/Exerc._____
  Weight_____ Reps _____/_____/_____
6) Machine/Exerc._____
  Weight_____ Reps _____/_____/_____
7) Machine/Exerc._____
  Weight_____ Reps _____/_____/_____
8) Machine/Exerc._____
  Weight_____ Reps _____/_____/_____
Resistance Tr. Total Time_____

CARDIO WALKING:
Treadmill: Distance _____
  Time _____ Speed _____
  Time walked without support _____
Elliptical: Distance _____Time _____
  Reversed direction every _____ minutes
  Time walked without support _____
Stepper: Distance _____Time _____
  Time walked without support _____
Track: Distance _____Time _____
  Speed or pace (if recorded) _____
  Time walked without support _____
  Fastest lap _____
  Fastest lap without support_____
Total Cardio Walking Time:_____
Max. Heart Rate Noted:_____

RECOVERY PLAN: _____

Week No. _____ Day No.:_____

Exercises/Drills Done:
_____Time_____
_____Time_____
_____Time_____
_____Time_____
_____Time_____
_____Time_____
_____Time_____
_____Time_____
_____Time_____
_____Time_____
Total Time Spent_____

NUTRITION PLAN:
Nutrient-rich foods eaten | quantity:
BREAKFAST:
_____ | _____
_____ | _____
_____ | _____
_____ | _____
Drinks:_____
LUNCH:
_____ | _____
_____ | _____
_____ | _____
_____ | _____
_____ | _____
_____ | _____
Drinks:_____
Snacks:_____
DINNER:
_____ | _____
_____ | _____
_____ | _____
_____ | _____
_____ | _____
_____ | _____
Drinks:_____
Snacks:_____

RECOVERY PLAN: _____

Week No. _____ Day No.:_____

Exercises/Drills Done:
_____Time_____
_____Time_____
_____Time_____
_____Time_____
_____Time_____
_____Time_____
_____Time_____
_____Time_____
_____Time_____
_____Time_____
Total Time Spent_____

SUPPLEMENTS TAKEN:
_____ | _____
_____ | _____
_____ | _____
_____ | _____
_____ | _____
Supplements I Need to Buy:
_____ | _____
_____ | _____

MEDICINES TAKEN:
_____ | _____
_____ | _____
_____ | _____
_____ | _____
_____ | _____
_____ | _____

YOGA TRAINING:
Exercises:_____
_____
_____
_____
_____
Total Yoga Time: _____
Notes:_____

RECOVERY BASICS:
☐ **Were physical exercise targets (time and total no. of reps) met?**
☐ **Did I focus well on exercises?**
☐ **Did I work intensively + aggressively?**
☐ **Did I push myself to increase difficulty?**

NOTES, SUCCESSES, BREAKTHROUGHS, PROGRESS!
_____
_____
_____
_____
_____
_____

Daily Worksheet

Day of the Week:	Date:	Day No.	Max. Heart Rate:	A.M. Weight:	A.M. Blood Pressure: _____ OVER _____

Glasses of water drunk today (check): ○ ○ ○ ○ ○ ○ ○ ○

WALKING Plan No. _____

Week No.: _____ **Day No.:** _____

CORE WORK:

Total Time _____

RESISTANCE TRAINING:

1) Machine/Exerc._____
   Weight_____ Reps _____/_____/_____

2) Machine/Exerc._____
   Weight_____ Reps _____/_____/_____

3) Machine/Exerc._____
   Weight_____ Reps _____/_____/_____

4) Machine/Exerc._____
   Weight_____ Reps _____/_____/_____

5) Machine/Exerc._____
   Weight_____ Reps _____/_____/_____

6) Machine/Exerc._____
   Weight_____ Reps _____/_____/_____

7) Machine/Exerc._____
   Weight_____ Reps _____/_____/_____

8) Machine/Exerc._____
   Weight_____ Reps _____/_____/_____

Resistance Tr. Total Time_____

CARDIO WALKING:

Treadmill: Distance _____
   Time _____ Speed _____
   Time walked without support _____

Elliptical: Distance _____Time _____
   Reversed direction every _____ minutes
   Time walked without support _____

Stepper: Distance _____Time _____
   Time walked without support _____

Track: Distance _____Time _____
   Speed or pace (if recorded) _____
   Time walked without support _____
   Fastest lap _____
   Fastest lap without support_____

Total Cardio Walking Time:_____
Max. Heart Rate Noted:_____

RECOVERY BASICS:

☐ **Were physical exercise targets (time and total no. of reps) met?**
☐ **Did I focus well on exercises?**
☐ **Did I work intensively + aggressively?**
☐ **Did I push myself to increase difficulty?**

RECOVERY PLAN: _____

Week No. _____ **Day No.:**_____

Exercises/Drills Done:

_____Time_____
_____Time_____
_____Time_____
_____Time_____
_____Time_____
_____Time_____
_____Time_____
_____Time_____
_____Time_____

Total Time Spent_____

NUTRITION PLAN:

Nutrient-rich foods eaten | quantity:

BREAKFAST:
_____ | _____
_____ | _____
_____ | _____
_____ | _____

Drinks:_____

LUNCH:
_____ | _____
_____ | _____
_____ | _____
_____ | _____
_____ | _____

Drinks:_____
Snacks:_____

DINNER:
_____ | _____
_____ | _____
_____ | _____
_____ | _____
_____ | _____
_____ | _____

Drinks:_____
Snacks:_____

RECOVERY PLAN: _____

Week No. _____ **Day No.:**_____

Exercises/Drills Done:

_____Time_____
_____Time_____
_____Time_____
_____Time_____
_____Time_____
_____Time_____
_____Time_____
_____Time_____
_____Time_____

Total Time Spent_____

SUPPLEMENTS TAKEN:

_____ | _____
_____ | _____
_____ | _____
_____ | _____
_____ | _____

Supplements I Need to Buy:
_____ | _____
_____ | _____

MEDICINES TAKEN:

_____ | _____
_____ | _____
_____ | _____
_____ | _____
_____ | _____
_____ | _____

YOGA TRAINING:

Exercises:_____
_____
_____
_____
_____
_____

Total Yoga Time: _____
Notes:_____

NOTES, SUCCESSES, BREAKTHROUGHS, PROGRESS!

_____
_____
_____
_____
_____

Daily Worksheet

Day of the Week:	Date:	Day No.	Max. Heart Rate:	A.M. Weight:	A.M. Blood Pressure: _____ OVER _____

Glasses of water drunk today (check): ○ ○ ○ ○ ○ ○ ○ ○

WALKING Plan No. _____

Week No.: _____ **Day No.:** _____

CORE WORK:

Total Time _____

RESISTANCE TRAINING:

1) Machine/Exerc. _____
   Weight _____ Reps _____/_____/_____
2) Machine/Exerc. _____
   Weight _____ Reps _____/_____/_____
3) Machine/Exerc. _____
   Weight _____ Reps _____/_____/_____
4) Machine/Exerc. _____
   Weight _____ Reps _____/_____/_____
5) Machine/Exerc. _____
   Weight _____ Reps _____/_____/_____
6) Machine/Exerc. _____
   Weight _____ Reps _____/_____/_____
7) Machine/Exerc. _____
   Weight _____ Reps _____/_____/_____
8) Machine/Exerc. _____
   Weight _____ Reps _____/_____/_____

Resistance Tr. Total Time _____

CARDIO WALKING:

Treadmill: Distance _____
   Time _____ Speed _____
   Time walked without support _____
Elliptical: Distance _____ Time _____
   Reversed direction every _____ minutes
   Time walked without support _____
Stepper: Distance _____ Time _____
   Time walked without support _____
Track: Distance _____ Time _____
   Speed or pace (if recorded) _____
   Time walked without support _____
   Fastest lap _____
   Fastest lap without support _____
Total Cardio Walking Time: _____
Max. Heart Rate Noted: _____

RECOVERY BASICS:
☐ Were physical exercise targets (time
   and total no. of reps) met?
☐ Did I focus well on exercises?
☐ Did I work intensively + aggressively?
☐ Did I push myself to increase difficulty?

RECOVERY PLAN: _____

Week No. _____ **Day No.:** _____

Exercises/Drills Done:
_____ Time _____
_____ Time _____
_____ Time _____
_____ Time _____
_____ Time _____
_____ Time _____
_____ Time _____
_____ Time _____
_____ Time _____
_____ Time _____

Total Time Spent _____

NUTRITION PLAN:

Nutrient-rich foods eaten | quantity:

BREAKFAST:
_____ | _____
_____ | _____
_____ | _____
_____ | _____

Drinks: _____

LUNCH:
_____ | _____
_____ | _____
_____ | _____
_____ | _____
_____ | _____
_____ | _____

Drinks: _____
Snacks: _____

DINNER:
_____ | _____
_____ | _____
_____ | _____
_____ | _____
_____ | _____
_____ | _____

Drinks: _____
Snacks: _____

RECOVERY PLAN: _____

Week No. _____ **Day No.:** _____

Exercises/Drills Done:
_____ Time _____
_____ Time _____
_____ Time _____
_____ Time _____
_____ Time _____
_____ Time _____
_____ Time _____
_____ Time _____
_____ Time _____
_____ Time _____

Total Time Spent _____

SUPPLEMENTS TAKEN:
_____ | _____
_____ | _____
_____ | _____
_____ | _____
_____ | _____

Supplements I Need to Buy:
_____ | _____
_____ | _____

MEDICINES TAKEN:
_____ | _____
_____ | _____
_____ | _____
_____ | _____
_____ | _____
_____ | _____

YOGA TRAINING:

Exercises: _____
_____
_____
_____
_____
_____

Total Yoga Time: _____
Notes: _____

NOTES, SUCCESSES, BREAKTHROUGHS, PROGRESS!
_____
_____
_____
_____
_____

Start of Week Worksheet—Week No. 2

Date: Week Beginning Monday, _____, 20___

> Not continuing to seek recovery from stroke when your rehab is over is like not going back onto the field to play the second half of a football game because you are so far behind. The game is not over. You can still win. It is not time to quit—it is not time to be conservative—it is also not time to be frantic. It is time to be more methodical, more aggressive and tougher than you have ever been before.
>
> Roger Maxwell

Start of Week Statistics:

MEASUREMENTS—MEN:	MEASUREMENTS—WOMEN:	WEIGHT: _____
Waist:_____ Chest:_____	Waist:_____ Hips:_____	BLOOD PRESSURE:
Upper Leg: ____ Upper Arm:_____	Upper Leg: ____ Upper Arm:____	_____ over _____

Fill out the following information to guide you during the coming week.

Last week's successes and progress:_____

_____

_____

How well I am physically functioning right now: _____

_____

_____

Goals and expectations for this week:_____

_____

_____

Skills or exercises I want to especially focus on improving this week:_____

_____

_____

Shopping List: brain nutrient foods to add to diet this week:

_____   _____

_____   _____

If my weight or blood pressure are high, plan to reduce them (current/continuing):

_____

Daily Worksheet

Day of the Week:	Date:	Day No.	Max. Heart Rate:	A.M. Weight:	A.M. Blood Pressure: _____ OVER _____

Glasses of water drunk today (check): ○ ○ ○ ○ ○ ○ ○ ○

WALKING Plan No. _____

Week No.:_____ **Day No.:**_____

CORE WORK:

Total Time _____

RESISTANCE TRAINING:

1) Machine/Exerc._____

　Weight_____ Reps _____/_____/_____

2) Machine/Exerc._____

　Weight_____ Reps _____/_____/_____

3) Machine/Exerc._____

　Weight_____ Reps _____/_____/_____

4) Machine/Exerc._____

　Weight_____ Reps _____/_____/_____

5) Machine/Exerc._____

　Weight_____ Reps _____/_____/_____

6) Machine/Exerc._____

　Weight_____ Reps _____/_____/_____

7) Machine/Exerc._____

　Weight_____ Reps _____/_____/_____

8) Machine/Exerc._____

　Weight_____ Reps _____/_____/_____

Resistance Tr. Total Time_____

CARDIO WALKING:

Treadmill: Distance _____

　Time _____ Speed _____

　Time walked without support _____

Elliptical: Distance _____Time _____

　Reversed direction every _____ minutes

　Time walked without support _____

Stepper: Distance _____Time _____

　Time walked without support _____

Track: Distance _____Time _____

　Speed or pace (if recorded) _____

　Time walked without support _____

　Fastest lap _____

　Fastest lap without support_____

Total Cardio Walking Time:_____

Max. Heart Rate Noted:_____

RECOVERY BASICS:

☐ **Were physical exercise targets (time and total no. of reps) met?**

☐ **Did I focus well on exercises?**

☐ **Did I work intensively + aggressively?**

☐ **Did I push myself to increase difficulty?**

RECOVERY PLAN: _____

Week No. _____ **Day No.:**_____

Exercises/Drills Done:

_____Time_____

_____Time_____

_____Time_____

_____Time_____

_____Time_____

_____Time_____

_____Time_____

_____Time_____

_____Time_____

_____Time_____

Total Time Spent_____

NUTRITION PLAN:

Nutrient-rich foods eaten ┃ quantity:

BREAKFAST:

_____┃_____

_____┃_____

_____┃_____

_____┃_____

Drinks:_____

LUNCH:

_____┃_____

_____┃_____

_____┃_____

_____┃_____

_____┃_____

_____┃_____

Drinks:_____

Snacks:_____

DINNER:

_____┃_____

_____┃_____

_____┃_____

_____┃_____

_____┃_____

_____┃_____

Drinks:_____

Snacks:_____

RECOVERY PLAN: _____

Week No. _____ **Day No.:**_____

Exercises/Drills Done:

_____Time_____

_____Time_____

_____Time_____

_____Time_____

_____Time_____

_____Time_____

_____Time_____

_____Time_____

_____Time_____

_____Time_____

Total Time Spent_____

SUPPLEMENTS TAKEN:

_____┃_____

_____┃_____

_____┃_____

_____┃_____

_____┃_____

_____┃_____

Supplements I Need to Buy:

_____┃_____

_____┃_____

MEDICINES TAKEN:

_____┃_____

_____┃_____

_____┃_____

_____┃_____

_____┃_____

_____┃_____

YOGA TRAINING:

Exercises:_____

_____

_____

_____

_____

Total Yoga Time: _____

Notes:_____

NOTES, SUCCESSES, BREAKTHROUGHS, PROGRESS!

_____

_____

_____

_____

_____

Daily Worksheet

Day of the Week:	Date:	Day No.	Max. Heart Rate:	A.M. Weight:	A.M. Blood Pressure: _____ OVER _____

Glasses of water drunk today (check): ○ ○ ○ ○ ○ ○ ○ ○

WALKING Plan No. _____

Week No.:_____ Day No.:_____

CORE WORK:

Total Time _____

RESISTANCE TRAINING:

1) Machine/Exerc._____

   Weight_____ Reps _____/_____/_____

2) Machine/Exerc._____

   Weight_____ Reps _____/_____/_____

3) Machine/Exerc._____

   Weight_____ Reps _____/_____/_____

4) Machine/Exerc._____

   Weight_____ Reps _____/_____/_____

5) Machine/Exerc._____

   Weight_____ Reps _____/_____/_____

6) Machine/Exerc._____

   Weight_____ Reps _____/_____/_____

7) Machine/Exerc._____

   Weight_____ Reps _____/_____/_____

8) Machine/Exerc._____

   Weight_____ Reps _____/_____/_____

Resistance Tr. Total Time_____

CARDIO WALKING:

Treadmill: Distance _____

   Time _____ Speed _____

   Time walked without support _____

Elliptical: Distance _____Time _____

   Reversed direction every _____ minutes

   Time walked without support _____

Stepper: Distance _____Time _____

   Time walked without support _____

Track: Distance _____Time _____

   Speed or pace (if recorded) _____

   Time walked without support _____

   Fastest lap _____

   Fastest lap without support_____

Total Cardio Walking Time:_____

Max. Heart Rate Noted:_____

RECOVERY PLAN: _____

Week No. _____ Day No.:_____

Exercises/Drills Done:

_____Time_____

_____Time_____

_____Time_____

_____Time_____

_____Time_____

_____Time_____

_____Time_____

_____Time_____

_____Time_____

Total Time Spent_____

NUTRITION PLAN:

Nutrient-rich foods eaten | quantity:

BREAKFAST:

_____ | _____

_____ | _____

_____ | _____

_____ | _____

Drinks:_____

LUNCH:

_____ | _____

_____ | _____

_____ | _____

_____ | _____

_____ | _____

Drinks:_____

Snacks:_____

DINNER:

_____ | _____

_____ | _____

_____ | _____

_____ | _____

_____ | _____

_____ | _____

Drinks:_____

Snacks:_____

RECOVERY PLAN: _____

Week No. _____ Day No.:_____

Exercises/Drills Done:

_____Time_____

_____Time_____

_____Time_____

_____Time_____

_____Time_____

_____Time_____

_____Time_____

_____Time_____

_____Time_____

Total Time Spent_____

SUPPLEMENTS TAKEN:

_____ | _____

_____ | _____

_____ | _____

_____ | _____

_____ | _____

_____ | _____

Supplements I Need to Buy:

_____ | _____

_____ | _____

MEDICINES TAKEN:

_____ | _____

_____ | _____

_____ | _____

_____ | _____

_____ | _____

_____ | _____

YOGA TRAINING:

Exercises:_____

_____

_____

_____

Total Yoga Time: _____

Notes:_____

RECOVERY BASICS:

☐ **Were physical exercise targets (time and total no. of reps) met?**

☐ **Did I focus well on exercises?**

☐ **Did I work intensively + aggressively?**

☐ **Did I push myself to increase difficulty?**

NOTES, SUCCESSES, BREAKTHROUGHS, PROGRESS!

_____

_____

_____

_____

_____

Daily Worksheet

Day of the Week:	Date:	Day No.	Max. Heart Rate:	A.M. Weight:	A.M. Blood Pressure: _____ OVER _____

Glasses of water drunk today (check): ○ ○ ○ ○ ○ ○ ○ ○

WALKING Plan No. _____

Week No.:_____ **Day No.:**_____

CORE WORK:
Total Time _____

RESISTANCE TRAINING:

1) Machine/Exerc._____
   Weight_____ Reps ____/_____/_____
2) Machine/Exerc._____
   Weight_____ Reps ____/_____/_____
3) Machine/Exerc._____
   Weight_____ Reps ____/_____/_____
4) Machine/Exerc._____
   Weight_____ Reps ____/_____/_____
5) Machine/Exerc._____
   Weight_____ Reps ____/_____/_____
6) Machine/Exerc._____
   Weight_____ Reps ____/_____/_____
7) Machine/Exerc._____
   Weight_____ Reps ____/_____/_____
8) Machine/Exerc._____
   Weight_____ Reps ____/_____/_____

Resistance Tr. Total Time_____

CARDIO WALKING:

Treadmill: Distance _____
   Time _____ Speed _____
   Time walked without support _____
Elliptical: Distance _____Time _____
   Reversed direction every _____ minutes
   Time walked without support _____
Stepper: Distance _____Time _____
   Time walked without support _____
Track: Distance _____Time _____
   Speed or pace (if recorded) _____
   Time walked without support _____
   Fastest lap _____
   Fastest lap without support_____

Total Cardio Walking Time:_____
Max. Heart Rate Noted:_____

RECOVERY BASICS:
☐ **Were physical exercise targets (time and total no. of reps) met?**
☐ **Did I focus well on exercises?**
☐ **Did I work intensively + aggressively?**
☐ **Did I push myself to increase difficulty?**

RECOVERY PLAN: _____
Week No. _____ **Day No.:**_____

Exercises/Drills Done:
_____Time_____
_____Time_____
_____Time_____
_____Time_____
_____Time_____
_____Time_____
_____Time_____
_____Time_____
_____Time_____

Total Time Spent_____

NUTRITION PLAN:
Nutrient-rich foods eaten | quantity:
BREAKFAST:
_____ | _____
_____ | _____
_____ | _____
_____ | _____
Drinks:_____
LUNCH:
_____ | _____
_____ | _____
_____ | _____
_____ | _____
_____ | _____
_____ | _____
Drinks:_____
Snacks:_____
DINNER:
_____ | _____
_____ | _____
_____ | _____
_____ | _____
_____ | _____
_____ | _____
Drinks:_____
Snacks:_____

RECOVERY PLAN: _____
Week No. _____ **Day No.:**_____

Exercises/Drills Done:
_____Time_____
_____Time_____
_____Time_____
_____Time_____
_____Time_____
_____Time_____
_____Time_____
_____Time_____
_____Time_____

Total Time Spent_____

SUPPLEMENTS TAKEN:
_____ | _____
_____ | _____
_____ | _____
_____ | _____
_____ | _____
_____ | _____

Supplements I Need to Buy:
_____ | _____
_____ | _____

MEDICINES TAKEN:
_____ | _____
_____ | _____
_____ | _____
_____ | _____
_____ | _____
_____ | _____

YOGA TRAINING:
Exercises:_____
_____
_____
_____
_____
_____
Total Yoga Time: _____
Notes:_____

NOTES, SUCCESSES, BREAKTHROUGHS, PROGRESS!
_____
_____
_____
_____
_____
_____

Daily Worksheet

Day of the Week:	Date:	Day No.	Max. Heart Rate:	A.M. Weight:	A.M. Blood Pressure: _____ OVER _____

Glasses of water drunk today (check): ○ ○ ○ ○ ○ ○ ○ ○

WALKING Plan No. _____

Week No.:_____ Day No.:_____

CORE WORK:

Total Time _____

RESISTANCE TRAINING:

1) Machine/Exerc._____

  Weight_____ Reps _____/_____/_____

2) Machine/Exerc._____

  Weight_____ Reps _____/_____/_____

3) Machine/Exerc._____

  Weight_____ Reps _____/_____/_____

4) Machine/Exerc._____

  Weight_____ Reps _____/_____/_____

5) Machine/Exerc._____

  Weight_____ Reps _____/_____/_____

6) Machine/Exerc._____

  Weight_____ Reps _____/_____/_____

7) Machine/Exerc._____

  Weight_____ Reps _____/_____/_____

8) Machine/Exerc._____

  Weight_____ Reps _____/_____/_____

Resistance Tr. Total Time_____

CARDIO WALKING:

Treadmill: Distance _____

  Time _____ Speed _____

  Time walked without support _____

Elliptical: Distance _____Time _____

  Reversed direction every _____ minutes

  Time walked without support _____

Stepper: Distance _____Time _____

  Time walked without support _____

Track: Distance _____Time _____

  Speed or pace (if recorded) _____

  Time walked without support _____

  Fastest lap _____

  Fastest lap without support_____

Total Cardio Walking Time:_____

Max. Heart Rate Noted:_____

RECOVERY PLAN: _____

Week No. _____ Day No.:_____

Exercises/Drills Done:

_____Time_____

_____Time_____

_____Time_____

_____Time_____

_____Time_____

_____Time_____

_____Time_____

_____Time_____

_____Time_____

Total Time Spent_____

NUTRITION PLAN:

Nutrient-rich foods eaten | quantity:

BREAKFAST:

_____|_____

_____|_____

_____|_____

_____|_____

Drinks:_____

LUNCH:

_____|_____

_____|_____

_____|_____

_____|_____

_____|_____

Drinks:_____

Snacks:_____

DINNER:

_____|_____

_____|_____

_____|_____

_____|_____

_____|_____

_____|_____

Drinks:_____

Snacks:_____

RECOVERY PLAN: _____

Week No. _____ Day No.:_____

Exercises/Drills Done:

_____Time_____

_____Time_____

_____Time_____

_____Time_____

_____Time_____

_____Time_____

_____Time_____

_____Time_____

_____Time_____

Total Time Spent_____

SUPPLEMENTS TAKEN:

_____|_____

_____|_____

_____|_____

_____|_____

_____|_____

Supplements I Need to Buy:

_____|_____

_____|_____

MEDICINES TAKEN:

_____|_____

_____|_____

_____|_____

_____|_____

_____|_____

_____|_____

YOGA TRAINING:

Exercises:_____

_____

_____

_____

_____

Total Yoga Time: _____

Notes:_____

RECOVERY BASICS:

☐ **Were physical exercise targets (time and total no. of reps) met?**

☐ **Did I focus well on exercises?**

☐ **Did I work intensively + aggressively?**

☐ **Did I push myself to increase difficulty?**

NOTES, SUCCESSES, BREAKTHROUGHS, PROGRESS!

_____

_____

_____

_____

_____

Daily Worksheet

Day of the Week:	Date:	Day No.	Max. Heart Rate:	A.M. Weight:	A.M. Blood Pressure: _____ OVER _____

Glasses of water drunk today (check): ○ ○ ○ ○ ○ ○ ○ ○

WALKING Plan No. _____

Week No.:_____   Day No.:_____

CORE WORK:
Total Time _____

RESISTANCE TRAINING:
1) Machine/Exerc._____

Weight_____ Reps _____/_____/_____

2) Machine/Exerc._____

Weight_____ Reps _____/_____/_____

3) Machine/Exerc._____

Weight_____ Reps _____/_____/_____

4) Machine/Exerc._____

Weight_____ Reps _____/_____/_____

5) Machine/Exerc._____

Weight_____ Reps _____/_____/_____

6) Machine/Exerc._____

Weight_____ Reps _____/_____/_____

7) Machine/Exerc._____

Weight_____ Reps _____/_____/_____

8) Machine/Exerc._____

Weight_____ Reps _____/_____/_____

Resistance Tr. Total Time_____

CARDIO WALKING:
Treadmill: Distance _____

Time _____ Speed _____

Time walked without support _____

Elliptical: Distance _____Time _____

Reversed direction every _____ minutes

Time walked without support _____

Stepper: Distance _____Time _____

Time walked without support _____

Track: Distance _____Time _____

Speed or pace (if recorded) _____

Time walked without support _____

Fastest lap _____

Fastest lap without support_____

Total Cardio Walking Time:_____

Max. Heart Rate Noted:_____

RECOVERY BASICS:
☐ **Were physical exercise targets (time and total no. of reps) met?**

☐ **Did I focus well on exercises?**

☐ **Did I work intensively + aggressively?**

☐ **Did I push myself to increase difficulty?**

RECOVERY PLAN: _____

Week No. _____   Day No.:_____

Exercises/Drills Done:
_____Time_____

_____Time_____

_____Time_____

_____Time_____

_____Time_____

_____Time_____

_____Time_____

_____Time_____

_____Time_____

Total Time Spent_____

NUTRITION PLAN:
Nutrient-rich foods eaten ǀ quantity:

BREAKFAST:

_____ ǀ _____

_____ ǀ _____

_____ ǀ _____

_____ ǀ _____

Drinks:_____

LUNCH:

_____ ǀ _____

_____ ǀ _____

_____ ǀ _____

_____ ǀ _____

_____ ǀ _____

_____ ǀ _____

Drinks:_____

Snacks:_____

DINNER:

_____ ǀ _____

_____ ǀ _____

_____ ǀ _____

_____ ǀ _____

_____ ǀ _____

_____ ǀ _____

_____ ǀ _____

Drinks:_____

Snacks:_____

RECOVERY PLAN: _____

Week No. _____   Day No.:_____

Exercises/Drills Done:
_____Time_____

_____Time_____

_____Time_____

_____Time_____

_____Time_____

_____Time_____

_____Time_____

_____Time_____

_____Time_____

Total Time Spent_____

SUPPLEMENTS TAKEN:
_____ ǀ _____

_____ ǀ _____

_____ ǀ _____

_____ ǀ _____

_____ ǀ _____

_____ ǀ _____

Supplements I Need to Buy:

_____ ǀ _____

_____ ǀ _____

MEDICINES TAKEN:
_____ ǀ _____

_____ ǀ _____

_____ ǀ _____

_____ ǀ _____

_____ ǀ _____

_____ ǀ _____

YOGA TRAINING:
Exercises:_____

_____

_____

_____

_____

Total Yoga Time: _____

Notes:_____

NOTES, SUCCESSES, BREAKTHROUGHS, PROGRESS!

_____

_____

_____

_____

_____

Daily Worksheet

Day of the Week:	Date:	Day No.	Max. Heart Rate:	A.M. Weight:	A.M. Blood Pressure: _____ OVER _____

Glasses of water drunk today (check): ○ ○ ○ ○ ○ ○ ○ ○

WALKING Plan No. _____

Week No.: _____ **Day No.:** _____

CORE WORK:

Total Time _____

RESISTANCE TRAINING:

1) Machine/Exerc. _____
  Weight_____ Reps _____/_____/_____

2) Machine/Exerc. _____
  Weight_____ Reps _____/_____/_____

3) Machine/Exerc. _____
  Weight_____ Reps _____/_____/_____

4) Machine/Exerc. _____
  Weight_____ Reps _____/_____/_____

5) Machine/Exerc. _____
  Weight_____ Reps _____/_____/_____

6) Machine/Exerc. _____
  Weight_____ Reps _____/_____/_____

7) Machine/Exerc. _____
  Weight_____ Reps _____/_____/_____

8) Machine/Exerc. _____
  Weight_____ Reps _____/_____/_____

Resistance Tr. Total Time _____

CARDIO WALKING:

Treadmill: Distance _____
  Time _____ Speed _____
  Time walked without support _____

Elliptical: Distance _____ Time _____
  Reversed direction every _____ minutes
  Time walked without support _____

Stepper: Distance _____ Time _____
  Time walked without support _____

Track: Distance _____ Time _____
  Speed or pace (if recorded) _____
  Time walked without support _____
  Fastest lap _____
  Fastest lap without support _____

Total Cardio Walking Time: _____

Max. Heart Rate Noted: _____

RECOVERY BASICS:

☐ **Were physical exercise targets (time and total no. of reps) met?**
☐ **Did I focus well on exercises?**
☐ **Did I work intensively + aggressively?**
☐ **Did I push myself to increase difficulty?**

RECOVERY PLAN: _____

Week No. _____ **Day No.:** _____

Exercises/Drills Done:

_____ Time _____
_____ Time _____
_____ Time _____
_____ Time _____
_____ Time _____
_____ Time _____
_____ Time _____
_____ Time _____
_____ Time _____
_____ Time _____

Total Time Spent _____

NUTRITION PLAN:

Nutrient-rich foods eaten | quantity:

BREAKFAST:
_____ | _____
_____ | _____
_____ | _____
_____ | _____

Drinks: _____

LUNCH:
_____ | _____
_____ | _____
_____ | _____
_____ | _____
_____ | _____
_____ | _____

Drinks: _____
Snacks: _____

DINNER:
_____ | _____
_____ | _____
_____ | _____
_____ | _____
_____ | _____
_____ | _____
_____ | _____

Drinks: _____
Snacks: _____

RECOVERY PLAN: _____

Week No. _____ **Day No.:** _____

Exercises/Drills Done:

_____ Time _____
_____ Time _____
_____ Time _____
_____ Time _____
_____ Time _____
_____ Time _____
_____ Time _____
_____ Time _____
_____ Time _____
_____ Time _____

Total Time Spent _____

SUPPLEMENTS TAKEN:

_____ | _____
_____ | _____
_____ | _____
_____ | _____
_____ | _____

Supplements I Need to Buy:

_____ | _____
_____ | _____

MEDICINES TAKEN:

_____ | _____
_____ | _____
_____ | _____
_____ | _____
_____ | _____

YOGA TRAINING:

Exercises: _____
_____
_____
_____
_____

Total Yoga Time: _____
Notes: _____

NOTES, SUCCESSES, BREAKTHROUGHS, PROGRESS!

_____
_____
_____
_____
_____

Daily Worksheet

Day of the Week:	Date:	Day No.	Max. Heart Rate:	A.M. Weight:	A.M. Blood Pressure: _____ OVER _____

Glasses of water drunk today (check): ○ ○ ○ ○ ○ ○ ○ ○

WALKING Plan No. _____

Week No.:_____ **Day No.:**_____

CORE WORK:

Total Time _____

RESISTANCE TRAINING:

1) Machine/Exerc._____

 Weight_____ Reps _____/_____/_____

2) Machine/Exerc._____

 Weight_____ Reps _____/_____/_____

3) Machine/Exerc._____

 Weight_____ Reps _____/_____/_____

4) Machine/Exerc._____

 Weight_____ Reps _____/_____/_____

5) Machine/Exerc._____

 Weight_____ Reps _____/_____/_____

6) Machine/Exerc._____

 Weight_____ Reps _____/_____/_____

7) Machine/Exerc._____

 Weight_____ Reps _____/_____/_____

8) Machine/Exerc._____

 Weight_____ Reps _____/_____/_____

Resistance Tr. Total Time_____

CARDIO WALKING:

Treadmill: Distance _____

 Time _____ Speed _____

 Time walked without support _____

Elliptical: Distance _____Time _____

 Reversed direction every _____ minutes

 Time walked without support _____

Stepper: Distance _____Time _____

 Time walked without support _____

Track: Distance _____Time _____

 Speed or pace (if recorded) _____

 Time walked without support _____

 Fastest lap _____

 Fastest lap without support_____

Total Cardio Walking Time:_____

Max. Heart Rate Noted:_____

RECOVERY BASICS:

☐ Were physical exercise targets (time and total no. of reps) met?

☐ Did I focus well on exercises?

☐ Did I work intensively + aggressively?

☐ Did I push myself to increase difficulty?

RECOVERY PLAN: _____

Week No. _____ **Day No.:**_____

Exercises/Drills Done:

_____Time_____

_____Time_____

_____Time_____

_____Time_____

_____Time_____

_____Time_____

_____Time_____

_____Time_____

_____Time_____

_____Time_____

Total Time Spent_____

NUTRITION PLAN:

Nutrient-rich foods eaten | quantity:

BREAKFAST:

_____ | _____

_____ | _____

_____ | _____

_____ | _____

Drinks:_____

LUNCH:

_____ | _____

_____ | _____

_____ | _____

_____ | _____

_____ | _____

Drinks:_____

Snacks:_____

DINNER:

_____ | _____

_____ | _____

_____ | _____

_____ | _____

_____ | _____

_____ | _____

Drinks:_____

Snacks:_____

RECOVERY PLAN: _____

Week No. _____ **Day No.:**_____

Exercises/Drills Done:

_____Time_____

_____Time_____

_____Time_____

_____Time_____

_____Time_____

_____Time_____

_____Time_____

_____Time_____

_____Time_____

_____Time_____

Total Time Spent_____

SUPPLEMENTS TAKEN:

_____ | _____

_____ | _____

_____ | _____

_____ | _____

_____ | _____

_____ | _____

Supplements I Need to Buy:

_____ | _____

_____ | _____

MEDICINES TAKEN:

_____ | _____

_____ | _____

_____ | _____

_____ | _____

_____ | _____

_____ | _____

YOGA TRAINING:

Exercises:_____

_____

_____

_____

_____

_____

Total Yoga Time: _____

Notes:_____

NOTES, SUCCESSES, BREAKTHROUGHS, PROGRESS!

_____

_____

_____

_____

_____

Start of Week Worksheet—Week No. 3

Date: Week Beginning Monday, _____, 20___

It doesn't matter how many people disagree with what you want to do. The only important thing is what you believe to be true, and the choices you make to realize your goals and dreams. What you then do is your choice alone. In other words: All real success and achievement result from your own choices, not those of others who may try to make your choices for you. YOU ARE THE ONE WHO CAUSES YOUR OWN SUCCESS.

Kirk Mango and Daveda Lamont from *Becoming a True Champion*

Start of Week Statistics:

MEASUREMENTS—MEN:	MEASUREMENTS—WOMEN:	WEIGHT: _____
Waist:_____ Chest:_____	Waist:_____ Hips:_____	BLOOD PRESSURE:
Upper Leg: ___ Upper Arm:____	Upper Leg: ___ Upper Arm:____	_____ over _____

Fill out the following information to guide you during the coming week.

Last week's successes and progress:_____

_____

_____

How well I am physically functioning right now: _____

_____

_____

Goals and expectations for this week:_____

_____

_____

Skills or exercises I want to especially focus on improving this week:_____

_____

_____

Shopping List: brain nutrient foods to add to diet this week:

_____   _____

_____   _____

If my weight or blood pressure are high, plan to reduce them (current/continuing):

_____

Daily Worksheet

Day of the Week:	Date:	Day No.	Max. Heart Rate:	A.M. Weight:	A.M. Blood Pressure: _____ OVER _____

Glasses of water drunk today (check): ○ ○ ○ ○ ○ ○ ○ ○

WALKING Plan No. _____

Week No.:_____ Day No.:_____

CORE WORK:

Total Time _____

RESISTANCE TRAINING:

1) Machine/Exerc._____

Weight_____ Reps _____/_____/_____

2) Machine/Exerc._____

Weight_____ Reps _____/_____/_____

3) Machine/Exerc._____

Weight_____ Reps _____/_____/_____

4) Machine/Exerc._____

Weight_____ Reps _____/_____/_____

5) Machine/Exerc._____

Weight_____ Reps _____/_____/_____

6) Machine/Exerc._____

Weight_____ Reps _____/_____/_____

7) Machine/Exerc._____

Weight_____ Reps _____/_____/_____

8) Machine/Exerc._____

Weight_____ Reps _____/_____/_____

Resistance Tr. Total Time_____

CARDIO WALKING:

Treadmill: Distance _____

Time _____ Speed _____

Time walked without support _____

Elliptical: Distance _____Time _____

Reversed direction every _____ minutes

Time walked without support _____

Stepper: Distance _____Time _____

Time walked without support _____

Track: Distance _____Time _____

Speed or pace (if recorded) _____

Time walked without support _____

Fastest lap _____

Fastest lap without support_____

Total Cardio Walking Time:_____

Max. Heart Rate Noted:_____

RECOVERY BASICS:

☐ Were physical exercise targets (time and total no. of reps) met?

☐ Did I focus well on exercises?

☐ Did I work intensively + aggressively?

☐ Did I push myself to increase difficulty?

RECOVERY PLAN: _____

Week No. _____ Day No.:_____

Exercises/Drills Done:

_____Time_____

_____Time_____

_____Time_____

_____Time_____

_____Time_____

_____Time_____

_____Time_____

_____Time_____

_____Time_____

_____Time_____

Total Time Spent_____

NUTRITION PLAN:

Nutrient-rich foods eaten | quantity:

BREAKFAST:

_____ | _____

_____ | _____

_____ | _____

_____ | _____

_____ | _____

Drinks:_____

LUNCH:

_____ | _____

_____ | _____

_____ | _____

_____ | _____

_____ | _____

Drinks:_____

Snacks:_____

DINNER:

_____ | _____

_____ | _____

_____ | _____

_____ | _____

_____ | _____

_____ | _____

Drinks:_____

Snacks:_____

RECOVERY PLAN: _____

Week No. _____ Day No.:_____

Exercises/Drills Done:

_____Time_____

_____Time_____

_____Time_____

_____Time_____

_____Time_____

_____Time_____

_____Time_____

_____Time_____

_____Time_____

_____Time_____

Total Time Spent_____

SUPPLEMENTS TAKEN:

_____ | _____

_____ | _____

_____ | _____

_____ | _____

_____ | _____

_____ | _____

Supplements I Need to Buy:

_____ | _____

_____ | _____

MEDICINES TAKEN:

_____ | _____

_____ | _____

_____ | _____

_____ | _____

_____ | _____

_____ | _____

_____ | _____

YOGA TRAINING:

Exercises:_____

_____

_____

_____

_____

Total Yoga Time: _____

Notes:_____

NOTES, SUCCESSES, BREAKTHROUGHS, PROGRESS!

_____

_____

_____

_____

_____

Daily Worksheet

Day of the Week:	Date:	Day No.	Max. Heart Rate:	A.M. Weight:	A.M. Blood Pressure: _____ OVER _____

Glasses of water drunk today (check): ○ ○ ○ ○ ○ ○ ○ ○

WALKING Plan No. _____

Week No.:_____   Day No.:_____

CORE WORK:

Total Time _____

RESISTANCE TRAINING:

1) Machine/Exerc._____
   Weight_____ Reps _____/_____/_____
2) Machine/Exerc._____
   Weight_____ Reps _____/_____/_____
3) Machine/Exerc._____
   Weight_____ Reps _____/_____/_____
4) Machine/Exerc._____
   Weight_____ Reps _____/_____/_____
5) Machine/Exerc._____
   Weight_____ Reps _____/_____/_____
6) Machine/Exerc._____
   Weight_____ Reps _____/_____/_____
7) Machine/Exerc._____
   Weight_____ Reps _____/_____/_____
8) Machine/Exerc._____
   Weight_____ Reps _____/_____/_____

Resistance Tr. Total Time_____

CARDIO WALKING:

Treadmill: Distance _____
   Time _____ Speed _____
   Time walked without support _____
Elliptical: Distance _____Time _____
   Reversed direction every _____ minutes
   Time walked without support _____
Stepper: Distance _____Time _____
   Time walked without support _____
Track: Distance _____Time _____
   Speed or pace (if recorded) _____
   Time walked without support _____
   Fastest lap _____
   Fastest lap without support_____

Total Cardio Walking Time:_____
Max. Heart Rate Noted:_____

RECOVERY BASICS:
☐ Were physical exercise targets (time and total no. of reps) met?
☐ Did I focus well on exercises?
☐ Did I work intensively + aggressively?
☐ Did I push myself to increase difficulty?

RECOVERY PLAN: _____

Week No. _____   Day No.:_____

Exercises/Drills Done:

_____Time_____
_____Time_____
_____Time_____
_____Time_____
_____Time_____
_____Time_____
_____Time_____
_____Time_____
_____Time_____

Total Time Spent_____

NUTRITION PLAN:

Nutrient-rich foods eaten | quantity:
BREAKFAST:
_____ | _____
_____ | _____
_____ | _____
_____ | _____
Drinks:_____

LUNCH:
_____ | _____
_____ | _____
_____ | _____
_____ | _____
_____ | _____
Drinks:_____
Snacks:_____

DINNER:
_____ | _____
_____ | _____
_____ | _____
_____ | _____
_____ | _____
_____ | _____
Drinks:_____
Snacks:_____

RECOVERY PLAN: _____

Week No. _____   Day No.:_____

Exercises/Drills Done:

_____Time_____
_____Time_____
_____Time_____
_____Time_____
_____Time_____
_____Time_____
_____Time_____
_____Time_____
_____Time_____

Total Time Spent_____

SUPPLEMENTS TAKEN:

_____ | _____
_____ | _____
_____ | _____
_____ | _____
_____ | _____
_____ | _____

Supplements I Need to Buy:
_____ | _____
_____ | _____

MEDICINES TAKEN:
_____ | _____
_____ | _____
_____ | _____
_____ | _____
_____ | _____
_____ | _____

YOGA TRAINING:
Exercises:_____
_____
_____
_____
_____

Total Yoga Time: _____
Notes:_____

NOTES, SUCCESSES, BREAKTHROUGHS, PROGRESS!

_____
_____
_____
_____
_____

Daily Worksheet

Day of the Week:	Date:	Day No.	Max. Heart Rate:	A.M. Weight:	A.M. Blood Pressure: _____ OVER _____

Glasses of water drunk today (check): ○ ○ ○ ○ ○ ○ ○ ○

WALKING Plan No. _____

Week No.: _____ **Day No.:** _____

CORE WORK:

Total Time _____

RESISTANCE TRAINING:

1) Machine/Exerc. _____

   Weight _____ Reps _____/_____/_____

2) Machine/Exerc. _____

   Weight _____ Reps _____/_____/_____

3) Machine/Exerc. _____

   Weight _____ Reps _____/_____/_____

4) Machine/Exerc. _____

   Weight _____ Reps _____/_____/_____

5) Machine/Exerc. _____

   Weight _____ Reps _____/_____/_____

6) Machine/Exerc. _____

   Weight _____ Reps _____/_____/_____

7) Machine/Exerc. _____

   Weight _____ Reps _____/_____/_____

8) Machine/Exerc. _____

   Weight _____ Reps _____/_____/_____

Resistance Tr. Total Time _____

CARDIO WALKING:

Treadmill: Distance _____

   Time _____ Speed _____

   Time walked without support _____

Elliptical: Distance _____ Time _____

   Reversed direction every _____ minutes

   Time walked without support _____

Stepper: Distance _____ Time _____

   Time walked without support _____

Track: Distance _____ Time _____

   Speed or pace (if recorded) _____

   Time walked without support _____

   Fastest lap _____

   Fastest lap without support _____

Total Cardio Walking Time: _____

Max. Heart Rate Noted: _____

RECOVERY PLAN: _____

Week No. _____ **Day No.:** _____

Exercises/Drills Done:

_____ Time _____

_____ Time _____

_____ Time _____

_____ Time _____

_____ Time _____

_____ Time _____

_____ Time _____

_____ Time _____

_____ Time _____

Total Time Spent _____

NUTRITION PLAN:

Nutrient-rich foods eaten | quantity:

BREAKFAST:

_____ | _____

_____ | _____

_____ | _____

_____ | _____

Drinks: _____

LUNCH:

_____ | _____

_____ | _____

_____ | _____

_____ | _____

_____ | _____

Drinks: _____

Snacks: _____

DINNER:

_____ | _____

_____ | _____

_____ | _____

_____ | _____

_____ | _____

_____ | _____

Drinks: _____

Snacks: _____

RECOVERY PLAN: _____

Week No. _____ **Day No.:** _____

Exercises/Drills Done:

_____ Time _____

_____ Time _____

_____ Time _____

_____ Time _____

_____ Time _____

_____ Time _____

_____ Time _____

_____ Time _____

_____ Time _____

Total Time Spent _____

SUPPLEMENTS TAKEN:

_____ | _____

_____ | _____

_____ | _____

_____ | _____

_____ | _____

Supplements I Need to Buy:

_____ | _____

_____ | _____

MEDICINES TAKEN:

_____ | _____

_____ | _____

_____ | _____

_____ | _____

_____ | _____

YOGA TRAINING:

Exercises: _____

_____

_____

_____

Total Yoga Time: _____

Notes: _____

RECOVERY BASICS:

☐ **Were physical exercise targets (time and total no. of reps) met?**

☐ **Did I focus well on exercises?**

☐ **Did I work intensively + aggressively?**

☐ **Did I push myself to increase difficulty?**

NOTES, SUCCESSES, BREAKTHROUGHS, PROGRESS!

_____

_____

_____

_____

_____

Daily Worksheet

Day of the Week:	Date:	Day No.	Max. Heart Rate:	A.M. Weight:	A.M. Blood Pressure: _____ OVER _____

Glasses of water drunk today (check): ○ ○ ○ ○ ○ ○ ○ ○

WALKING Plan No. _____
Week No.: _____ **Day No.:** _____

CORE WORK:
Total Time _____

RESISTANCE TRAINING:

1) Machine/Exerc. _____
Weight _____ Reps _____ / _____ / _____

2) Machine/Exerc. _____
Weight _____ Reps _____ / _____ / _____

3) Machine/Exerc. _____
Weight _____ Reps _____ / _____ / _____

4) Machine/Exerc. _____
Weight _____ Reps _____ / _____ / _____

5) Machine/Exerc. _____
Weight _____ Reps _____ / _____ / _____

6) Machine/Exerc. _____
Weight _____ Reps _____ / _____ / _____

7) Machine/Exerc. _____
Weight _____ Reps _____ / _____ / _____

8) Machine/Exerc. _____
Weight _____ Reps _____ / _____ / _____

Resistance Tr. Total Time _____

CARDIO WALKING:

Treadmill: Distance _____
Time _____ Speed _____
Time walked without support _____

Elliptical: Distance _____ Time _____
Reversed direction every _____ minutes
Time walked without support _____

Stepper: Distance _____ Time _____
Time walked without support _____

Track: Distance _____ Time _____
Speed or pace (if recorded) _____
Time walked without support _____
Fastest lap _____
Fastest lap without support _____

Total Cardio Walking Time: _____
Max. Heart Rate Noted: _____

RECOVERY BASICS:
☐ **Were physical exercise targets (time and total no. of reps) met?**
☐ **Did I focus well on exercises?**
☐ **Did I work intensively + aggressively?**
☐ **Did I push myself to increase difficulty?**

RECOVERY PLAN: _____
Week No. _____ **Day No.:** _____

Exercises/Drills Done:
_____ Time _____
_____ Time _____
_____ Time _____
_____ Time _____
_____ Time _____
_____ Time _____
_____ Time _____
_____ Time _____
_____ Time _____
_____ Time _____

Total Time Spent _____

NUTRITION PLAN:
Nutrient-rich foods eaten | quantity:
BREAKFAST:
_____ | _____
_____ | _____
_____ | _____
_____ | _____
Drinks: _____
LUNCH:
_____ | _____
_____ | _____
_____ | _____
_____ | _____
_____ | _____
Drinks: _____
Snacks: _____
DINNER:
_____ | _____
_____ | _____
_____ | _____
_____ | _____
_____ | _____
Drinks: _____
Snacks: _____

NOTES, SUCCESSES, BREAKTHROUGHS, PROGRESS!
_____
_____
_____
_____
_____

RECOVERY PLAN: _____
Week No. _____ **Day No.:** _____

Exercises/Drills Done:
_____ Time _____
_____ Time _____
_____ Time _____
_____ Time _____
_____ Time _____
_____ Time _____
_____ Time _____
_____ Time _____
_____ Time _____
_____ Time _____

Total Time Spent _____

SUPPLEMENTS TAKEN:
_____ | _____
_____ | _____
_____ | _____
_____ | _____
_____ | _____
_____ | _____

Supplements I Need to Buy:
_____ | _____
_____ | _____

MEDICINES TAKEN:
_____ | _____
_____ | _____
_____ | _____
_____ | _____
_____ | _____

YOGA TRAINING:
Exercises: _____
_____
_____
_____
_____
_____

Total Yoga Time: _____
Notes: _____

Daily Worksheet

Day of the Week:	Date:	Day No.	Max. Heart Rate:	A.M. Weight:	A.M. Blood Pressure: _____ OVER _____

Glasses of water drunk today (check): ○ ○ ○ ○ ○ ○ ○ ○

WALKING Plan No. _____

Week No.:_____ Day No.:_____

CORE WORK:

Total Time _____

RESISTANCE TRAINING:

1) Machine/Exerc._____

  Weight_____ Reps _____/_____/_____

2) Machine/Exerc._____

  Weight_____ Reps _____/_____/_____

3) Machine/Exerc._____

  Weight_____ Reps _____/_____/_____

4) Machine/Exerc._____

  Weight_____ Reps _____/_____/_____

5) Machine/Exerc._____

  Weight_____ Reps _____/_____/_____

6) Machine/Exerc._____

  Weight_____ Reps _____/_____/_____

7) Machine/Exerc._____

  Weight_____ Reps _____/_____/_____

8) Machine/Exerc._____

  Weight_____ Reps _____/_____/_____

Resistance Tr. Total Time_____

CARDIO WALKING:

Treadmill: Distance _____

  Time _____ Speed _____

  Time walked without support _____

Elliptical: Distance _____Time _____

  Reversed direction every _____ minutes

  Time walked without support _____

Stepper: Distance _____Time _____

  Time walked without support _____

Track: Distance _____Time _____

  Speed or pace (if recorded) _____

  Time walked without support _____

  Fastest lap _____

  Fastest lap without support_____

Total Cardio Walking Time:_____

Max. Heart Rate Noted:_____

RECOVERY BASICS:

☐ Were physical exercise targets (time and total no. of reps) met?

☐ Did I focus well on exercises?

☐ Did I work intensively + aggressively?

☐ Did I push myself to increase difficulty?

RECOVERY PLAN: _____

Week No. _____ Day No.:_____

Exercises/Drills Done:

_____Time_____

_____Time_____

_____Time_____

_____Time_____

_____Time_____

_____Time_____

_____Time_____

_____Time_____

_____Time_____

Total Time Spent_____

NUTRITION PLAN:

Nutrient-rich foods eaten | quantity:

BREAKFAST:

_____ | _____

_____ | _____

_____ | _____

_____ | _____

Drinks:_____

LUNCH:

_____ | _____

_____ | _____

_____ | _____

_____ | _____

_____ | _____

Drinks:_____

Snacks:_____

DINNER:

_____ | _____

_____ | _____

_____ | _____

_____ | _____

_____ | _____

_____ | _____

Drinks:_____

Snacks:_____

NOTES, SUCCESSES, BREAKTHROUGHS, PROGRESS!

_____

_____

_____

_____

_____

_____

RECOVERY PLAN: _____

Week No. _____ Day No.:_____

Exercises/Drills Done:

_____Time_____

_____Time_____

_____Time_____

_____Time_____

_____Time_____

_____Time_____

_____Time_____

_____Time_____

_____Time_____

Total Time Spent_____

SUPPLEMENTS TAKEN:

_____ | _____

_____ | _____

_____ | _____

_____ | _____

_____ | _____

Supplements I Need to Buy:

_____ | _____

_____ | _____

MEDICINES TAKEN:

_____ | _____

_____ | _____

_____ | _____

_____ | _____

_____ | _____

_____ | _____

YOGA TRAINING:

Exercises:_____

_____

_____

_____

_____

Total Yoga Time: _____

Notes:_____

Daily Worksheet

Day of the Week:	Date:	Day No.	Max. Heart Rate:	A.M. Weight:	A.M. Blood Pressure: _____ OVER _____

Glasses of water drunk today (check): ○ ○ ○ ○ ○ ○ ○ ○

WALKING Plan No. _____

Week No.:_____ Day No.:_____

CORE WORK:

Total Time _____

RESISTANCE TRAINING:

1) Machine/Exerc._____

   Weight_____ Reps _____/_____/_____

2) Machine/Exerc._____

   Weight_____ Reps _____/_____/_____

3) Machine/Exerc._____

   Weight_____ Reps _____/_____/_____

4) Machine/Exerc._____

   Weight_____ Reps _____/_____/_____

5) Machine/Exerc._____

   Weight_____ Reps _____/_____/_____

6) Machine/Exerc._____

   Weight_____ Reps _____/_____/_____

7) Machine/Exerc._____

   Weight_____ Reps _____/_____/_____

8) Machine/Exerc._____

   Weight_____ Reps _____/_____/_____

Resistance Tr. Total Time_____

CARDIO WALKING:

Treadmill: Distance _____

   Time _____ Speed _____

   Time walked without support _____

Elliptical: Distance _____Time _____

   Reversed direction every _____ minutes

   Time walked without support _____

Stepper: Distance _____Time _____

   Time walked without support _____

Track: Distance _____Time _____

   Speed or pace (if recorded) _____

   Time walked without support _____

   Fastest lap _____

   Fastest lap without support_____

Total Cardio Walking Time:_____

Max. Heart Rate Noted:_____

RECOVERY BASICS:

☐ **Were physical exercise targets (time and total no. of reps) met?**

☐ **Did I focus well on exercises?**

☐ **Did I work intensively + aggressively?**

☐ **Did I push myself to increase difficulty?**

RECOVERY PLAN: _____

Week No. _____ Day No.:_____

Exercises/Drills Done:

_____Time_____

_____Time_____

_____Time_____

_____Time_____

_____Time_____

_____Time_____

_____Time_____

_____Time_____

_____Time_____

Total Time Spent_____

NUTRITION PLAN:

Nutrient-rich foods eaten | quantity:

BREAKFAST:

_____|_____

_____|_____

_____|_____

_____|_____

Drinks:_____

LUNCH:

_____|_____

_____|_____

_____|_____

_____|_____

_____|_____

Drinks:_____

Snacks:_____

DINNER:

_____|_____

_____|_____

_____|_____

_____|_____

_____|_____

_____|_____

Drinks:_____

Snacks:_____

NOTES, SUCCESSES, BREAKTHROUGHS, PROGRESS!

_____

_____

_____

_____

_____

RECOVERY PLAN: _____

Week No. _____ Day No.:_____

Exercises/Drills Done:

_____Time_____

_____Time_____

_____Time_____

_____Time_____

_____Time_____

_____Time_____

_____Time_____

_____Time_____

_____Time_____

Total Time Spent_____

SUPPLEMENTS TAKEN:

_____|_____

_____|_____

_____|_____

_____|_____

_____|_____

_____|_____

Supplements I Need to Buy:

_____|_____

_____|_____

MEDICINES TAKEN:

_____|_____

_____|_____

_____|_____

_____|_____

_____|_____

_____|_____

YOGA TRAINING:

Exercises:_____

_____

_____

_____

Total Yoga Time: _____

Notes:_____

Daily Worksheet

Day of the Week:	Date:	Day No.	Max. Heart Rate:	A.M. Weight:	A.M. Blood Pressure: _____ OVER _____

Glasses of water drunk today (check): ○ ○ ○ ○ ○ ○ ○ ○

WALKING Plan No. _____

Week No.: _____   **Day No.:** _____

CORE WORK:

Total Time _____

RESISTANCE TRAINING:

1) Machine/Exerc. _____
  Weight _____ Reps _____/_____/_____
2) Machine/Exerc. _____
  Weight _____ Reps _____/_____/_____
3) Machine/Exerc. _____
  Weight _____ Reps _____/_____/_____
4) Machine/Exerc. _____
  Weight _____ Reps _____/_____/_____
5) Machine/Exerc. _____
  Weight _____ Reps _____/_____/_____
6) Machine/Exerc. _____
  Weight _____ Reps _____/_____/_____
7) Machine/Exerc. _____
  Weight _____ Reps _____/_____/_____
8) Machine/Exerc. _____
  Weight _____ Reps _____/_____/_____

Resistance Tr. Total Time _____

CARDIO WALKING:

Treadmill: Distance _____
  Time _____ Speed _____
  Time walked without support _____
Elliptical: Distance _____ Time _____
  Reversed direction every _____ minutes
  Time walked without support _____
Stepper: Distance _____ Time _____
  Time walked without support _____
Track: Distance _____ Time _____
  Speed or pace (if recorded) _____
  Time walked without support _____
  Fastest lap _____
  Fastest lap without support _____

Total Cardio Walking Time: _____
Max. Heart Rate Noted: _____

RECOVERY PLAN: _____

Week No. _____   **Day No.:** _____

Exercises/Drills Done:

_____ Time _____
_____ Time _____
_____ Time _____
_____ Time _____
_____ Time _____
_____ Time _____
_____ Time _____
_____ Time _____
_____ Time _____
_____ Time _____
_____ Time _____

Total Time Spent _____

NUTRITION PLAN:

Nutrient-rich foods eaten | quantity:

BREAKFAST:

_____ | _____
_____ | _____
_____ | _____
_____ | _____
_____ | _____

Drinks: _____

LUNCH:

_____ | _____
_____ | _____
_____ | _____
_____ | _____
_____ | _____
_____ | _____

Drinks: _____
Snacks: _____

DINNER:

_____ | _____
_____ | _____
_____ | _____
_____ | _____
_____ | _____
_____ | _____

Drinks: _____
Snacks: _____

RECOVERY PLAN: _____

Week No. _____   **Day No.:** _____

Exercises/Drills Done:

_____ Time _____
_____ Time _____
_____ Time _____
_____ Time _____
_____ Time _____
_____ Time _____
_____ Time _____
_____ Time _____
_____ Time _____
_____ Time _____
_____ Time _____

Total Time Spent _____

SUPPLEMENTS TAKEN:

_____ | _____
_____ | _____
_____ | _____
_____ | _____
_____ | _____
_____ | _____

Supplements I Need to Buy:

_____ | _____
_____ | _____

MEDICINES TAKEN:

_____ | _____
_____ | _____
_____ | _____
_____ | _____
_____ | _____
_____ | _____

YOGA TRAINING:

Exercises: _____
_____
_____
_____
_____
_____

Total Yoga Time: _____
Notes: _____

RECOVERY BASICS:

☐ **Were physical exercise targets (time and total no. of reps) met?**
☐ **Did I focus well on exercises?**
☐ **Did I work intensively + aggressively?**
☐ **Did I push myself to increase difficulty?**

NOTES, SUCCESSES, BREAKTHROUGHS, PROGRESS!

_____
_____
_____
_____
_____
_____
_____

Start of Week Worksheet—Week No. 4

Date: Week Beginning Monday, _____, 20___

> Remember to realize that you have achieved something if you got through the day even "pretty well"! Each day is one step further on the road to recovery.
>
> Kathy Maxwell

Start of Week Statistics:

MEASUREMENTS—MEN:	MEASUREMENTS—WOMEN:	WEIGHT: _____
Waist:_____ Chest:_____	Waist:_____ Hips:_____	BLOOD PRESSURE:
Upper Leg: ____ Upper Arm:_____	Upper Leg: ____ Upper Arm:____	_____ over _____

Fill out the following information to guide you during the coming week.

Last week's successes and progress:_____

_____

_____

How well I am physically functioning right now: _____

_____

_____

Goals and expectations for this week:_____

_____

_____

Skills or exercises I want to especially focus on improving this week:_____

_____

_____

Shopping List: brain nutrient foods to add to diet this week:

_____   _____

_____   _____

If my weight or blood pressure are high, plan to reduce them (current/continuing):

_____

_____

Daily Worksheet

Day of the Week:	Date:	Day No.	Max. Heart Rate:	A.M. Weight:	A.M. Blood Pressure: _____ OVER _____

Glasses of water drunk today (check): ○ ○ ○ ○ ○ ○ ○ ○

WALKING Plan No. _____

Week No.:_____ **Day No.:**_____

CORE WORK:

Total Time _____

RESISTANCE TRAINING:

1) Machine/Exerc._____

   Weight_____ Reps _____/_____/_____

2) Machine/Exerc._____

   Weight_____ Reps _____/_____/_____

3) Machine/Exerc._____

   Weight_____ Reps _____/_____/_____

4) Machine/Exerc._____

   Weight_____ Reps _____/_____/_____

5) Machine/Exerc._____

   Weight_____ Reps _____/_____/_____

6) Machine/Exerc._____

   Weight_____ Reps _____/_____/_____

7) Machine/Exerc._____

   Weight_____ Reps _____/_____/_____

8) Machine/Exerc._____

   Weight_____ Reps _____/_____/_____

Resistance Tr. Total Time_____

CARDIO WALKING:

Treadmill: Distance _____

   Time _____ Speed _____

   Time walked without support _____

Elliptical: Distance _____Time _____

   Reversed direction every _____ minutes

   Time walked without support _____

Stepper: Distance _____Time _____

   Time walked without support _____

Track: Distance _____Time _____

   Speed or pace (if recorded) _____

   Time walked without support _____

   Fastest lap _____

   Fastest lap without support_____

Total Cardio Walking Time:_____

Max. Heart Rate Noted:_____

RECOVERY PLAN: _____

Week No. _____ **Day No.:**_____

Exercises/Drills Done:

_____Time_____

_____Time_____

_____Time_____

_____Time_____

_____Time_____

_____Time_____

_____Time_____

_____Time_____

Total Time Spent_____

NUTRITION PLAN:

Nutrient-rich foods eaten | quantity:

BREAKFAST:

_____ | _____

_____ | _____

_____ | _____

_____ | _____

Drinks:_____

LUNCH:

_____ | _____

_____ | _____

_____ | _____

_____ | _____

_____ | _____

Drinks:_____

Snacks:_____

DINNER:

_____ | _____

_____ | _____

_____ | _____

_____ | _____

_____ | _____

_____ | _____

Drinks:_____

Snacks:_____

RECOVERY PLAN: _____

Week No. _____ **Day No.:**_____

Exercises/Drills Done:

_____Time_____

_____Time_____

_____Time_____

_____Time_____

_____Time_____

_____Time_____

_____Time_____

_____Time_____

Total Time Spent_____

SUPPLEMENTS TAKEN:

_____ | _____

_____ | _____

_____ | _____

_____ | _____

_____ | _____

Supplements I Need to Buy:

_____ | _____

_____ | _____

MEDICINES TAKEN:

_____ | _____

_____ | _____

_____ | _____

_____ | _____

_____ | _____

_____ | _____

YOGA TRAINING:

Exercises:_____

_____

_____

_____

_____

_____

Total Yoga Time: _____

Notes:_____

RECOVERY BASICS:

☐ **Were physical exercise targets (time and total no. of reps) met?**

☐ **Did I focus well on exercises?**

☐ **Did I work intensively + aggressively?**

☐ **Did I push myself to increase difficulty?**

NOTES, SUCCESSES, BREAKTHROUGHS, PROGRESS!

_____

_____

_____

_____

_____

_____

Daily Worksheet

Day of the Week:	Date:	Day No.	Max. Heart Rate:	A.M. Weight:	A.M. Blood Pressure: _____ OVER _____

Glasses of water drunk today (check): ○ ○ ○ ○ ○ ○ ○ ○

WALKING Plan No. _____

Week No.:_____ Day No.:_____

CORE WORK:

Total Time _____

RESISTANCE TRAINING:

1) Machine/Exerc._____

   Weight_____ Reps _____/_____/_____

2) Machine/Exerc._____

   Weight_____ Reps _____/_____/_____

3) Machine/Exerc._____

   Weight_____ Reps _____/_____/_____

4) Machine/Exerc._____

   Weight_____ Reps _____/_____/_____

5) Machine/Exerc._____

   Weight_____ Reps _____/_____/_____

6) Machine/Exerc._____

   Weight_____ Reps _____/_____/_____

7) Machine/Exerc._____

   Weight_____ Reps _____/_____/_____

8) Machine/Exerc._____

   Weight_____ Reps _____/_____/_____

Resistance Tr. Total Time_____

CARDIO WALKING:

Treadmill: Distance _____

   Time _____ Speed _____

   Time walked without support _____

Elliptical: Distance _____Time _____

   Reversed direction every _____ minutes

   Time walked without support _____

Stepper: Distance _____Time _____

   Time walked without support _____

Track: Distance _____Time _____

   Speed or pace (if recorded) _____

   Time walked without support _____

   Fastest lap _____

   Fastest lap without support_____

Total Cardio Walking Time:_____

Max. Heart Rate Noted:_____

RECOVERY BASICS:

☐ **Were physical exercise targets (time and total no. of reps) met?**

☐ **Did I focus well on exercises?**

☐ **Did I work intensively + aggressively?**

☐ **Did I push myself to increase difficulty?**

RECOVERY PLAN: _____

Week No. _____ Day No.:_____

Exercises/Drills Done:

_____Time_____

_____Time_____

_____Time_____

_____Time_____

_____Time_____

_____Time_____

_____Time_____

_____Time_____

_____Time_____

Total Time Spent_____

NUTRITION PLAN:

Nutrient-rich foods eaten | quantity:

BREAKFAST:

_____ | _____

_____ | _____

_____ | _____

_____ | _____

Drinks:_____

LUNCH:

_____ | _____

_____ | _____

_____ | _____

_____ | _____

_____ | _____

Drinks:_____

Snacks:_____

DINNER:

_____ | _____

_____ | _____

_____ | _____

_____ | _____

_____ | _____

_____ | _____

Drinks:_____

Snacks:_____

RECOVERY PLAN: _____

Week No. _____ Day No.:_____

Exercises/Drills Done:

_____Time_____

_____Time_____

_____Time_____

_____Time_____

_____Time_____

_____Time_____

_____Time_____

_____Time_____

_____Time_____

Total Time Spent_____

SUPPLEMENTS TAKEN:

_____ | _____

_____ | _____

_____ | _____

_____ | _____

Supplements I Need to Buy:

_____ | _____

_____ | _____

MEDICINES TAKEN:

_____ | _____

_____ | _____

_____ | _____

_____ | _____

_____ | _____

_____ | _____

YOGA TRAINING:

Exercises:_____

_____

_____

_____

_____

Total Yoga Time: _____

Notes:_____

NOTES, SUCCESSES, BREAKTHROUGHS, PROGRESS!

_____

_____

_____

_____

_____

Daily Worksheet

Day of the Week:	Date:	Day No.	Max. Heart Rate:	A.M. Weight:	A.M. Blood Pressure: _____ OVER _____

Glasses of water drunk today (check): ○ ○ ○ ○ ○ ○ ○ ○

WALKING Plan No. _____

Week No.:_____ Day No.:_____

CORE WORK:

Total Time _____

RESISTANCE TRAINING:

1) Machine/Exerc._____

　Weight_____ Reps _____/_____/_____

2) Machine/Exerc._____

　Weight_____ Reps _____/_____/_____

3) Machine/Exerc._____

　Weight_____ Reps _____/_____/_____

4) Machine/Exerc._____

　Weight_____ Reps _____/_____/_____

5) Machine/Exerc._____

　Weight_____ Reps _____/_____/_____

6) Machine/Exerc._____

　Weight_____ Reps _____/_____/_____

7) Machine/Exerc._____

　Weight_____ Reps _____/_____/_____

8) Machine/Exerc._____

　Weight_____ Reps _____/_____/_____

Resistance Tr. Total Time_____

CARDIO WALKING:

Treadmill: Distance _____

　Time _____ Speed _____

　Time walked without support _____

Elliptical: Distance _____Time _____

　Reversed direction every _____ minutes

　Time walked without support _____

Stepper: Distance _____Time _____

　Time walked without support _____

Track: Distance _____Time _____

　Speed or pace (if recorded) _____

　Time walked without support _____

　Fastest lap _____

　Fastest lap without support_____

Total Cardio Walking Time:_____

Max. Heart Rate Noted:_____

RECOVERY PLAN: _____

Week No. _____ Day No.:_____

Exercises/Drills Done:

_____Time_____

_____Time_____

_____Time_____

_____Time_____

_____Time_____

_____Time_____

_____Time_____

_____Time_____

_____Time_____

_____Time_____

Total Time Spent_____

NUTRITION PLAN:

Nutrient-rich foods eaten | quantity:

BREAKFAST:

_____ | _____

_____ | _____

_____ | _____

_____ | _____

Drinks:_____

LUNCH:

_____ | _____

_____ | _____

_____ | _____

_____ | _____

_____ | _____

Drinks:_____

Snacks:_____

DINNER:

_____ | _____

_____ | _____

_____ | _____

_____ | _____

_____ | _____

_____ | _____

Drinks:_____

Snacks:_____

RECOVERY PLAN: _____

Week No. _____ Day No.:_____

Exercises/Drills Done:

_____Time_____

_____Time_____

_____Time_____

_____Time_____

_____Time_____

_____Time_____

_____Time_____

_____Time_____

_____Time_____

_____Time_____

Total Time Spent_____

SUPPLEMENTS TAKEN:

_____ | _____

_____ | _____

_____ | _____

_____ | _____

_____ | _____

_____ | _____

Supplements I Need to Buy:

_____ | _____

_____ | _____

MEDICINES TAKEN:

_____ | _____

_____ | _____

_____ | _____

_____ | _____

_____ | _____

_____ | _____

YOGA TRAINING:

Exercises:_____

_____

_____

_____

_____

_____

Total Yoga Time: _____

Notes:_____

RECOVERY BASICS:

☐ **Were physical exercise targets (time and total no. of reps) met?**

☐ **Did I focus well on exercises?**

☐ **Did I work intensively + aggressively?**

☐ **Did I push myself to increase difficulty?**

NOTES, SUCCESSES, BREAKTHROUGHS, PROGRESS!

_____

_____

_____

_____

_____

Daily Worksheet

Day of the Week:	Date:	Day No.	Max. Heart Rate:	A.M. Weight:	A.M. Blood Pressure: _____ OVER _____

Glasses of water drunk today (check): ○ ○ ○ ○ ○ ○ ○ ○

WALKING Plan No. _____

Week No.:_____ **Day No.:**_____

CORE WORK:

Total Time _____

RESISTANCE TRAINING:

1) Machine/Exerc._____

   Weight_____ Reps _____/_____/_____

2) Machine/Exerc._____

   Weight_____ Reps _____/_____/_____

3) Machine/Exerc._____

   Weight_____ Reps _____/_____/_____

4) Machine/Exerc._____

   Weight_____ Reps _____/_____/_____

5) Machine/Exerc._____

   Weight_____ Reps _____/_____/_____

6) Machine/Exerc._____

   Weight_____ Reps _____/_____/_____

7) Machine/Exerc._____

   Weight_____ Reps _____/_____/_____

8) Machine/Exerc._____

   Weight_____ Reps _____/_____/_____

Resistance Tr. Total Time_____

CARDIO WALKING:

Treadmill: Distance _____

   Time _____ Speed _____

   Time walked without support _____

Elliptical: Distance _____Time _____

   Reversed direction every _____ minutes

   Time walked without support _____

Stepper: Distance _____Time _____

   Time walked without support _____

Track: Distance _____Time _____

   Speed or pace (if recorded) _____

   Time walked without support _____

   Fastest lap _____

   Fastest lap without support_____

Total Cardio Walking Time:_____

Max. Heart Rate Noted:_____

RECOVERY BASICS:

☐ **Were physical exercise targets (time and total no. of reps) met?**

☐ **Did I focus well on exercises?**

☐ **Did I work intensively + aggressively?**

☐ **Did I push myself to increase difficulty?**

RECOVERY PLAN: _____

Week No. _____ **Day No.:**_____

Exercises/Drills Done:

_____Time_____

_____Time_____

_____Time_____

_____Time_____

_____Time_____

_____Time_____

_____Time_____

_____Time_____

_____Time_____

Total Time Spent_____

NUTRITION PLAN:

Nutrient-rich foods eaten ǀ quantity:

BREAKFAST:

_____ǀ_____

_____ǀ_____

_____ǀ_____

_____ǀ_____

Drinks:_____

LUNCH:

_____ǀ_____

_____ǀ_____

_____ǀ_____

_____ǀ_____

_____ǀ_____

Drinks:_____

Snacks:_____

DINNER:

_____ǀ_____

_____ǀ_____

_____ǀ_____

_____ǀ_____

_____ǀ_____

_____ǀ_____

Drinks:_____

Snacks:_____

RECOVERY PLAN: _____

Week No. _____ **Day No.:**_____

Exercises/Drills Done:

_____Time_____

_____Time_____

_____Time_____

_____Time_____

_____Time_____

_____Time_____

_____Time_____

_____Time_____

_____Time_____

Total Time Spent_____

SUPPLEMENTS TAKEN:

_____ǀ_____

_____ǀ_____

_____ǀ_____

_____ǀ_____

_____ǀ_____

_____ǀ_____

Supplements I Need to Buy:

_____ǀ_____

_____ǀ_____

MEDICINES TAKEN:

_____ǀ_____

_____ǀ_____

_____ǀ_____

_____ǀ_____

_____ǀ_____

_____ǀ_____

YOGA TRAINING:

Exercises:_____

_____

_____

_____

Total Yoga Time: _____

Notes:_____

NOTES, SUCCESSES, BREAKTHROUGHS, PROGRESS!

_____

_____

_____

_____

Daily Worksheet

Day of the Week:	Date:	Day No.	Max. Heart Rate:	A.M. Weight:	A.M. Blood Pressure: _____ OVER _____

Glasses of water drunk today (check): ○ ○ ○ ○ ○ ○ ○ ○

WALKING Plan No. _____

Week No.:_____ Day No.:_____

CORE WORK:

Total Time _____

RESISTANCE TRAINING:

1) Machine/Exerc._____

   Weight_____ Reps _____/_____/_____

2) Machine/Exerc._____

   Weight_____ Reps _____/_____/_____

3) Machine/Exerc._____

   Weight_____ Reps _____/_____/_____

4) Machine/Exerc._____

   Weight_____ Reps _____/_____/_____

5) Machine/Exerc._____

   Weight_____ Reps _____/_____/_____

6) Machine/Exerc._____

   Weight_____ Reps _____/_____/_____

7) Machine/Exerc._____

   Weight_____ Reps _____/_____/_____

8) Machine/Exerc._____

   Weight_____ Reps _____/_____/_____

Resistance Tr. Total Time_____

CARDIO WALKING:

Treadmill: Distance _____

   Time _____ Speed _____

   Time walked without support _____

Elliptical: Distance _____Time _____

   Reversed direction every _____ minutes

   Time walked without support _____

Stepper: Distance _____Time _____

   Time walked without support _____

Track: Distance _____Time _____

   Speed or pace (if recorded) _____

   Time walked without support _____

   Fastest lap _____

   Fastest lap without support_____

Total Cardio Walking Time:_____

Max. Heart Rate Noted:_____

RECOVERY BASICS:

☐ Were physical exercise targets (time and total no. of reps) met?

☐ Did I focus well on exercises?

☐ Did I work intensively + aggressively?

☐ Did I push myself to increase difficulty?

RECOVERY PLAN: _____

Week No. _____ Day No.:_____

Exercises/Drills Done:

_____Time_____

_____Time_____

_____Time_____

_____Time_____

_____Time_____

_____Time_____

_____Time_____

_____Time_____

Total Time Spent_____

NUTRITION PLAN:

Nutrient-rich foods eaten | quantity:

BREAKFAST:

_____ | _____

_____ | _____

_____ | _____

_____ | _____

Drinks:_____

LUNCH:

_____ | _____

_____ | _____

_____ | _____

_____ | _____

_____ | _____

Drinks:_____

Snacks:_____

DINNER:

_____ | _____

_____ | _____

_____ | _____

_____ | _____

_____ | _____

_____ | _____

Drinks:_____

Snacks:_____

RECOVERY PLAN: _____

Week No. _____ Day No.:_____

Exercises/Drills Done:

_____Time_____

_____Time_____

_____Time_____

_____Time_____

_____Time_____

_____Time_____

_____Time_____

_____Time_____

Total Time Spent_____

SUPPLEMENTS TAKEN:

_____ | _____

_____ | _____

_____ | _____

_____ | _____

_____ | _____

_____ | _____

Supplements I Need to Buy:

_____ | _____

_____ | _____

MEDICINES TAKEN:

_____ | _____

_____ | _____

_____ | _____

_____ | _____

_____ | _____

_____ | _____

YOGA TRAINING:

Exercises:_____

_____

_____

_____

_____

_____

Total Yoga Time: _____

Notes:_____

NOTES, SUCCESSES, BREAKTHROUGHS, PROGRESS!

_____

_____

_____

_____

_____

Daily Worksheet

Day of the Week:	Date:	Day No.	Max. Heart Rate:	A.M. Weight:	A.M. Blood Pressure: _____ OVER _____

Glasses of water drunk today (check): ○ ○ ○ ○ ○ ○ ○ ○

WALKING Plan No. _____

Week No.:_____   Day No.:_____

CORE WORK:

Total Time _____

RESISTANCE TRAINING:

1) Machine/Exerc._____

    Weight_____ Reps _____/_____/_____

2) Machine/Exerc._____

    Weight_____ Reps _____/_____/_____

3) Machine/Exerc._____

    Weight_____ Reps _____/_____/_____

4) Machine/Exerc._____

    Weight_____ Reps _____/_____/_____

5) Machine/Exerc._____

    Weight_____ Reps _____/_____/_____

6) Machine/Exerc._____

    Weight_____ Reps _____/_____/_____

7) Machine/Exerc._____

    Weight_____ Reps _____/_____/_____

8) Machine/Exerc._____

    Weight_____ Reps _____/_____/_____

Resistance Tr. Total Time_____

CARDIO WALKING:

Treadmill: Distance _____

    Time _____ Speed _____

    Time walked without support _____

Elliptical: Distance _____Time _____

    Reversed direction every _____ minutes

    Time walked without support _____

Stepper: Distance _____Time _____

    Time walked without support _____

Track: Distance _____Time _____

    Speed or pace (if recorded) _____

    Time walked without support _____

    Fastest lap _____

    Fastest lap without support_____

Total Cardio Walking Time:_____

Max. Heart Rate Noted:_____

RECOVERY BASICS:

☐ **Were physical exercise targets (time and total no. of reps) met?**

☐ **Did I focus well on exercises?**

☐ **Did I work intensively + aggressively?**

☐ **Did I push myself to increase difficulty?**

RECOVERY PLAN: _____

Week No. _____   Day No.:_____

Exercises/Drills Done:

_____Time_____
_____Time_____
_____Time_____
_____Time_____
_____Time_____
_____Time_____
_____Time_____
_____Time_____
_____Time_____

Total Time Spent_____

NUTRITION PLAN:

Nutrient-rich foods eaten | quantity:

BREAKFAST:

_____ | _____
_____ | _____
_____ | _____
_____ | _____

Drinks:_____

LUNCH:

_____ | _____
_____ | _____
_____ | _____
_____ | _____
_____ | _____
_____ | _____

Drinks:_____

Snacks:_____

DINNER:

_____ | _____
_____ | _____
_____ | _____
_____ | _____
_____ | _____
_____ | _____

Drinks:_____

Snacks:_____

RECOVERY PLAN: _____

Week No. _____   Day No.:_____

Exercises/Drills Done:

_____Time_____
_____Time_____
_____Time_____
_____Time_____
_____Time_____
_____Time_____
_____Time_____
_____Time_____
_____Time_____

Total Time Spent_____

SUPPLEMENTS TAKEN:

_____ | _____
_____ | _____
_____ | _____
_____ | _____
_____ | _____

Supplements I Need to Buy:

_____ | _____
_____ | _____

MEDICINES TAKEN:

_____ | _____
_____ | _____
_____ | _____
_____ | _____
_____ | _____
_____ | _____

YOGA TRAINING:

Exercises:_____

_____

_____

_____

_____

Total Yoga Time: _____

Notes:_____

NOTES, SUCCESSES, BREAKTHROUGHS, PROGRESS!

_____

_____

_____

_____

_____

Daily Worksheet

Day of the Week:	Date:	Day No.	Max. Heart Rate:	A.M. Weight:	A.M. Blood Pressure: _____ OVER _____

Glasses of water drunk today (check): ○ ○ ○ ○ ○ ○ ○ ○

WALKING Plan No. _____

Week No.:_____ Day No.:_____

CORE WORK:
Total Time _____

RESISTANCE TRAINING:
1) Machine/Exerc._____
   Weight_____ Reps _____/_____/_____
2) Machine/Exerc._____
   Weight_____ Reps _____/_____/_____
3) Machine/Exerc._____
   Weight_____ Reps _____/_____/_____
4) Machine/Exerc._____
   Weight_____ Reps _____/_____/_____
5) Machine/Exerc._____
   Weight_____ Reps _____/_____/_____
6) Machine/Exerc._____
   Weight_____ Reps _____/_____/_____
7) Machine/Exerc._____
   Weight_____ Reps _____/_____/_____
8) Machine/Exerc._____
   Weight_____ Reps _____/_____/_____

Resistance Tr. Total Time_____

CARDIO WALKING:
Treadmill: Distance _____
   Time _____ Speed _____
   Time walked without support _____
Elliptical: Distance _____Time _____
   Reversed direction every _____ minutes
   Time walked without support _____
Stepper: Distance _____Time _____
   Time walked without support _____
Track: Distance _____Time _____
   Speed or pace (if recorded) _____
   Time walked without support _____
   Fastest lap _____
   Fastest lap without support_____
Total Cardio Walking Time:_____
Max. Heart Rate Noted:_____

RECOVERY BASICS:
☐ **Were physical exercise targets (time and total no. of reps) met?**
☐ **Did I focus well on exercises?**
☐ **Did I work intensively + aggressively?**
☐ **Did I push myself to increase difficulty?**

RECOVERY PLAN: _____

Week No. _____ Day No.:_____

Exercises/Drills Done:
_____Time_____
_____Time_____
_____Time_____
_____Time_____
_____Time_____
_____Time_____
_____Time_____
_____Time_____
_____Time_____
_____Time_____
_____Time_____

Total Time Spent_____

NUTRITION PLAN:
Nutrient-rich foods eaten | quantity:
BREAKFAST:
_____ | _____
_____ | _____
_____ | _____
_____ | _____
Drinks:_____
LUNCH:
_____ | _____
_____ | _____
_____ | _____
_____ | _____
_____ | _____
Drinks:_____
Snacks:_____
DINNER:
_____ | _____
_____ | _____
_____ | _____
_____ | _____
_____ | _____
_____ | _____
Drinks:_____
Snacks:_____

RECOVERY PLAN: _____

Week No. _____ Day No.:_____

Exercises/Drills Done:
_____Time_____
_____Time_____
_____Time_____
_____Time_____
_____Time_____
_____Time_____
_____Time_____
_____Time_____
_____Time_____
_____Time_____

Total Time Spent_____

SUPPLEMENTS TAKEN:
_____ | _____
_____ | _____
_____ | _____
_____ | _____
_____ | _____

Supplements I Need to Buy:
_____ | _____
_____ | _____

MEDICINES TAKEN:
_____ | _____
_____ | _____
_____ | _____
_____ | _____
_____ | _____
_____ | _____

YOGA TRAINING:
Exercises:_____
_____
_____
_____
_____
_____

Total Yoga Time: _____
Notes:_____

NOTES, SUCCESSES, BREAKTHROUGHS, PROGRESS!
_____
_____
_____
_____
_____

Start of Week Worksheet—Week No. 5

Date: Week Beginning Monday, _____, 20___

It is said that calm seas, which are easy to navigate, do not good sailors make. Rough seas, on the other hand, can make great sailors. Right now, your seas are rough and it may seem hard for you to move forward. But at the same time, you now have an opportunity to be great. We would like to help you do the right things to fulfill your potential. Let this book be your guide!

Roger Maxwell

Start of Week Statistics:

MEASUREMENTS—MEN:	MEASUREMENTS—WOMEN:	WEIGHT: _____
Waist:_____ Chest:_____	Waist:_____ Hips:_____	BLOOD PRESSURE:
Upper Leg: ____ Upper Arm:_____	Upper Leg: ____ Upper Arm:____	_____ over _____

Fill out the following information to guide you during the coming week.

Last week's successes and progress:_____
_____
_____

How well I am physically functioning right now: _____
_____
_____

Goals and expectations for this week:_____
_____
_____

Skills or exercises I want to especially focus on improving this week:_____
_____
_____

Shopping List: brain nutrient foods to add to diet this week:

_____   _____

_____   _____

If my weight or blood pressure are high, plan to reduce them (current/continuing):

_____

Daily Worksheet

Day of the Week:	Date:	Day No.	Max. Heart Rate:	A.M. Weight:	A.M. Blood Pressure: _____ OVER _____

Glasses of water drunk today (check): ○ ○ ○ ○ ○ ○ ○ ○

WALKING Plan No. _____

Week No.:_____   Day No.:_____

CORE WORK:
Total Time _____

RESISTANCE TRAINING:

1) Machine/Exerc._____

  Weight_____ Reps _____/_____/_____

2) Machine/Exerc._____

  Weight_____ Reps _____/_____/_____

3) Machine/Exerc._____

  Weight_____ Reps _____/_____/_____

4) Machine/Exerc._____

  Weight_____ Reps _____/_____/_____

5) Machine/Exerc._____

  Weight_____ Reps _____/_____/_____

6) Machine/Exerc._____

  Weight_____ Reps _____/_____/_____

7) Machine/Exerc._____

  Weight_____ Reps _____/_____/_____

8) Machine/Exerc._____

  Weight_____ Reps _____/_____/_____

Resistance Tr. Total Time_____

CARDIO WALKING:

Treadmill: Distance _____

  Time _____ Speed _____

  Time walked without support _____

Elliptical: Distance _____Time _____

  Reversed direction every _____ minutes

  Time walked without support _____

Stepper: Distance _____Time _____

  Time walked without support _____

Track: Distance _____Time _____

  Speed or pace (if recorded) _____

  Time walked without support _____

  Fastest lap _____

  Fastest lap without support_____

Total Cardio Walking Time:_____

Max. Heart Rate Noted:_____

RECOVERY PLAN: _____

Week No. _____   Day No.:_____

Exercises/Drills Done:

_____Time_____

_____Time_____

_____Time_____

_____Time_____

_____Time_____

_____Time_____

_____Time_____

_____Time_____

_____Time_____

Total Time Spent_____

NUTRITION PLAN:

Nutrient-rich foods eaten | quantity:

BREAKFAST:

_____|_____

_____|_____

_____|_____

_____|_____

Drinks:_____

LUNCH:

_____|_____

_____|_____

_____|_____

_____|_____

_____|_____

_____|_____

Drinks:_____

Snacks:_____

DINNER:

_____|_____

_____|_____

_____|_____

_____|_____

_____|_____

_____|_____

Drinks:_____

Snacks:_____

RECOVERY PLAN: _____

Week No. _____   Day No.:_____

Exercises/Drills Done:

_____Time_____

_____Time_____

_____Time_____

_____Time_____

_____Time_____

_____Time_____

_____Time_____

_____Time_____

_____Time_____

Total Time Spent_____

SUPPLEMENTS TAKEN:

_____|_____

_____|_____

_____|_____

_____|_____

_____|_____

Supplements I Need to Buy:

_____|_____

_____|_____

MEDICINES TAKEN:

_____|_____

_____|_____

_____|_____

_____|_____

_____|_____

YOGA TRAINING:

Exercises:_____

_____

_____

_____

_____

Total Yoga Time: _____

Notes:_____

RECOVERY BASICS:
☐ Were physical exercise targets (time and total no. of reps) met?
☐ Did I focus well on exercises?
☐ Did I work intensively + aggressively?
☐ Did I push myself to increase difficulty?

NOTES, SUCCESSES, BREAKTHROUGHS, PROGRESS!

_____

_____

_____

_____

_____

_____

Daily Worksheet

Day of the Week:	Date:	Day No.	Max. Heart Rate:	A.M. Weight:	A.M. Blood Pressure: _____ OVER _____

Glasses of water drunk today (check): ◯ ◯ ◯ ◯ ◯ ◯ ◯ ◯

WALKING Plan No. _____

Week No.:_____ Day No.:_____

CORE WORK:

Total Time _____

RESISTANCE TRAINING:

1) Machine/Exerc._____

   Weight_____ Reps ____/_____/_____

2) Machine/Exerc._____

   Weight_____ Reps ____/_____/_____

3) Machine/Exerc._____

   Weight_____ Reps ____/_____/_____

4) Machine/Exerc._____

   Weight_____ Reps ____/_____/_____

5) Machine/Exerc._____

   Weight_____ Reps ____/_____/_____

6) Machine/Exerc._____

   Weight_____ Reps ____/_____/_____

7) Machine/Exerc._____

   Weight_____ Reps ____/_____/_____

8) Machine/Exerc._____

   Weight_____ Reps ____/_____/_____

Resistance Tr. Total Time_____

CARDIO WALKING:

Treadmill: Distance _____

   Time _____ Speed _____

   Time walked without support _____

Elliptical: Distance _____Time _____

   Reversed direction every _____ minutes

   Time walked without support _____

Stepper: Distance _____Time _____

   Time walked without support _____

Track: Distance _____Time _____

   Speed or pace (if recorded) _____

   Time walked without support _____

   Fastest lap _____

   Fastest lap without support_____

Total Cardio Walking Time:_____

Max. Heart Rate Noted:_____

RECOVERY BASICS:

☐ **Were physical exercise targets (time and total no. of reps) met?**

☐ **Did I focus well on exercises?**

☐ **Did I work intensively + aggressively?**

☐ **Did I push myself to increase difficulty?**

RECOVERY PLAN: _____

Week No. _____ Day No.:_____

Exercises/Drills Done:

_____Time_____

_____Time_____

_____Time_____

_____Time_____

_____Time_____

_____Time_____

_____Time_____

_____Time_____

_____Time_____

Total Time Spent_____

NUTRITION PLAN:

Nutrient-rich foods eaten | quantity:

BREAKFAST:

_____ | _____

_____ | _____

_____ | _____

_____ | _____

Drinks:_____

LUNCH:

_____ | _____

_____ | _____

_____ | _____

_____ | _____

_____ | _____

Drinks:_____

Snacks:_____

DINNER:

_____ | _____

_____ | _____

_____ | _____

_____ | _____

_____ | _____

_____ | _____

Drinks:_____

Snacks:_____

NOTES, SUCCESSES, BREAKTHROUGHS, PROGRESS!

_____

_____

_____

_____

_____

RECOVERY PLAN: _____

Week No. _____ Day No.:_____

Exercises/Drills Done:

_____Time_____

_____Time_____

_____Time_____

_____Time_____

_____Time_____

_____Time_____

_____Time_____

_____Time_____

_____Time_____

Total Time Spent_____

SUPPLEMENTS TAKEN:

_____ | _____

_____ | _____

_____ | _____

_____ | _____

_____ | _____

Supplements I Need to Buy:

_____ | _____

_____ | _____

MEDICINES TAKEN:

_____ | _____

_____ | _____

_____ | _____

_____ | _____

_____ | _____

_____ | _____

YOGA TRAINING:

Exercises:_____

_____

_____

_____

_____

Total Yoga Time: _____

Notes:_____

Daily Worksheet

Day of the Week:	Date:	Day No.	Max. Heart Rate:	A.M. Weight:	A.M. Blood Pressure: _____ OVER _____

Glasses of water drunk today (check): ○ ○ ○ ○ ○ ○ ○ ○

WALKING Plan No. _____

Week No.:_____ Day No.:_____

CORE WORK:

Total Time _____

RESISTANCE TRAINING:

1) Machine/Exerc._____

   Weight_____ Reps _____/_____/_____

2) Machine/Exerc._____

   Weight_____ Reps _____/_____/_____

3) Machine/Exerc._____

   Weight_____ Reps _____/_____/_____

4) Machine/Exerc._____

   Weight_____ Reps _____/_____/_____

5) Machine/Exerc._____

   Weight_____ Reps _____/_____/_____

6) Machine/Exerc._____

   Weight_____ Reps _____/_____/_____

7) Machine/Exerc._____

   Weight_____ Reps _____/_____/_____

8) Machine/Exerc._____

   Weight_____ Reps _____/_____/_____

Resistance Tr. Total Time_____

CARDIO WALKING:

Treadmill: Distance _____

   Time _____ Speed _____

   Time walked without support _____

Elliptical: Distance _____Time _____

   Reversed direction every _____ minutes

   Time walked without support _____

Stepper: Distance _____Time _____

   Time walked without support _____

Track: Distance _____Time _____

   Speed or pace (if recorded) _____

   Time walked without support _____

   Fastest lap _____

   Fastest lap without support_____

Total Cardio Walking Time:_____

Max. Heart Rate Noted:_____

RECOVERY PLAN: _____

Week No. _____ Day No.:_____

Exercises/Drills Done:

_____Time_____
_____Time_____
_____Time_____
_____Time_____
_____Time_____
_____Time_____
_____Time_____
_____Time_____
_____Time_____

Total Time Spent_____

NUTRITION PLAN:

Nutrient-rich foods eaten | quantity:

BREAKFAST:

_____|_____
_____|_____
_____|_____
_____|_____
_____|_____

Drinks:_____

LUNCH:

_____|_____
_____|_____
_____|_____
_____|_____
_____|_____
_____|_____

Drinks:_____

Snacks:_____

DINNER:

_____|_____
_____|_____
_____|_____
_____|_____
_____|_____
_____|_____

Drinks:_____

Snacks:_____

RECOVERY PLAN: _____

Week No. _____ Day No.:_____

Exercises/Drills Done:

_____Time_____
_____Time_____
_____Time_____
_____Time_____
_____Time_____
_____Time_____
_____Time_____
_____Time_____
_____Time_____

Total Time Spent_____

SUPPLEMENTS TAKEN:

_____|_____
_____|_____
_____|_____
_____|_____
_____|_____

Supplements I Need to Buy:

_____|_____
_____|_____

MEDICINES TAKEN:

_____|_____
_____|_____
_____|_____
_____|_____
_____|_____

YOGA TRAINING:

Exercises:_____
_____
_____
_____
_____

Total Yoga Time: _____

Notes:_____

RECOVERY BASICS:

☐ **Were physical exercise targets (time and total no. of reps) met?**

☐ **Did I focus well on exercises?**

☐ **Did I work intensively + aggressively?**

☐ **Did I push myself to increase difficulty?**

NOTES, SUCCESSES, BREAKTHROUGHS, PROGRESS!

_____
_____
_____
_____
_____

Daily Worksheet

Day of the Week:	Date:	Day No.	Max. Heart Rate:	A.M. Weight:	A.M. Blood Pressure: _____ OVER _____

Glasses of water drunk today (check): ○ ○ ○ ○ ○ ○ ○ ○

WALKING Plan No. _____

Week No.:_____ Day No.:_____

CORE WORK:

Total Time _____

RESISTANCE TRAINING:

1) Machine/Exerc._____

   Weight_____ Reps _____/_____/_____

2) Machine/Exerc._____

   Weight_____ Reps _____/_____/_____

3) Machine/Exerc._____

   Weight_____ Reps _____/_____/_____

4) Machine/Exerc._____

   Weight_____ Reps _____/_____/_____

5) Machine/Exerc._____

   Weight_____ Reps _____/_____/_____

6) Machine/Exerc._____

   Weight_____ Reps _____/_____/_____

7) Machine/Exerc._____

   Weight_____ Reps _____/_____/_____

8) Machine/Exerc._____

   Weight_____ Reps _____/_____/_____

Resistance Tr. Total Time_____

CARDIO WALKING:

Treadmill: Distance _____

   Time _____ Speed _____

   Time walked without support _____

Elliptical: Distance _____Time _____

   Reversed direction every _____ minutes

   Time walked without support _____

Stepper: Distance _____Time _____

   Time walked without support _____

Track: Distance _____Time _____

   Speed or pace (if recorded) _____

   Time walked without support _____

   Fastest lap _____

   Fastest lap without support_____

Total Cardio Walking Time:_____

Max. Heart Rate Noted:_____

RECOVERY PLAN: _____

Week No. _____ Day No.:_____

Exercises/Drills Done:

_____Time_____

_____Time_____

_____Time_____

_____Time_____

_____Time_____

_____Time_____

_____Time_____

_____Time_____

_____Time_____

Total Time Spent_____

NUTRITION PLAN:

Nutrient-rich foods eaten | quantity:

BREAKFAST:

_____ | _____

_____ | _____

_____ | _____

_____ | _____

Drinks:_____

LUNCH:

_____ | _____

_____ | _____

_____ | _____

_____ | _____

_____ | _____

Drinks:_____

Snacks:_____

DINNER:

_____ | _____

_____ | _____

_____ | _____

_____ | _____

_____ | _____

_____ | _____

Drinks:_____

Snacks:_____

RECOVERY PLAN: _____

Week No. _____ Day No.:_____

Exercises/Drills Done:

_____Time_____

_____Time_____

_____Time_____

_____Time_____

_____Time_____

_____Time_____

_____Time_____

_____Time_____

_____Time_____

Total Time Spent_____

SUPPLEMENTS TAKEN:

_____ | _____

_____ | _____

_____ | _____

_____ | _____

_____ | _____

Supplements I Need to Buy:

_____ | _____

_____ | _____

MEDICINES TAKEN:

_____ | _____

_____ | _____

_____ | _____

_____ | _____

_____ | _____

_____ | _____

_____ | _____

YOGA TRAINING:

Exercises:_____

_____

_____

_____

_____

Total Yoga Time: _____

Notes:_____

RECOVERY BASICS:

☐ **Were physical exercise targets (time and total no. of reps) met?**

☐ **Did I focus well on exercises?**

☐ **Did I work intensively + aggressively?**

☐ **Did I push myself to increase difficulty?**

NOTES, SUCCESSES, BREAKTHROUGHS, PROGRESS!

_____

_____

_____

_____

_____

_____

Daily Worksheet

Day of the Week:	Date:	Day No.	Max. Heart Rate:	A.M. Weight:	A.M. Blood Pressure: _____ OVER _____

Glasses of water drunk today (check): ◯ ◯ ◯ ◯ ◯ ◯ ◯ ◯

WALKING Plan No. _____

Week No.: _____ **Day No.:** _____

CORE WORK:
Total Time _____

RESISTANCE TRAINING:

1) Machine/Exerc. _____
   Weight _____ Reps _____/_____/_____

2) Machine/Exerc. _____
   Weight _____ Reps _____/_____/_____

3) Machine/Exerc. _____
   Weight _____ Reps _____/_____/_____

4) Machine/Exerc. _____
   Weight _____ Reps _____/_____/_____

5) Machine/Exerc. _____
   Weight _____ Reps _____/_____/_____

6) Machine/Exerc. _____
   Weight _____ Reps _____/_____/_____

7) Machine/Exerc. _____
   Weight _____ Reps _____/_____/_____

8) Machine/Exerc. _____
   Weight _____ Reps _____/_____/_____

Resistance Tr. Total Time _____

CARDIO WALKING:

Treadmill: Distance _____
   Time _____ Speed _____
   Time walked without support _____

Elliptical: Distance _____ Time _____
   Reversed direction every _____ minutes
   Time walked without support _____

Stepper: Distance _____ Time _____
   Time walked without support _____

Track: Distance _____ Time _____
   Speed or pace (if recorded) _____
   Time walked without support _____
   Fastest lap _____
   Fastest lap without support _____

Total Cardio Walking Time: _____

Max. Heart Rate Noted: _____

RECOVERY PLAN: _____

Week No. _____ **Day No.:** _____

Exercises/Drills Done:
_____Time_____
_____Time_____
_____Time_____
_____Time_____
_____Time_____
_____Time_____
_____Time_____
_____Time_____
_____Time_____

Total Time Spent _____

NUTRITION PLAN:

Nutrient-rich foods eaten | quantity:

BREAKFAST:
_____ | _____
_____ | _____
_____ | _____
_____ | _____

Drinks: _____

LUNCH:
_____ | _____
_____ | _____
_____ | _____
_____ | _____
_____ | _____
_____ | _____

Drinks: _____
Snacks: _____

DINNER:
_____ | _____
_____ | _____
_____ | _____
_____ | _____
_____ | _____
_____ | _____

Drinks: _____
Snacks: _____

RECOVERY PLAN: _____

Week No. _____ **Day No.:** _____

Exercises/Drills Done:
_____Time_____
_____Time_____
_____Time_____
_____Time_____
_____Time_____
_____Time_____
_____Time_____
_____Time_____
_____Time_____

Total Time Spent _____

SUPPLEMENTS TAKEN:
_____ | _____
_____ | _____
_____ | _____
_____ | _____
_____ | _____
_____ | _____

Supplements I Need to Buy:
_____ | _____
_____ | _____

MEDICINES TAKEN:
_____ | _____
_____ | _____
_____ | _____
_____ | _____
_____ | _____
_____ | _____

YOGA TRAINING:
Exercises: _____
_____
_____
_____
_____
_____

Total Yoga Time: _____
Notes: _____

RECOVERY BASICS:
☐ Were physical exercise targets (time and total no. of reps) met?
☐ Did I focus well on exercises?
☐ Did I work intensively + aggressively?
☐ Did I push myself to increase difficulty?

NOTES, SUCCESSES, BREAKTHROUGHS, PROGRESS!
_____
_____
_____
_____
_____
_____

Daily Worksheet

Day of the Week:	Date:	Day No.	Max. Heart Rate:	A.M. Weight:	A.M. Blood Pressure: _____ OVER _____

Glasses of water drunk today (check): ○ ○ ○ ○ ○ ○ ○ ○

WALKING Plan No. _____
Week No.: _____ **Day No.:** _____

CORE WORK:
Total Time _____

RESISTANCE TRAINING:
1) Machine/Exerc. _____
　Weight _____ Reps _____/_____/_____
2) Machine/Exerc. _____
　Weight _____ Reps _____/_____/_____
3) Machine/Exerc. _____
　Weight _____ Reps _____/_____/_____
4) Machine/Exerc. _____
　Weight _____ Reps _____/_____/_____
5) Machine/Exerc. _____
　Weight _____ Reps _____/_____/_____
6) Machine/Exerc. _____
　Weight _____ Reps _____/_____/_____
7) Machine/Exerc. _____
　Weight _____ Reps _____/_____/_____
8) Machine/Exerc. _____
　Weight _____ Reps _____/_____/_____
Resistance Tr. Total Time _____

CARDIO WALKING:
Treadmill: Distance _____
　Time _____ Speed _____
　Time walked without support _____
Elliptical: Distance _____ Time _____
　Reversed direction every _____ minutes
　Time walked without support _____
Stepper: Distance _____ Time _____
　Time walked without support _____
Track: Distance _____ Time _____
　Speed or pace (if recorded) _____
　Time walked without support _____
　Fastest lap _____
　Fastest lap without support _____
Total Cardio Walking Time: _____
Max. Heart Rate Noted: _____

RECOVERY PLAN: _____
Week No. _____ **Day No.:** _____

Exercises/Drills Done:
_____Time_____
_____Time_____
_____Time_____
_____Time_____
_____Time_____
_____Time_____
_____Time_____
_____Time_____
_____Time_____
_____Time_____
Total Time Spent _____

NUTRITION PLAN:
Nutrient-rich foods eaten | quantity:
BREAKFAST:
_____|_____
_____|_____
_____|_____
_____|_____
Drinks: _____
LUNCH:
_____|_____
_____|_____
_____|_____
_____|_____
_____|_____
Drinks: _____
Snacks: _____
DINNER:
_____|_____
_____|_____
_____|_____
_____|_____
_____|_____
Drinks: _____
Snacks: _____

RECOVERY PLAN: _____
Week No. _____ **Day No.:** _____

Exercises/Drills Done:
_____Time_____
_____Time_____
_____Time_____
_____Time_____
_____Time_____
_____Time_____
_____Time_____
_____Time_____
_____Time_____
Total Time Spent _____

SUPPLEMENTS TAKEN:
_____|_____
_____|_____
_____|_____
_____|_____
_____|_____
Supplements I Need to Buy:
_____|_____
_____|_____

MEDICINES TAKEN:
_____|_____
_____|_____
_____|_____
_____|_____
_____|_____

YOGA TRAINING:
Exercises: _____
_____
_____
_____
_____
Total Yoga Time: _____
Notes: _____

RECOVERY BASICS:
☐ **Were physical exercise targets (time and total no. of reps) met?**
☐ **Did I focus well on exercises?**
☐ **Did I work intensively + aggressively?**
☐ **Did I push myself to increase difficulty?**

NOTES, SUCCESSES, BREAKTHROUGHS, PROGRESS!
_____
_____
_____
_____
_____
_____

Daily Worksheet

Day of the Week:	Date:	Day No.	Max. Heart Rate:	A.M. Weight:	A.M. Blood Pressure: _____ OVER _____

Glasses of water drunk today (check): ○ ○ ○ ○ ○ ○ ○ ○

WALKING Plan No. _____

Week No.:_____ Day No.:_____

CORE WORK:

Total Time _____

RESISTANCE TRAINING:

1) Machine/Exerc._____

Weight_____ Reps _____/_____/_____

2) Machine/Exerc._____

Weight_____ Reps _____/_____/_____

3) Machine/Exerc._____

Weight_____ Reps _____/_____/_____

4) Machine/Exerc._____

Weight_____ Reps _____/_____/_____

5) Machine/Exerc._____

Weight_____ Reps _____/_____/_____

6) Machine/Exerc._____

Weight_____ Reps _____/_____/_____

7) Machine/Exerc._____

Weight_____ Reps _____/_____/_____

8) Machine/Exerc._____

Weight_____ Reps _____/_____/_____

Resistance Tr. Total Time_____

CARDIO WALKING:

Treadmill: Distance _____

Time _____ Speed _____

Time walked without support _____

Elliptical: Distance _____Time _____

Reversed direction every _____ minutes

Time walked without support _____

Stepper: Distance _____Time _____

Time walked without support _____

Track: Distance _____Time _____

Speed or pace (if recorded) _____

Time walked without support _____

Fastest lap _____

Fastest lap without support_____

Total Cardio Walking Time:_____

Max. Heart Rate Noted:_____

RECOVERY PLAN: _____

Week No. _____ Day No.:_____

Exercises/Drills Done:

_____Time_____

_____Time_____

_____Time_____

_____Time_____

_____Time_____

_____Time_____

_____Time_____

_____Time_____

_____Time_____

Total Time Spent_____

NUTRITION PLAN:

Nutrient-rich foods eaten | quantity:

BREAKFAST:

_____ | _____

_____ | _____

_____ | _____

_____ | _____

Drinks:_____

LUNCH:

_____ | _____

_____ | _____

_____ | _____

_____ | _____

_____ | _____

Drinks:_____

Snacks:_____

DINNER:

_____ | _____

_____ | _____

_____ | _____

_____ | _____

_____ | _____

_____ | _____

Drinks:_____

Snacks:_____

RECOVERY PLAN: _____

Week No. _____ Day No.:_____

Exercises/Drills Done:

_____Time_____

_____Time_____

_____Time_____

_____Time_____

_____Time_____

_____Time_____

_____Time_____

_____Time_____

_____Time_____

Total Time Spent_____

SUPPLEMENTS TAKEN:

_____ | _____

_____ | _____

_____ | _____

_____ | _____

_____ | _____

Supplements I Need to Buy:

_____ | _____

_____ | _____

MEDICINES TAKEN:

_____ | _____

_____ | _____

_____ | _____

_____ | _____

_____ | _____

_____ | _____

YOGA TRAINING:

Exercises:_____

_____

_____

_____

_____

Total Yoga Time: _____

Notes:_____

RECOVERY BASICS:

☐ **Were physical exercise targets (time and total no. of reps) met?**

☐ **Did I focus well on exercises?**

☐ **Did I work intensively + aggressively?**

☐ **Did I push myself to increase difficulty?**

NOTES, SUCCESSES, BREAKTHROUGHS, PROGRESS!

_____

_____

_____

_____

_____

Start of Week Worksheet—Week No. 6

Date: Week Beginning Monday, _____, 20___

> ...There were times during some of my practice sessions when nothing was going well and it didn't seem like I would be able to accomplish my daily training objective within a reasonable amount of time. What I did in situations like this was discipline myself to simply finish the number of repetitions I had committed myself to.... I basically pushed myself through my workout. You might think that nothing would be gained by doing this—yet my training the following day was almost always better. It was as if my body had learned or improved from my pushing through the workout, even though I did not subjectively feel like I had done anything worthwhile that day.
>
> Kirk Mango from *Becoming a True Champion*

Start of Week Statistics:

MEASUREMENTS—MEN:	MEASUREMENTS—WOMEN:	WEIGHT: _____
Waist:_____ Chest:_____	Waist:_____ Hips:_____	BLOOD PRESSURE:
Upper Leg: ____ Upper Arm:_____	Upper Leg: ____ Upper Arm:____	_____ over _____

Fill out the following information to guide you during the coming week.

Last week's successes and progress:_____

_____

_____

How well I am physically functioning right now: _____

_____

_____

Goals and expectations for this week:_____

_____

_____

Skills or exercises I want to especially focus on improving this week:_____

_____

_____

Shopping List: brain nutrient foods to add to diet this week:

_____   _____

_____   _____

If my weight or blood pressure are high, plan to reduce them (current/continuing):

_____

223

Daily Worksheet

Day of the Week:	Date:	Day No.	Max. Heart Rate:	A.M. Weight:	A.M. Blood Pressure: _____ OVER _____

Glasses of water drunk today (check): ○ ○ ○ ○ ○ ○ ○ ○

WALKING Plan No. _____

Week No.: _____ **Day No.:** _____

CORE WORK:

Total Time _____

RESISTANCE TRAINING:

1) Machine/Exerc. _____

Weight _____ Reps _____/_____/_____

2) Machine/Exerc. _____

Weight _____ Reps _____/_____/_____

3) Machine/Exerc. _____

Weight _____ Reps _____/_____/_____

4) Machine/Exerc. _____

Weight _____ Reps _____/_____/_____

5) Machine/Exerc. _____

Weight _____ Reps _____/_____/_____

6) Machine/Exerc. _____

Weight _____ Reps _____/_____/_____

7) Machine/Exerc. _____

Weight _____ Reps _____/_____/_____

8) Machine/Exerc. _____

Weight _____ Reps _____/_____/_____

Resistance Tr. Total Time _____

CARDIO WALKING:

Treadmill: Distance _____

Time _____ Speed _____

Time walked without support _____

Elliptical: Distance _____ Time _____

Reversed direction every _____ minutes

Time walked without support _____

Stepper: Distance _____ Time _____

Time walked without support _____

Track: Distance _____ Time _____

Speed or pace (if recorded) _____

Time walked without support _____

Fastest lap _____

Fastest lap without support _____

Total Cardio Walking Time: _____

Max. Heart Rate Noted: _____

RECOVERY PLAN: _____

Week No. _____ **Day No.:** _____

Exercises/Drills Done:

_____ Time _____

_____ Time _____

_____ Time _____

_____ Time _____

_____ Time _____

_____ Time _____

_____ Time _____

_____ Time _____

_____ Time _____

_____ Time _____

Total Time Spent _____

NUTRITION PLAN:

Nutrient-rich foods eaten | quantity:

BREAKFAST:

_____ | _____

_____ | _____

_____ | _____

_____ | _____

Drinks: _____

LUNCH:

_____ | _____

_____ | _____

_____ | _____

_____ | _____

_____ | _____

Drinks: _____

Snacks: _____

DINNER:

_____ | _____

_____ | _____

_____ | _____

_____ | _____

_____ | _____

_____ | _____

Drinks: _____

Snacks: _____

RECOVERY PLAN: _____

Week No. _____ **Day No.:** _____

Exercises/Drills Done:

_____ Time _____

_____ Time _____

_____ Time _____

_____ Time _____

_____ Time _____

_____ Time _____

_____ Time _____

_____ Time _____

_____ Time _____

_____ Time _____

Total Time Spent _____

SUPPLEMENTS TAKEN:

_____ | _____

_____ | _____

_____ | _____

_____ | _____

_____ | _____

Supplements I Need to Buy:

_____ | _____

_____ | _____

MEDICINES TAKEN:

_____ | _____

_____ | _____

_____ | _____

_____ | _____

_____ | _____

_____ | _____

YOGA TRAINING:

Exercises: _____

_____

_____

_____

_____

_____

Total Yoga Time: _____

Notes: _____

RECOVERY BASICS:

☐ Were physical exercise targets (time and total no. of reps) met?

☐ Did I focus well on exercises?

☐ Did I work intensively + aggressively?

☐ Did I push myself to increase difficulty?

NOTES, SUCCESSES, BREAKTHROUGHS, PROGRESS!

_____

_____

_____

_____

_____

Daily Worksheet

Day of the Week:	Date:	Day No.	Max. Heart Rate:	A.M. Weight:	A.M. Blood Pressure: _____ OVER _____

Glasses of water drunk today (check): ○ ○ ○ ○ ○ ○ ○ ○

WALKING Plan No. _____

Week No.:_____ Day No.:_____

CORE WORK:

Total Time _____

RESISTANCE TRAINING:

1) Machine/Exerc._____

   Weight_____ Reps _____/_____/_____

2) Machine/Exerc._____

   Weight_____ Reps _____/_____/_____

3) Machine/Exerc._____

   Weight_____ Reps _____/_____/_____

4) Machine/Exerc._____

   Weight_____ Reps _____/_____/_____

5) Machine/Exerc._____

   Weight_____ Reps _____/_____/_____

6) Machine/Exerc._____

   Weight_____ Reps _____/_____/_____

7) Machine/Exerc._____

   Weight_____ Reps _____/_____/_____

8) Machine/Exerc._____

   Weight_____ Reps _____/_____/_____

Resistance Tr. Total Time_____

CARDIO WALKING:

Treadmill: Distance _____

   Time _____ Speed _____

   Time walked without support _____

Elliptical: Distance _____Time _____

   Reversed direction every _____ minutes

   Time walked without support _____

Stepper: Distance _____Time _____

   Time walked without support _____

Track: Distance _____Time _____

   Speed or pace (if recorded) _____

   Time walked without support _____

   Fastest lap _____

   Fastest lap without support_____

Total Cardio Walking Time:_____

Max. Heart Rate Noted:_____

RECOVERY PLAN: _____

Week No. _____ Day No.:_____

Exercises/Drills Done:

_____Time_____

_____Time_____

_____Time_____

_____Time_____

_____Time_____

_____Time_____

_____Time_____

_____Time_____

_____Time_____

_____Time_____

Total Time Spent_____

NUTRITION PLAN:

Nutrient-rich foods eaten | quantity:

BREAKFAST:

_____ | _____

_____ | _____

_____ | _____

_____ | _____

Drinks:_____

LUNCH:

_____ | _____

_____ | _____

_____ | _____

_____ | _____

_____ | _____

Drinks:_____

Snacks:_____

DINNER:

_____ | _____

_____ | _____

_____ | _____

_____ | _____

_____ | _____

_____ | _____

Drinks:_____

Snacks:_____

RECOVERY PLAN: _____

Week No. _____ Day No.:_____

Exercises/Drills Done:

_____Time_____

_____Time_____

_____Time_____

_____Time_____

_____Time_____

_____Time_____

_____Time_____

_____Time_____

_____Time_____

_____Time_____

Total Time Spent_____

SUPPLEMENTS TAKEN:

_____ | _____

_____ | _____

_____ | _____

_____ | _____

_____ | _____

_____ | _____

Supplements I Need to Buy:

_____ | _____

_____ | _____

MEDICINES TAKEN:

_____ | _____

_____ | _____

_____ | _____

_____ | _____

_____ | _____

_____ | _____

YOGA TRAINING:

Exercises:_____

_____

_____

_____

Total Yoga Time: _____

Notes:_____

RECOVERY BASICS:

☐ **Were physical exercise targets (time and total no. of reps) met?**

☐ **Did I focus well on exercises?**

☐ **Did I work intensively + aggressively?**

☐ **Did I push myself to increase difficulty?**

NOTES, SUCCESSES, BREAKTHROUGHS, PROGRESS!

_____

_____

_____

_____

_____

Daily Worksheet

Day of the Week:	Date:	Day No.	Max. Heart Rate:	A.M. Weight:	A.M. Blood Pressure: _____ OVER _____

Glasses of water drunk today (check): ○ ○ ○ ○ ○ ○ ○ ○

WALKING Plan No. _____
Week No.:_____ Day No.:_____

CORE WORK:
Total Time _____

RESISTANCE TRAINING:

1) Machine/Exerc._____
Weight_____ Reps _____/_____/_____

2) Machine/Exerc._____
Weight_____ Reps _____/_____/_____

3) Machine/Exerc._____
Weight_____ Reps _____/_____/_____

4) Machine/Exerc._____
Weight_____ Reps _____/_____/_____

5) Machine/Exerc._____
Weight_____ Reps _____/_____/_____

6) Machine/Exerc._____
Weight_____ Reps _____/_____/_____

7) Machine/Exerc._____
Weight_____ Reps _____/_____/_____

8) Machine/Exerc._____
Weight_____ Reps _____/_____/_____

Resistance Tr. Total Time_____

CARDIO WALKING:

Treadmill: Distance _____
Time _____ Speed _____
Time walked without support _____

Elliptical: Distance _____Time _____
Reversed direction every _____ minutes
Time walked without support _____

Stepper: Distance _____Time _____
Time walked without support _____

Track: Distance _____Time _____
Speed or pace (if recorded) _____
Time walked without support _____
Fastest lap _____
Fastest lap without support_____

Total Cardio Walking Time:_____
Max. Heart Rate Noted:_____

RECOVERY PLAN: _____
Week No. _____ Day No.:_____

Exercises/Drills Done:
_____Time_____
_____Time_____
_____Time_____
_____Time_____
_____Time_____
_____Time_____
_____Time_____
_____Time_____
_____Time_____
_____Time_____

Total Time Spent_____

NUTRITION PLAN:

Nutrient-rich foods eaten | quantity:
BREAKFAST:
_____ | _____
_____ | _____
_____ | _____
_____ | _____
Drinks:_____

LUNCH:
_____ | _____
_____ | _____
_____ | _____
_____ | _____
_____ | _____
Drinks:_____
Snacks:_____

DINNER:
_____ | _____
_____ | _____
_____ | _____
_____ | _____
_____ | _____
_____ | _____
Drinks:_____
Snacks:_____

RECOVERY PLAN: _____
Week No. _____ Day No.:_____

Exercises/Drills Done:
_____Time_____
_____Time_____
_____Time_____
_____Time_____
_____Time_____
_____Time_____
_____Time_____
_____Time_____
_____Time_____

Total Time Spent_____

SUPPLEMENTS TAKEN:
_____ | _____
_____ | _____
_____ | _____
_____ | _____
_____ | _____

Supplements I Need to Buy:
_____ | _____
_____ | _____

MEDICINES TAKEN:
_____ | _____
_____ | _____
_____ | _____
_____ | _____
_____ | _____
_____ | _____

YOGA TRAINING:
Exercises:_____
_____
_____
_____
_____

Total Yoga Time: _____
Notes:_____

RECOVERY BASICS:
☐ **Were physical exercise targets (time and total no. of reps) met?**
☐ **Did I focus well on exercises?**
☐ **Did I work intensively + aggressively?**
☐ **Did I push myself to increase difficulty?**

NOTES, SUCCESSES, BREAKTHROUGHS, PROGRESS!
_____
_____
_____
_____

Daily Worksheet

Day of the Week:	Date:	Day No.	Max. Heart Rate:	A.M. Weight:	A.M. Blood Pressure: _____ OVER _____

Glasses of water drunk today (check): ○ ○ ○ ○ ○ ○ ○ ○

WALKING Plan No. _____

Week No.:_____ Day No.:_____

CORE WORK:

Total Time _____

RESISTANCE TRAINING:

1) Machine/Exerc._____

  Weight_____ Reps _____/_____/_____

2) Machine/Exerc._____

  Weight_____ Reps _____/_____/_____

3) Machine/Exerc._____

  Weight_____ Reps _____/_____/_____

4) Machine/Exerc._____

  Weight_____ Reps _____/_____/_____

5) Machine/Exerc._____

  Weight_____ Reps _____/_____/_____

6) Machine/Exerc._____

  Weight_____ Reps _____/_____/_____

7) Machine/Exerc._____

  Weight_____ Reps _____/_____/_____

8) Machine/Exerc._____

  Weight_____ Reps _____/_____/_____

Resistance Tr. Total Time_____

CARDIO WALKING:

Treadmill: Distance _____

  Time _____ Speed _____

  Time walked without support _____

Elliptical: Distance _____Time _____

  Reversed direction every _____ minutes

  Time walked without support _____

Stepper: Distance _____Time _____

  Time walked without support _____

Track: Distance _____Time _____

  Speed or pace (if recorded) _____

  Time walked without support _____

  Fastest lap _____

  Fastest lap without support_____

Total Cardio Walking Time:_____

Max. Heart Rate Noted:_____

RECOVERY BASICS:

☐ **Were physical exercise targets (time and total no. of reps) met?**

☐ **Did I focus well on exercises?**

☐ **Did I work intensively + aggressively?**

☐ **Did I push myself to increase difficulty?**

RECOVERY PLAN: _____

Week No. _____ Day No.:_____

Exercises/Drills Done:

_____Time_____

_____Time_____

_____Time_____

_____Time_____

_____Time_____

_____Time_____

_____Time_____

_____Time_____

Total Time Spent_____

NUTRITION PLAN:

Nutrient-rich foods eaten | quantity:

BREAKFAST:

_____ | _____

_____ | _____

_____ | _____

_____ | _____

Drinks:_____

LUNCH:

_____ | _____

_____ | _____

_____ | _____

_____ | _____

_____ | _____

Drinks:_____

Snacks:_____

DINNER:

_____ | _____

_____ | _____

_____ | _____

_____ | _____

_____ | _____

_____ | _____

Drinks:_____

Snacks:_____

RECOVERY PLAN: _____

Week No. _____ Day No.:_____

Exercises/Drills Done:

_____Time_____

_____Time_____

_____Time_____

_____Time_____

_____Time_____

_____Time_____

_____Time_____

_____Time_____

Total Time Spent_____

SUPPLEMENTS TAKEN:

_____ | _____

_____ | _____

_____ | _____

_____ | _____

_____ | _____

Supplements I Need to Buy:

_____ | _____

_____ | _____

MEDICINES TAKEN:

_____ | _____

_____ | _____

_____ | _____

_____ | _____

_____ | _____

_____ | _____

YOGA TRAINING:

Exercises:_____

_____

_____

_____

_____

Total Yoga Time: _____

Notes:_____

NOTES, SUCCESSES, BREAKTHROUGHS, PROGRESS!

_____

_____

_____

_____

_____

Daily Worksheet

Day of the Week:	Date:	Day No.	Max. Heart Rate:	A.M. Weight:	A.M. Blood Pressure: _____ OVER _____

Glasses of water drunk today (check): ○ ○ ○ ○ ○ ○ ○ ○

WALKING Plan No. _____

Week No.:_____ Day No.:_____

CORE WORK:
Total Time _____

RESISTANCE TRAINING:

1) Machine/Exerc._____
   Weight_____ Reps _____/_____/_____

2) Machine/Exerc._____
   Weight_____ Reps _____/_____/_____

3) Machine/Exerc._____
   Weight_____ Reps _____/_____/_____

4) Machine/Exerc._____
   Weight_____ Reps _____/_____/_____

5) Machine/Exerc._____
   Weight_____ Reps _____/_____/_____

6) Machine/Exerc._____
   Weight_____ Reps _____/_____/_____

7) Machine/Exerc._____
   Weight_____ Reps _____/_____/_____

8) Machine/Exerc._____
   Weight_____ Reps _____/_____/_____

Resistance Tr. Total Time_____

CARDIO WALKING:

Treadmill: Distance _____
   Time _____ Speed _____
   Time walked without support _____

Elliptical: Distance _____Time _____
   Reversed direction every _____ minutes
   Time walked without support _____

Stepper: Distance _____Time _____
   Time walked without support _____

Track: Distance _____Time _____
   Speed or pace (if recorded) _____
   Time walked without support _____
   Fastest lap _____
   Fastest lap without support_____

Total Cardio Walking Time:_____

Max. Heart Rate Noted:_____

RECOVERY BASICS:
☐ Were physical exercise targets (time and total no. of reps) met?
☐ Did I focus well on exercises?
☐ Did I work intensively + aggressively?
☐ Did I push myself to increase difficulty?

RECOVERY PLAN: _____

Week No. _____ Day No.:_____

Exercises/Drills Done:
_____Time_____
_____Time_____
_____Time_____
_____Time_____
_____Time_____
_____Time_____
_____Time_____
_____Time_____
_____Time_____
_____Time_____

Total Time Spent_____

NUTRITION PLAN:

Nutrient-rich foods eaten | quantity:

BREAKFAST:
_____|_____
_____|_____
_____|_____
_____|_____

Drinks:_____

LUNCH:
_____|_____
_____|_____
_____|_____
_____|_____
_____|_____
_____|_____

Drinks:_____
Snacks:_____

DINNER:
_____|_____
_____|_____
_____|_____
_____|_____
_____|_____
_____|_____
_____|_____

Drinks:_____
Snacks:_____

RECOVERY PLAN: _____

Week No. _____ Day No.:_____

Exercises/Drills Done:
_____Time_____
_____Time_____
_____Time_____
_____Time_____
_____Time_____
_____Time_____
_____Time_____
_____Time_____
_____Time_____

Total Time Spent_____

SUPPLEMENTS TAKEN:
_____|_____
_____|_____
_____|_____
_____|_____
_____|_____

Supplements I Need to Buy:
_____|_____
_____|_____

MEDICINES TAKEN:
_____|_____
_____|_____
_____|_____
_____|_____
_____|_____
_____|_____

YOGA TRAINING:
Exercises:_____
_____
_____
_____
_____

Total Yoga Time: _____
Notes:_____

NOTES, SUCCESSES, BREAKTHROUGHS, PROGRESS!
_____
_____
_____
_____
_____

Daily Worksheet

Day of the Week:	Date:	Day No.	Max. Heart Rate:	A.M. Weight:	A.M. Blood Pressure: _____ OVER _____

Glasses of water drunk today (check): ○ ○ ○ ○ ○ ○ ○ ○

WALKING Plan No. _____

Week No.:_____ Day No.:_____

CORE WORK:

Total Time _____

RESISTANCE TRAINING:

1) Machine/Exerc. _____
   Weight_____ Reps _____/_____/_____

2) Machine/Exerc. _____
   Weight_____ Reps _____/_____/_____

3) Machine/Exerc. _____
   Weight_____ Reps _____/_____/_____

4) Machine/Exerc. _____
   Weight_____ Reps _____/_____/_____

5) Machine/Exerc. _____
   Weight_____ Reps _____/_____/_____

6) Machine/Exerc. _____
   Weight_____ Reps _____/_____/_____

7) Machine/Exerc. _____
   Weight_____ Reps _____/_____/_____

8) Machine/Exerc. _____
   Weight_____ Reps _____/_____/_____

Resistance Tr. Total Time _____

CARDIO WALKING:

Treadmill: Distance _____
   Time _____ Speed _____
   Time walked without support _____

Elliptical: Distance _____ Time _____
   Reversed direction every _____ minutes
   Time walked without support _____

Stepper: Distance _____ Time _____
   Time walked without support _____

Track: Distance _____ Time _____
   Speed or pace (if recorded) _____
   Time walked without support _____
   Fastest lap _____
   Fastest lap without support_____

Total Cardio Walking Time: _____
Max. Heart Rate Noted: _____

RECOVERY BASICS:

☐ **Were physical exercise targets (time and total no. of reps) met?**
☐ **Did I focus well on exercises?**
☐ **Did I work intensively + aggressively?**
☐ **Did I push myself to increase difficulty?**

RECOVERY PLAN: _____

Week No. _____ Day No.:_____

Exercises/Drills Done:

_____Time_____
_____Time_____
_____Time_____
_____Time_____
_____Time_____
_____Time_____
_____Time_____
_____Time_____
_____Time_____

Total Time Spent _____

NUTRITION PLAN:

Nutrient-rich foods eaten | quantity:

BREAKFAST:
_____ | _____
_____ | _____
_____ | _____
_____ | _____

Drinks: _____

LUNCH:
_____ | _____
_____ | _____
_____ | _____
_____ | _____
_____ | _____
_____ | _____

Drinks: _____
Snacks: _____

DINNER:
_____ | _____
_____ | _____
_____ | _____
_____ | _____
_____ | _____
_____ | _____

Drinks: _____
Snacks: _____

NOTES, SUCCESSES, BREAKTHROUGHS, PROGRESS!

_____
_____
_____
_____
_____
_____

RECOVERY PLAN: _____

Week No. _____ Day No.:_____

Exercises/Drills Done:

_____Time_____
_____Time_____
_____Time_____
_____Time_____
_____Time_____
_____Time_____
_____Time_____
_____Time_____
_____Time_____

Total Time Spent _____

SUPPLEMENTS TAKEN:

_____ | _____
_____ | _____
_____ | _____
_____ | _____
_____ | _____
_____ | _____

Supplements I Need to Buy:
_____ | _____
_____ | _____

MEDICINES TAKEN:

_____ | _____
_____ | _____
_____ | _____
_____ | _____
_____ | _____
_____ | _____

YOGA TRAINING:

Exercises: _____
_____
_____
_____
_____
_____

Total Yoga Time: _____
Notes: _____

Daily Worksheet

Day of the Week:	Date:	Day No.	Max. Heart Rate:	A.M. Weight:	A.M. Blood Pressure: _____ OVER _____

Glasses of water drunk today (check): ◯ ◯ ◯ ◯ ◯ ◯ ◯ ◯

WALKING Plan No. _____

Week No.:_____ Day No.:_____

CORE WORK:
Total Time _____

RESISTANCE TRAINING:
1) Machine/Exerc._____
  Weight_____ Reps _____/_____/_____
2) Machine/Exerc._____
  Weight_____ Reps _____/_____/_____
3) Machine/Exerc._____
  Weight_____ Reps _____/_____/_____
4) Machine/Exerc._____
  Weight_____ Reps _____/_____/_____
5) Machine/Exerc._____
  Weight_____ Reps _____/_____/_____
6) Machine/Exerc._____
  Weight_____ Reps _____/_____/_____
7) Machine/Exerc._____
  Weight_____ Reps _____/_____/_____
8) Machine/Exerc._____
  Weight_____ Reps _____/_____/_____

Resistance Tr. Total Time_____

CARDIO WALKING:
Treadmill: Distance _____
  Time _____ Speed _____
  Time walked without support _____
Elliptical: Distance _____ Time _____
  Reversed direction every _____ minutes
  Time walked without support _____
Stepper: Distance _____ Time _____
  Time walked without support _____
Track: Distance _____ Time _____
  Speed or pace (if recorded) _____
  Time walked without support _____
  Fastest lap _____
  Fastest lap without support_____
Total Cardio Walking Time:_____
Max. Heart Rate Noted:_____

RECOVERY BASICS:
☐ **Were physical exercise targets (time and total no. of reps) met?**
☐ **Did I focus well on exercises?**
☐ **Did I work intensively + aggressively?**
☐ **Did I push myself to increase difficulty?**

RECOVERY PLAN: _____

Week No. _____ Day No.:_____

Exercises/Drills Done:
_____Time_____
_____Time_____
_____Time_____
_____Time_____
_____Time_____
_____Time_____
_____Time_____
_____Time_____
_____Time_____
_____Time_____

Total Time Spent_____

NUTRITION PLAN:
Nutrient-rich foods eaten | quantity:
BREAKFAST:
_____ | _____
_____ | _____
_____ | _____
_____ | _____
Drinks:_____
LUNCH:
_____ | _____
_____ | _____
_____ | _____
_____ | _____
_____ | _____
Drinks:_____
Snacks:_____
DINNER:
_____ | _____
_____ | _____
_____ | _____
_____ | _____
_____ | _____
_____ | _____
Drinks:_____
Snacks:_____

RECOVERY PLAN: _____

Week No. _____ Day No.:_____

Exercises/Drills Done:
_____Time_____
_____Time_____
_____Time_____
_____Time_____
_____Time_____
_____Time_____
_____Time_____
_____Time_____
_____Time_____

Total Time Spent_____

SUPPLEMENTS TAKEN:
_____ | _____
_____ | _____
_____ | _____
_____ | _____
_____ | _____

Supplements I Need to Buy:
_____ | _____
_____ | _____

MEDICINES TAKEN:
_____ | _____
_____ | _____
_____ | _____
_____ | _____
_____ | _____
_____ | _____

YOGA TRAINING:
Exercises:_____
_____
_____
_____
Total Yoga Time: _____
Notes:_____

NOTES, SUCCESSES, BREAKTHROUGHS, PROGRESS!
_____
_____
_____
_____
_____

Start of Week Worksheet—Week No. 7

Date: **Week Beginning Monday, _____, 20___**

Numerous scientific studies show that people can recover from stroke and virtually all of the widely publicized limitations on recovery from stroke are pure myth. It has been scientifically shown that:

1. People don't need much brain to thrive (hemispherectomy studies prove this.)
2. People can grow new brain cells throughout their lives (adult neurogenesis studies prove this).
3. People, of all ages, can form new pathways in this brain (brain plasticity studies prove this). You're never too old to learn new things!
4. People, even if elderly, can function perfectly despite "brain disease" (cognitive reserve studies prove this). YOU CAN RECOVER from stroke. People have learned—and my experience proves—good exercise and nutrition work together, so YOU WILL RECOVER from stroke.

Roger Maxwell

Start of Week Statistics:

MEASUREMENTS—MEN:	MEASUREMENTS—WOMEN:	WEIGHT: _____
Waist:_____ Chest:_____	Waist:_____ Hips:_____	**BLOOD PRESSURE:**
Upper Leg: ____ Upper Arm:_____	Upper Leg: ____ Upper Arm:____	_____ over _____

Fill out the following information to guide you during the coming week.

Last week's successes and progress:_____

_____

_____

How well I am physically functioning right now: _____

_____

_____

Goals and expectations for this week:_____

_____

_____

Skills or exercises I want to especially focus on improving this week:_____

_____

_____

Shopping List: brain nutrient foods to add to diet this week:

_____   _____

_____   _____

If my weight or blood pressure are high, plan to reduce them (current/continuing):

_____

231

Daily Worksheet

Day of the Week:	Date:	Day No.	Max. Heart Rate:	A.M. Weight:	A.M. Blood Pressure: _____ OVER _____

Glasses of water drunk today (check): ○ ○ ○ ○ ○ ○ ○ ○

WALKING Plan No. _____

Week No.: _____ **Day No.:** _____

CORE WORK:

Total Time _____

RESISTANCE TRAINING:

1) Machine/Exerc. _____
   Weight _____ Reps _____/_____/_____
2) Machine/Exerc. _____
   Weight _____ Reps _____/_____/_____
3) Machine/Exerc. _____
   Weight _____ Reps _____/_____/_____
4) Machine/Exerc. _____
   Weight _____ Reps _____/_____/_____
5) Machine/Exerc. _____
   Weight _____ Reps _____/_____/_____
6) Machine/Exerc. _____
   Weight _____ Reps _____/_____/_____
7) Machine/Exerc. _____
   Weight _____ Reps _____/_____/_____
8) Machine/Exerc. _____
   Weight _____ Reps _____/_____/_____

Resistance Tr. Total Time _____

CARDIO WALKING:

Treadmill: Distance _____
   Time _____ Speed _____
   Time walked without support _____
Elliptical: Distance _____ Time _____
   Reversed direction every _____ minutes
   Time walked without support _____
Stepper: Distance _____ Time _____
   Time walked without support _____
Track: Distance _____ Time _____
   Speed or pace (if recorded) _____
   Time walked without support _____
   Fastest lap _____
   Fastest lap without support _____
Total Cardio Walking Time: _____
Max. Heart Rate Noted: _____

RECOVERY PLAN: _____

Week No. _____ **Day No.:** _____

Exercises/Drills Done:

_____ Time _____
_____ Time _____
_____ Time _____
_____ Time _____
_____ Time _____
_____ Time _____
_____ Time _____
_____ Time _____
_____ Time _____

Total Time Spent _____

NUTRITION PLAN:

Nutrient-rich foods eaten | quantity:

BREAKFAST:
_____ | _____
_____ | _____
_____ | _____
_____ | _____
Drinks: _____

LUNCH:
_____ | _____
_____ | _____
_____ | _____
_____ | _____
_____ | _____
Drinks: _____
Snacks: _____

DINNER:
_____ | _____
_____ | _____
_____ | _____
_____ | _____
_____ | _____
_____ | _____
Drinks: _____
Snacks: _____

RECOVERY PLAN: _____

Week No. _____ **Day No.:** _____

Exercises/Drills Done:

_____ Time _____
_____ Time _____
_____ Time _____
_____ Time _____
_____ Time _____
_____ Time _____
_____ Time _____
_____ Time _____
_____ Time _____

Total Time Spent _____

SUPPLEMENTS TAKEN:

_____ | _____
_____ | _____
_____ | _____
_____ | _____
_____ | _____

Supplements I Need to Buy:
_____ | _____
_____ | _____

MEDICINES TAKEN:

_____ | _____
_____ | _____
_____ | _____
_____ | _____
_____ | _____
_____ | _____

YOGA TRAINING:

Exercises: _____
_____
_____
_____
_____
Total Yoga Time: _____
Notes: _____

RECOVERY BASICS:

☐ Were physical exercise targets (time and total no. of reps) met?
☐ Did I focus well on exercises?
☐ Did I work intensively + aggressively?
☐ Did I push myself to increase difficulty?

NOTES, SUCCESSES, BREAKTHROUGHS, PROGRESS!

_____
_____
_____
_____
_____

Daily Worksheet

Day of the Week:	Date:	Day No.	Max. Heart Rate:	A.M. Weight:	A.M. Blood Pressure: _____ OVER _____

Glasses of water drunk today (check): ○ ○ ○ ○ ○ ○ ○ ○

WALKING Plan No. _____

Week No.:_____ Day No.:_____

CORE WORK:

Total Time _____

RESISTANCE TRAINING:

1) **Machine/Exerc.**_____

   Weight_____ Reps _____/_____/_____

2) **Machine/Exerc.**_____

   Weight_____ Reps _____/_____/_____

3) **Machine/Exerc.**_____

   Weight_____ Reps _____/_____/_____

4) **Machine/Exerc.**_____

   Weight_____ Reps _____/_____/_____

5) **Machine/Exerc.**_____

   Weight_____ Reps _____/_____/_____

6) **Machine/Exerc.**_____

   Weight_____ Reps _____/_____/_____

7) **Machine/Exerc.**_____

   Weight_____ Reps _____/_____/_____

8) **Machine/Exerc.**_____

   Weight_____ Reps _____/_____/_____

Resistance Tr. Total Time_____

CARDIO WALKING:

Treadmill: Distance _____

   Time _____ Speed _____

   Time walked without support _____

Elliptical: Distance _____Time _____

   Reversed direction every _____ minutes

   Time walked without support _____

Stepper: Distance _____Time _____

   Time walked without support _____

Track: Distance _____Time _____

   Speed or pace (if recorded) _____

   Time walked without support _____

   Fastest lap _____

   Fastest lap without support_____

Total Cardio Walking Time:_____

Max. Heart Rate Noted:_____

RECOVERY BASICS:

☐ **Were physical exercise targets (time and total no. of reps) met?**

☐ **Did I focus well on exercises?**

☐ **Did I work intensively + aggressively?**

☐ **Did I push myself to increase difficulty?**

RECOVERY PLAN: _____

Week No. _____ Day No.:_____

Exercises/Drills Done:

_____Time_____

_____Time_____

_____Time_____

_____Time_____

_____Time_____

_____Time_____

_____Time_____

_____Time_____

_____Time_____

Total Time Spent_____

NUTRITION PLAN:

Nutrient-rich foods eaten | quantity:

BREAKFAST:

_____ | _____

_____ | _____

_____ | _____

_____ | _____

Drinks:_____

LUNCH:

_____ | _____

_____ | _____

_____ | _____

_____ | _____

_____ | _____

Drinks:_____

Snacks:_____

DINNER:

_____ | _____

_____ | _____

_____ | _____

_____ | _____

_____ | _____

_____ | _____

Drinks:_____

Snacks:_____

RECOVERY PLAN: _____

Week No. _____ Day No.:_____

Exercises/Drills Done:

_____Time_____

_____Time_____

_____Time_____

_____Time_____

_____Time_____

_____Time_____

_____Time_____

_____Time_____

_____Time_____

Total Time Spent_____

SUPPLEMENTS TAKEN:

_____ | _____

_____ | _____

_____ | _____

_____ | _____

_____ | _____

_____ | _____

Supplements I Need to Buy:

_____ | _____

_____ | _____

MEDICINES TAKEN:

_____ | _____

_____ | _____

_____ | _____

_____ | _____

_____ | _____

_____ | _____

YOGA TRAINING:

Exercises:_____

_____

_____

_____

_____

Total Yoga Time: _____

Notes:_____

NOTES, SUCCESSES, BREAKTHROUGHS, PROGRESS!

_____

_____

_____

_____

_____

Daily Worksheet

Day of the Week:	Date:	Day No.	Max. Heart Rate:	A.M. Weight:	A.M. Blood Pressure: _____ OVER _____

Glasses of water drunk today (check): ○ ○ ○ ○ ○ ○ ○ ○

WALKING Plan No. _____

Week No.:_____ **Day No.:**_____

CORE WORK:

Total Time _____

RESISTANCE TRAINING:

1) Machine/Exerc._____
   Weight_____ Reps ____/____/____

2) Machine/Exerc._____
   Weight_____ Reps ____/____/____

3) Machine/Exerc._____
   Weight_____ Reps ____/____/____

4) Machine/Exerc._____
   Weight_____ Reps ____/____/____

5) Machine/Exerc._____
   Weight_____ Reps ____/____/____

6) Machine/Exerc._____
   Weight_____ Reps ____/____/____

7) Machine/Exerc._____
   Weight_____ Reps ____/____/____

8) Machine/Exerc._____
   Weight_____ Reps ____/____/____

Resistance Tr. Total Time_____

CARDIO WALKING:

Treadmill: Distance _____
   Time _____ Speed _____
   Time walked without support _____

Elliptical: Distance _____Time _____
   Reversed direction every _____ minutes
   Time walked without support _____

Stepper: Distance _____Time _____
   Time walked without support _____

Track: Distance _____Time _____
   Speed or pace (if recorded) _____
   Time walked without support _____
   Fastest lap _____
   Fastest lap without support_____

Total Cardio Walking Time:_____
Max. Heart Rate Noted:_____

RECOVERY PLAN: _____

Week No. _____ **Day No.:**_____

Exercises/Drills Done:

_____Time_____
_____Time_____
_____Time_____
_____Time_____
_____Time_____
_____Time_____
_____Time_____
_____Time_____
_____Time_____
_____Time_____

Total Time Spent_____

NUTRITION PLAN:

Nutrient-rich foods eaten | quantity:

BREAKFAST:

_____ | _____
_____ | _____
_____ | _____
_____ | _____

Drinks:_____

LUNCH:

_____ | _____
_____ | _____
_____ | _____
_____ | _____
_____ | _____
_____ | _____

Drinks:_____
Snacks:_____

DINNER:

_____ | _____
_____ | _____
_____ | _____
_____ | _____
_____ | _____
_____ | _____

Drinks:_____
Snacks:_____

RECOVERY PLAN: _____

Week No. _____ **Day No.:**_____

Exercises/Drills Done:

_____Time_____
_____Time_____
_____Time_____
_____Time_____
_____Time_____
_____Time_____
_____Time_____
_____Time_____
_____Time_____
_____Time_____

Total Time Spent_____

SUPPLEMENTS TAKEN:

_____ | _____
_____ | _____
_____ | _____
_____ | _____
_____ | _____

Supplements I Need to Buy:

_____ | _____
_____ | _____

MEDICINES TAKEN:

_____ | _____
_____ | _____
_____ | _____
_____ | _____
_____ | _____

YOGA TRAINING:

Exercises:_____
_____
_____
_____
_____
_____

Total Yoga Time: _____
Notes:_____

RECOVERY BASICS:

☐ **Were physical exercise targets (time and total no. of reps) met?**
☐ **Did I focus well on exercises?**
☐ **Did I work intensively + aggressively?**
☐ **Did I push myself to increase difficulty?**

NOTES, SUCCESSES, BREAKTHROUGHS, PROGRESS!

_____
_____
_____
_____
_____

Daily Worksheet

Day of the Week:	Date:	Day No.	Max. Heart Rate:	A.M. Weight:	A.M. Blood Pressure: _____ OVER _____

Glasses of water drunk today (check): ○ ○ ○ ○ ○ ○ ○ ○

WALKING Plan No. _____
Week No.:_____ **Day No.:**_____

CORE WORK:
Total Time _____

RESISTANCE TRAINING:
1) Machine/Exerc._____
  Weight_____ Reps _____/_____/_____
2) Machine/Exerc._____
  Weight_____ Reps _____/_____/_____
3) Machine/Exerc._____
  Weight_____ Reps _____/_____/_____
4) Machine/Exerc._____
  Weight_____ Reps _____/_____/_____
5) Machine/Exerc._____
  Weight_____ Reps _____/_____/_____
6) Machine/Exerc._____
  Weight_____ Reps _____/_____/_____
7) Machine/Exerc._____
  Weight_____ Reps _____/_____/_____
8) Machine/Exerc._____
  Weight_____ Reps _____/_____/_____
Resistance Tr. Total Time_____

CARDIO WALKING:
Treadmill: Distance _____
  Time _____ Speed _____
  Time walked without support _____
Elliptical: Distance _____Time _____
  Reversed direction every _____ minutes
  Time walked without support _____
Stepper: Distance _____Time _____
  Time walked without support _____
Track: Distance _____Time _____
  Speed or pace (if recorded) _____
  Time walked without support _____
  Fastest lap _____
  Fastest lap without support_____
Total Cardio Walking Time:_____
Max. Heart Rate Noted:_____

RECOVERY BASICS:
☐ **Were physical exercise targets (time and total no. of reps) met?**
☐ **Did I focus well on exercises?**
☐ **Did I work intensively + aggressively?**
☐ **Did I push myself to increase difficulty?**

RECOVERY PLAN: _____
Week No. _____ **Day No.:**_____

Exercises/Drills Done:
_____Time_____
_____Time_____
_____Time_____
_____Time_____
_____Time_____
_____Time_____
_____Time_____
_____Time_____
_____Time_____
Total Time Spent_____

NUTRITION PLAN:
Nutrient-rich foods eaten | quantity:
BREAKFAST:
_____ | _____
_____ | _____
_____ | _____
_____ | _____
Drinks:_____
LUNCH:
_____ | _____
_____ | _____
_____ | _____
_____ | _____
_____ | _____
Drinks:_____
Snacks:_____
DINNER:
_____ | _____
_____ | _____
_____ | _____
_____ | _____
_____ | _____
_____ | _____
Drinks:_____
Snacks:_____

RECOVERY PLAN: _____
Week No. _____ **Day No.:**_____

Exercises/Drills Done:
_____Time_____
_____Time_____
_____Time_____
_____Time_____
_____Time_____
_____Time_____
_____Time_____
_____Time_____
_____Time_____
Total Time Spent_____

SUPPLEMENTS TAKEN:
_____ | _____
_____ | _____
_____ | _____
_____ | _____
_____ | _____
_____ | _____
Supplements I Need to Buy:
_____ | _____
_____ | _____

MEDICINES TAKEN:
_____ | _____
_____ | _____
_____ | _____
_____ | _____
_____ | _____
_____ | _____

YOGA TRAINING:
Exercises:_____
_____
_____
_____
_____
_____
Total Yoga Time: _____
Notes:_____

NOTES, SUCCESSES, BREAKTHROUGHS, PROGRESS!
_____
_____
_____
_____
_____

Daily Worksheet

Day of the Week:	Date:	Day No.	Max. Heart Rate:	A.M. Weight:	A.M. Blood Pressure: _____ OVER _____

Glasses of water drunk today (check): ○ ○ ○ ○ ○ ○ ○ ○

WALKING Plan No. _____

Week No.:_____ Day No.:_____

CORE WORK:
Total Time _____

RESISTANCE TRAINING:
1) Machine/Exerc._____
   Weight_____ Reps _____/_____/_____
2) Machine/Exerc._____
   Weight_____ Reps _____/_____/_____
3) Machine/Exerc._____
   Weight_____ Reps _____/_____/_____
4) Machine/Exerc._____
   Weight_____ Reps _____/_____/_____
5) Machine/Exerc._____
   Weight_____ Reps _____/_____/_____
6) Machine/Exerc._____
   Weight_____ Reps _____/_____/_____
7) Machine/Exerc._____
   Weight_____ Reps _____/_____/_____
8) Machine/Exerc._____
   Weight_____ Reps _____/_____/_____
Resistance Tr. Total Time_____

CARDIO WALKING:
Treadmill: Distance _____
   Time _____ Speed _____
   Time walked without support _____
Elliptical: Distance _____Time _____
   Reversed direction every _____ minutes
   Time walked without support _____
Stepper: Distance _____Time _____
   Time walked without support _____
Track: Distance _____Time _____
   Speed or pace (if recorded) _____
   Time walked without support _____
   Fastest lap _____
   Fastest lap without support_____
Total Cardio Walking Time:_____
Max. Heart Rate Noted:_____

RECOVERY BASICS:
☐ Were physical exercise targets (time and total no. of reps) met?
☐ Did I focus well on exercises?
☐ Did I work intensively + aggressively?
☐ Did I push myself to increase difficulty?

RECOVERY PLAN: _____

Week No. _____ Day No.:_____

Exercises/Drills Done:
_____Time_____
_____Time_____
_____Time_____
_____Time_____
_____Time_____
_____Time_____
_____Time_____
_____Time_____
_____Time_____
Total Time Spent_____

NUTRITION PLAN:
Nutrient-rich foods eaten | quantity:
BREAKFAST:
_____ | _____
_____ | _____
_____ | _____
_____ | _____
Drinks:_____
LUNCH:
_____ | _____
_____ | _____
_____ | _____
_____ | _____
_____ | _____
Drinks:_____
Snacks:_____
DINNER:
_____ | _____
_____ | _____
_____ | _____
_____ | _____
_____ | _____
_____ | _____
Drinks:_____
Snacks:_____

RECOVERY PLAN: _____

Week No. _____ Day No.:_____

Exercises/Drills Done:
_____Time_____
_____Time_____
_____Time_____
_____Time_____
_____Time_____
_____Time_____
_____Time_____
_____Time_____
_____Time_____
Total Time Spent_____

SUPPLEMENTS TAKEN:
_____ | _____
_____ | _____
_____ | _____
_____ | _____
_____ | _____
Supplements I Need to Buy:
_____ | _____
_____ | _____

MEDICINES TAKEN:
_____ | _____
_____ | _____
_____ | _____
_____ | _____
_____ | _____
_____ | _____

YOGA TRAINING:
Exercises:_____
_____
_____
_____
_____
_____
Total Yoga Time: _____
Notes:_____

NOTES, SUCCESSES, BREAKTHROUGHS, PROGRESS!
_____
_____
_____
_____
_____
_____

Daily Worksheet

Day of the Week:	Date:	Day No.	Max. Heart Rate:	A.M. Weight:	A.M. Blood Pressure: _____ OVER _____

Glasses of water drunk today (check): ○ ○ ○ ○ ○ ○ ○ ○

WALKING Plan No. _____

Week No.:_____ **Day No.:**_____

CORE WORK:

Total Time _____

RESISTANCE TRAINING:

1) **Machine/Exerc.**_____
   Weight_____ Reps _____/_____/_____
2) **Machine/Exerc.**_____
   Weight_____ Reps _____/_____/_____
3) **Machine/Exerc.**_____
   Weight_____ Reps _____/_____/_____
4) **Machine/Exerc.**_____
   Weight_____ Reps _____/_____/_____
5) **Machine/Exerc.**_____
   Weight_____ Reps _____/_____/_____
6) **Machine/Exerc.**_____
   Weight_____ Reps _____/_____/_____
7) **Machine/Exerc.**_____
   Weight_____ Reps _____/_____/_____
8) **Machine/Exerc.**_____
   Weight_____ Reps _____/_____/_____

Resistance Tr. Total Time_____

CARDIO WALKING:

Treadmill: Distance _____
   Time _____ Speed _____
   Time walked without support _____
Elliptical: Distance _____Time _____
   Reversed direction every _____ minutes
   Time walked without support _____
Stepper: Distance _____Time _____
   Time walked without support _____
Track: Distance _____Time _____
   Speed or pace (if recorded) _____
   Time walked without support _____
   Fastest lap _____
   Fastest lap without support_____

Total Cardio Walking Time:_____
Max. Heart Rate Noted:_____

RECOVERY BASICS:

☐ **Were physical exercise targets (time and total no. of reps) met?**
☐ **Did I focus well on exercises?**
☐ **Did I work intensively + aggressively?**
☐ **Did I push myself to increase difficulty?**

RECOVERY PLAN: _____

Week No. _____ **Day No.:**_____

Exercises/Drills Done:

_____Time_____
_____Time_____
_____Time_____
_____Time_____
_____Time_____
_____Time_____
_____Time_____
_____Time_____
_____Time_____

Total Time Spent_____

NUTRITION PLAN:

Nutrient-rich foods eaten | quantity:
BREAKFAST:
_____ | _____
_____ | _____
_____ | _____
_____ | _____
Drinks:_____

LUNCH:
_____ | _____
_____ | _____
_____ | _____
_____ | _____
_____ | _____
Drinks:_____
Snacks:_____

DINNER:
_____ | _____
_____ | _____
_____ | _____
_____ | _____
_____ | _____
Drinks:_____
Snacks:_____

NOTES, SUCCESSES, BREAKTHROUGHS, PROGRESS!

_____
_____
_____
_____
_____

RECOVERY PLAN: _____

Week No. _____ **Day No.:**_____

Exercises/Drills Done:

_____Time_____
_____Time_____
_____Time_____
_____Time_____
_____Time_____
_____Time_____
_____Time_____
_____Time_____
_____Time_____

Total Time Spent_____

SUPPLEMENTS TAKEN:

_____ | _____
_____ | _____
_____ | _____
_____ | _____
_____ | _____
_____ | _____

Supplements I Need to Buy:
_____ | _____
_____ | _____

MEDICINES TAKEN:
_____ | _____
_____ | _____
_____ | _____
_____ | _____
_____ | _____
_____ | _____

YOGA TRAINING:

Exercises:_____
_____
_____
_____
_____

Total Yoga Time: _____
Notes:_____

Daily Worksheet

Day of the Week:	Date:	Day No.	Max. Heart Rate:	A.M. Weight:	A.M. Blood Pressure: _____ OVER _____

Glasses of water drunk today (check): ○ ○ ○ ○ ○ ○ ○ ○

WALKING Plan No. _____

Week No.:_____ Day No.:_____

CORE WORK:
Total Time _____

RESISTANCE TRAINING:
1) Machine/Exerc._____
   Weight_____ Reps _____/_____/_____
2) Machine/Exerc._____
   Weight_____ Reps _____/_____/_____
3) Machine/Exerc._____
   Weight_____ Reps _____/_____/_____
4) Machine/Exerc._____
   Weight_____ Reps _____/_____/_____
5) Machine/Exerc._____
   Weight_____ Reps _____/_____/_____
6) Machine/Exerc._____
   Weight_____ Reps _____/_____/_____
7) Machine/Exerc._____
   Weight_____ Reps _____/_____/_____
8) Machine/Exerc._____
   Weight_____ Reps _____/_____/_____

Resistance Tr. Total Time_____

CARDIO WALKING:
Treadmill: Distance _____
   Time _____ Speed _____
   Time walked without support _____
Elliptical: Distance _____Time _____
   Reversed direction every _____ minutes
   Time walked without support _____
Stepper: Distance _____Time _____
   Time walked without support _____
Track: Distance _____Time _____
   Speed or pace (if recorded) _____
   Time walked without support _____
   Fastest lap _____
   Fastest lap without support_____
Total Cardio Walking Time:_____
Max. Heart Rate Noted:_____

RECOVERY BASICS:
☐ **Were physical exercise targets (time and total no. of reps) met?**
☐ **Did I focus well on exercises?**
☐ **Did I work intensively + aggressively?**
☐ **Did I push myself to increase difficulty?**

RECOVERY PLAN: _____

Week No. _____ Day No.:_____

Exercises/Drills Done:
_____Time_____
_____Time_____
_____Time_____
_____Time_____
_____Time_____
_____Time_____
_____Time_____
_____Time_____
_____Time_____
_____Time_____

Total Time Spent_____

NUTRITION PLAN:
Nutrient-rich foods eaten | quantity:
BREAKFAST:
_____ | _____
_____ | _____
_____ | _____
_____ | _____
Drinks:_____
LUNCH:
_____ | _____
_____ | _____
_____ | _____
_____ | _____
_____ | _____
Drinks:_____
Snacks:_____

DINNER:
_____ | _____
_____ | _____
_____ | _____
_____ | _____
_____ | _____
_____ | _____
Drinks:_____
Snacks:_____

RECOVERY PLAN: _____

Week No. _____ Day No.:_____

Exercises/Drills Done:
_____Time_____
_____Time_____
_____Time_____
_____Time_____
_____Time_____
_____Time_____
_____Time_____
_____Time_____
_____Time_____
_____Time_____

Total Time Spent_____

SUPPLEMENTS TAKEN:
_____ | _____
_____ | _____
_____ | _____
_____ | _____
_____ | _____

Supplements I Need to Buy:
_____ | _____
_____ | _____

MEDICINES TAKEN:
_____ | _____
_____ | _____
_____ | _____
_____ | _____
_____ | _____

YOGA TRAINING:
Exercises:_____
_____
_____
_____
_____
Total Yoga Time: _____
Notes:_____

NOTES, SUCCESSES, BREAKTHROUGHS, PROGRESS!
_____
_____
_____
_____
_____

Start of Week Worksheet—Week No. 8

Date: Week Beginning Monday, _____, 20___

Commitment is demonstrated through the consistency with which you apply effort to whatever task, concept, objective, or goal you have decided on. This means working on your goals every day, and devoting as much daily time as necessary to the effort. To accomplish consistency and dedication, a person may need to force himself or herself to honor and be loyal to the commitment they have made. This, of course, takes discipline.

Kirk Mango and Daveda Lamont
from Becoming a True Champion

Start of Week Statistics:

MEASUREMENTS—MEN:	MEASUREMENTS—WOMEN:	WEIGHT: _____
Waist:_____ Chest:_____	Waist:_____ Hips:_____	BLOOD PRESSURE:
Upper Leg: ____ Upper Arm:_____	Upper Leg: ____ Upper Arm:____	_____ over _____

Fill out the following information to guide you during the coming week.

Last week's successes and progress:_____

_____

_____

How well I am physically functioning right now: _____

_____

_____

Goals and expectations for this week:_____

_____

_____

Skills or exercises I want to especially focus on improving this week:_____

_____

_____

Shopping List: brain nutrient foods to add to diet this week:

_____   _____

_____   _____

If my weight or blood pressure are high, plan to reduce them (current/continuing):

_____

Daily Worksheet

Day of the Week:	Date:	Day No.	Max. Heart Rate:	A.M. Weight:	A.M. Blood Pressure: _____ OVER _____

Glasses of water drunk today (check): ○ ○ ○ ○ ○ ○ ○ ○

WALKING Plan No. _____

Week No.:_____ Day No.:_____

CORE WORK:
Total Time _____

RESISTANCE TRAINING:

1) Machine/Exerc._____
   Weight_____ Reps _____/_____/_____

2) Machine/Exerc._____
   Weight_____ Reps _____/_____/_____

3) Machine/Exerc._____
   Weight_____ Reps _____/_____/_____

4) Machine/Exerc._____
   Weight_____ Reps _____/_____/_____

5) Machine/Exerc._____
   Weight_____ Reps _____/_____/_____

6) Machine/Exerc._____
   Weight_____ Reps _____/_____/_____

7) Machine/Exerc._____
   Weight_____ Reps _____/_____/_____

8) Machine/Exerc._____
   Weight_____ Reps _____/_____/_____

Resistance Tr. Total Time_____

CARDIO WALKING:

Treadmill: Distance _____
   Time _____ Speed _____
   Time walked without support _____

Elliptical: Distance _____Time _____
   Reversed direction every _____ minutes
   Time walked without support _____

Stepper: Distance _____Time _____
   Time walked without support _____

Track: Distance _____Time _____
   Speed or pace (if recorded) _____
   Time walked without support _____
   Fastest lap _____
   Fastest lap without support_____

Total Cardio Walking Time:_____

Max. Heart Rate Noted:_____

RECOVERY PLAN: _____

Week No. _____ Day No.:_____

Exercises/Drills Done:
_____Time_____
_____Time_____
_____Time_____
_____Time_____
_____Time_____
_____Time_____
_____Time_____
_____Time_____

Total Time Spent_____

NUTRITION PLAN:

Nutrient-rich foods eaten | quantity:

BREAKFAST:
_____ | _____
_____ | _____
_____ | _____
_____ | _____

Drinks:_____

LUNCH:
_____ | _____
_____ | _____
_____ | _____
_____ | _____
_____ | _____

Drinks:_____
Snacks:_____

DINNER:
_____ | _____
_____ | _____
_____ | _____
_____ | _____
_____ | _____
_____ | _____

Drinks:_____
Snacks:_____

RECOVERY PLAN: _____

Week No. _____ Day No.:_____

Exercises/Drills Done:
_____Time_____
_____Time_____
_____Time_____
_____Time_____
_____Time_____
_____Time_____
_____Time_____
_____Time_____

Total Time Spent_____

SUPPLEMENTS TAKEN:
_____ | _____
_____ | _____
_____ | _____
_____ | _____
_____ | _____

Supplements I Need to Buy:
_____ | _____
_____ | _____

MEDICINES TAKEN:
_____ | _____
_____ | _____
_____ | _____
_____ | _____
_____ | _____

YOGA TRAINING:
Exercises:_____
_____
_____
_____

Total Yoga Time: _____
Notes:_____

RECOVERY BASICS:
☐ **Were physical exercise targets (time and total no. of reps) met?**
☐ **Did I focus well on exercises?**
☐ **Did I work intensively + aggressively?**
☐ **Did I push myself to increase difficulty?**

NOTES, SUCCESSES, BREAKTHROUGHS, PROGRESS!
_____
_____
_____
_____
_____

Daily Worksheet

Day of the Week:	Date:	Day No.	Max. Heart Rate:	A.M. Weight:	A.M. Blood Pressure: _____ OVER _____

Glasses of water drunk today (check): ○ ○ ○ ○ ○ ○ ○ ○

WALKING Plan No. _____

Week No.:_____ Day No.:_____

CORE WORK:

Total Time _____

RESISTANCE TRAINING:

1) Machine/Exerc._____

Weight_____ Reps _____/_____/_____

2) Machine/Exerc._____

Weight_____ Reps _____/_____/_____

3) Machine/Exerc._____

Weight_____ Reps _____/_____/_____

4) Machine/Exerc._____

Weight_____ Reps _____/_____/_____

5) Machine/Exerc._____

Weight_____ Reps _____/_____/_____

6) Machine/Exerc._____

Weight_____ Reps _____/_____/_____

7) Machine/Exerc._____

Weight_____ Reps _____/_____/_____

8) Machine/Exerc._____

Weight_____ Reps _____/_____/_____

Resistance Tr. Total Time_____

CARDIO WALKING:

Treadmill: Distance _____

Time _____ Speed _____

Time walked without support _____

Elliptical: Distance _____Time _____

Reversed direction every _____ minutes

Time walked without support _____

Stepper: Distance _____Time _____

Time walked without support _____

Track: Distance _____Time _____

Speed or pace (if recorded) _____

Time walked without support _____

Fastest lap _____

Fastest lap without support_____

Total Cardio Walking Time:_____

Max. Heart Rate Noted:_____

RECOVERY BASICS:

☐ **Were physical exercise targets (time and total no. of reps) met?**

☐ **Did I focus well on exercises?**

☐ **Did I work intensively + aggressively?**

☐ **Did I push myself to increase difficulty?**

RECOVERY PLAN: _____

Week No. _____ Day No.:_____

Exercises/Drills Done:

_____Time_____
_____Time_____
_____Time_____
_____Time_____
_____Time_____
_____Time_____
_____Time_____
_____Time_____
_____Time_____
_____Time_____

Total Time Spent_____

NUTRITION PLAN:

Nutrient-rich foods eaten | quantity:

BREAKFAST:

_____ | _____
_____ | _____
_____ | _____
_____ | _____

Drinks:_____

LUNCH:

_____ | _____
_____ | _____
_____ | _____
_____ | _____
_____ | _____

Drinks:_____

Snacks:_____

DINNER:

_____ | _____
_____ | _____
_____ | _____
_____ | _____
_____ | _____
_____ | _____

Drinks:_____

Snacks:_____

RECOVERY PLAN: _____

Week No. _____ Day No.:_____

Exercises/Drills Done:

_____Time_____
_____Time_____
_____Time_____
_____Time_____
_____Time_____
_____Time_____
_____Time_____
_____Time_____
_____Time_____
_____Time_____

Total Time Spent_____

SUPPLEMENTS TAKEN:

_____ | _____
_____ | _____
_____ | _____
_____ | _____
_____ | _____
_____ | _____

Supplements I Need to Buy:

_____ | _____
_____ | _____

MEDICINES TAKEN:

_____ | _____
_____ | _____
_____ | _____
_____ | _____
_____ | _____
_____ | _____

YOGA TRAINING:

Exercises:_____
_____
_____
_____

Total Yoga Time: _____

Notes:_____

NOTES, SUCCESSES, BREAKTHROUGHS, PROGRESS!

_____
_____
_____
_____

Daily Worksheet

Day of the Week:	Date:	Day No.	Max. Heart Rate:	A.M. Weight:	A.M. Blood Pressure: _____ OVER _____

Glasses of water drunk today (check): ○ ○ ○ ○ ○ ○ ○ ○

WALKING Plan No. _____

Week No.:_____ Day No.:_____

CORE WORK:

Total Time _____

RESISTANCE TRAINING:

1) Machine/Exerc._____

Weight_____ Reps _____/_____/_____

2) Machine/Exerc._____

Weight_____ Reps _____/_____/_____

3) Machine/Exerc._____

Weight_____ Reps _____/_____/_____

4) Machine/Exerc._____

Weight_____ Reps _____/_____/_____

5) Machine/Exerc._____

Weight_____ Reps _____/_____/_____

6) Machine/Exerc._____

Weight_____ Reps _____/_____/_____

7) Machine/Exerc._____

Weight_____ Reps _____/_____/_____

8) Machine/Exerc._____

Weight_____ Reps _____/_____/_____

Resistance Tr. Total Time_____

CARDIO WALKING:

Treadmill: Distance _____

Time _____ Speed _____

Time walked without support _____

Elliptical: Distance _____ Time _____

Reversed direction every _____ minutes

Time walked without support _____

Stepper: Distance _____ Time _____

Time walked without support _____

Track: Distance _____ Time _____

Speed or pace (if recorded) _____

Time walked without support _____

Fastest lap _____

Fastest lap without support_____

Total Cardio Walking Time:_____

Max. Heart Rate Noted:_____

RECOVERY BASICS:

☐ **Were physical exercise targets (time and total no. of reps) met?**

☐ **Did I focus well on exercises?**

☐ **Did I work intensively + aggressively?**

☐ **Did I push myself to increase difficulty?**

RECOVERY PLAN: _____

Week No. _____ Day No.:_____

Exercises/Drills Done:

_____Time_____

_____Time_____

_____Time_____

_____Time_____

_____Time_____

_____Time_____

_____Time_____

_____Time_____

_____Time_____

Total Time Spent_____

NUTRITION PLAN:

Nutrient-rich foods eaten | quantity:

BREAKFAST:

_____ | _____

_____ | _____

_____ | _____

_____ | _____

Drinks:_____

LUNCH:

_____ | _____

_____ | _____

_____ | _____

_____ | _____

_____ | _____

Drinks:_____

Snacks:_____

DINNER:

_____ | _____

_____ | _____

_____ | _____

_____ | _____

_____ | _____

_____ | _____

Drinks:_____

Snacks:_____

RECOVERY PLAN: _____

Week No. _____ Day No.:_____

Exercises/Drills Done:

_____Time_____

_____Time_____

_____Time_____

_____Time_____

_____Time_____

_____Time_____

_____Time_____

_____Time_____

_____Time_____

Total Time Spent_____

SUPPLEMENTS TAKEN:

_____ | _____

_____ | _____

_____ | _____

_____ | _____

_____ | _____

_____ | _____

Supplements I Need to Buy:

_____ | _____

_____ | _____

MEDICINES TAKEN:

_____ | _____

_____ | _____

_____ | _____

_____ | _____

_____ | _____

_____ | _____

YOGA TRAINING:

Exercises:_____

_____

_____

_____

_____

_____

Total Yoga Time: _____

Notes:_____

NOTES, SUCCESSES, BREAKTHROUGHS, PROGRESS!

_____

_____

_____

_____

_____

Daily Worksheet

Day of the Week:	Date:	Day No.	Max. Heart Rate:	A.M. Weight:	A.M. Blood Pressure: _____ OVER _____

Glasses of water drunk today (check): ◯ ◯ ◯ ◯ ◯ ◯ ◯ ◯

WALKING Plan No. _____
Week No.:_____   Day No.:_____

CORE WORK:
Total Time _____

RESISTANCE TRAINING:
1) Machine/Exerc._____
   Weight_____ Reps _____/_____/_____
2) Machine/Exerc._____
   Weight_____ Reps _____/_____/_____
3) Machine/Exerc._____
   Weight_____ Reps _____/_____/_____
4) Machine/Exerc._____
   Weight_____ Reps _____/_____/_____
5) Machine/Exerc._____
   Weight_____ Reps _____/_____/_____
6) Machine/Exerc._____
   Weight_____ Reps _____/_____/_____
7) Machine/Exerc._____
   Weight_____ Reps _____/_____/_____
8) Machine/Exerc._____
   Weight_____ Reps _____/_____/_____
Resistance Tr. Total Time_____

CARDIO WALKING:
Treadmill: Distance _____
   Time _____ Speed _____
   Time walked without support _____
Elliptical: Distance _____Time _____
   Reversed direction every _____ minutes
   Time walked without support _____
Stepper: Distance _____Time _____
   Time walked without support _____
Track: Distance _____Time _____
   Speed or pace (if recorded) _____
   Time walked without support _____
   Fastest lap _____
   Fastest lap without support_____
Total Cardio Walking Time:_____
Max. Heart Rate Noted:_____

RECOVERY BASICS:
☐ **Were physical exercise targets (time and total no. of reps) met?**
☐ **Did I focus well on exercises?**
☐ **Did I work intensively + aggressively?**
☐ **Did I push myself to increase difficulty?**

RECOVERY PLAN: _____
Week No. _____   Day No.:_____

Exercises/Drills Done:
_____Time_____
_____Time_____
_____Time_____
_____Time_____
_____Time_____
_____Time_____
_____Time_____
_____Time_____
_____Time_____
Total Time Spent_____

NUTRITION PLAN:
Nutrient-rich foods eaten | quantity:
BREAKFAST:
_____ | _____
_____ | _____
_____ | _____
_____ | _____
Drinks:_____
LUNCH:
_____ | _____
_____ | _____
_____ | _____
_____ | _____
_____ | _____
_____ | _____
Drinks:_____
Snacks:_____
DINNER:
_____ | _____
_____ | _____
_____ | _____
_____ | _____
_____ | _____
_____ | _____
Drinks:_____
Snacks:_____

RECOVERY PLAN: _____
Week No. _____   Day No.:_____

Exercises/Drills Done:
_____Time_____
_____Time_____
_____Time_____
_____Time_____
_____Time_____
_____Time_____
_____Time_____
_____Time_____
_____Time_____
Total Time Spent_____

SUPPLEMENTS TAKEN:
_____ | _____
_____ | _____
_____ | _____
_____ | _____
_____ | _____
_____ | _____
Supplements I Need to Buy:
_____ | _____
_____ | _____

MEDICINES TAKEN:
_____ | _____
_____ | _____
_____ | _____
_____ | _____
_____ | _____
_____ | _____

YOGA TRAINING:
Exercises:_____
_____
_____
_____
_____
_____
Total Yoga Time: _____
Notes:_____

NOTES, SUCCESSES, BREAKTHROUGHS, PROGRESS!
_____
_____
_____
_____
_____
_____
_____

Daily Worksheet

Day of the Week:	Date:	Day No.	Max. Heart Rate:	A.M. Weight:	A.M. Blood Pressure: _____ OVER _____

Glasses of water drunk today (check): ○ ○ ○ ○ ○ ○ ○ ○

WALKING Plan No. _____

Week No.:_____ Day No.:_____

CORE WORK:
Total Time _____

RESISTANCE TRAINING:
1) Machine/Exerc._____
  Weight_____ Reps _____/_____/_____
2) Machine/Exerc._____
  Weight_____ Reps _____/_____/_____
3) Machine/Exerc._____
  Weight_____ Reps _____/_____/_____
4) Machine/Exerc._____
  Weight_____ Reps _____/_____/_____
5) Machine/Exerc._____
  Weight_____ Reps _____/_____/_____
6) Machine/Exerc._____
  Weight_____ Reps _____/_____/_____
7) Machine/Exerc._____
  Weight_____ Reps _____/_____/_____
8) Machine/Exerc._____
  Weight_____ Reps _____/_____/_____
Resistance Tr. Total Time_____

CARDIO WALKING:
Treadmill: Distance _____
  Time _____ Speed _____
  Time walked without support _____
Elliptical: Distance _____Time _____
  Reversed direction every _____ minutes
  Time walked without support _____
Stepper: Distance _____Time _____
  Time walked without support _____
Track: Distance _____Time _____
  Speed or pace (if recorded) _____
  Time walked without support _____
  Fastest lap _____
  Fastest lap without support_____
Total Cardio Walking Time:_____
Max. Heart Rate Noted:_____

RECOVERY PLAN: _____

Week No. _____ Day No.:_____

Exercises/Drills Done:
_____Time_____
_____Time_____
_____Time_____
_____Time_____
_____Time_____
_____Time_____
_____Time_____
_____Time_____
_____Time_____
Total Time Spent_____

NUTRITION PLAN:
Nutrient-rich foods eaten | quantity:
BREAKFAST:
_____ | _____
_____ | _____
_____ | _____
_____ | _____
Drinks:_____
LUNCH:
_____ | _____
_____ | _____
_____ | _____
_____ | _____
_____ | _____
Drinks:_____
Snacks:_____

DINNER:
_____ | _____
_____ | _____
_____ | _____
_____ | _____
_____ | _____
_____ | _____
Drinks:_____
Snacks:_____

RECOVERY PLAN: _____

Week No. _____ Day No.:_____

Exercises/Drills Done:
_____Time_____
_____Time_____
_____Time_____
_____Time_____
_____Time_____
_____Time_____
_____Time_____
_____Time_____
_____Time_____
Total Time Spent_____

SUPPLEMENTS TAKEN:
_____ | _____
_____ | _____
_____ | _____
_____ | _____
_____ | _____
_____ | _____

Supplements I Need to Buy:
_____ | _____
_____ | _____

MEDICINES TAKEN:
_____ | _____
_____ | _____
_____ | _____
_____ | _____
_____ | _____
_____ | _____

YOGA TRAINING:
Exercises:_____
_____
_____
_____
_____
_____
Total Yoga Time: _____
Notes:_____

RECOVERY BASICS:
☐ **Were physical exercise targets (time and total no. of reps) met?**
☐ **Did I focus well on exercises?**
☐ **Did I work intensively + aggressively?**
☐ **Did I push myself to increase difficulty?**

NOTES, SUCCESSES, BREAKTHROUGHS, PROGRESS!
_____
_____
_____
_____
_____
_____

Daily Worksheet

Day of the Week:	Date:	Day No.	Max. Heart Rate:	A.M. Weight:	A.M. Blood Pressure: _____ OVER _____

Glasses of water drunk today (check): ○ ○ ○ ○ ○ ○ ○ ○

WALKING Plan No. _____

Week No.:_____ Day No.:_____

CORE WORK:

Total Time _____

RESISTANCE TRAINING:

1) Machine/Exerc._____

  Weight_____ Reps _____/_____/_____

2) Machine/Exerc._____

  Weight_____ Reps _____/_____/_____

3) Machine/Exerc._____

  Weight_____ Reps _____/_____/_____

4) Machine/Exerc._____

  Weight_____ Reps _____/_____/_____

5) Machine/Exerc._____

  Weight_____ Reps _____/_____/_____

6) Machine/Exerc._____

  Weight_____ Reps _____/_____/_____

7) Machine/Exerc._____

  Weight_____ Reps _____/_____/_____

8) Machine/Exerc._____

  Weight_____ Reps _____/_____/_____

Resistance Tr. Total Time_____

CARDIO WALKING:

Treadmill: Distance _____

  Time _____ Speed _____

  Time walked without support _____

Elliptical: Distance _____Time _____

  Reversed direction every _____ minutes

  Time walked without support _____

Stepper: Distance _____Time _____

  Time walked without support _____

Track: Distance _____Time _____

  Speed or pace (if recorded) _____

  Time walked without support _____

  Fastest lap _____

  Fastest lap without support_____

Total Cardio Walking Time:_____

Max. Heart Rate Noted:_____

RECOVERY BASICS:

☐ **Were physical exercise targets (time and total no. of reps) met?**

☐ **Did I focus well on exercises?**

☐ **Did I work intensively + aggressively?**

☐ **Did I push myself to increase difficulty?**

RECOVERY PLAN: _____

Week No. _____ Day No.:_____

Exercises/Drills Done:

_____Time_____

_____Time_____

_____Time_____

_____Time_____

_____Time_____

_____Time_____

_____Time_____

_____Time_____

_____Time_____

_____Time_____

Total Time Spent_____

NUTRITION PLAN:

Nutrient-rich foods eaten ⎮ quantity:

BREAKFAST:

_____⎮_____

_____⎮_____

_____⎮_____

_____⎮_____

Drinks:_____

LUNCH:

_____⎮_____

_____⎮_____

_____⎮_____

_____⎮_____

_____⎮_____

Drinks:_____

Snacks:_____

DINNER:

_____⎮_____

_____⎮_____

_____⎮_____

_____⎮_____

_____⎮_____

Drinks:_____

Snacks:_____

RECOVERY PLAN: _____

Week No. _____ Day No.:_____

Exercises/Drills Done:

_____Time_____

_____Time_____

_____Time_____

_____Time_____

_____Time_____

_____Time_____

_____Time_____

_____Time_____

_____Time_____

_____Time_____

Total Time Spent_____

SUPPLEMENTS TAKEN:

_____⎮_____

_____⎮_____

_____⎮_____

_____⎮_____

_____⎮_____

_____⎮_____

Supplements I Need to Buy:

_____⎮_____

_____⎮_____

MEDICINES TAKEN:

_____⎮_____

_____⎮_____

_____⎮_____

_____⎮_____

_____⎮_____

YOGA TRAINING:

Exercises:_____

_____

_____

_____

_____

_____

Total Yoga Time: _____

Notes:_____

NOTES, SUCCESSES, BREAKTHROUGHS, PROGRESS!

_____

_____

_____

_____

_____

Daily Worksheet

Day of the Week:	Date:	Day No.	Max. Heart Rate:	A.M. Weight:	A.M. Blood Pressure: _____ OVER _____

Glasses of water drunk today (check): ○ ○ ○ ○ ○ ○ ○ ○

WALKING Plan No. _____

Week No.:_____ **Day No.:**_____

CORE WORK:
Total Time _____

RESISTANCE TRAINING:

1) Machine/Exerc._____
  Weight_____ Reps _____/_____/_____
2) Machine/Exerc._____
  Weight_____ Reps _____/_____/_____
3) Machine/Exerc._____
  Weight_____ Reps _____/_____/_____
4) Machine/Exerc._____
  Weight_____ Reps _____/_____/_____
5) Machine/Exerc._____
  Weight_____ Reps _____/_____/_____
6) Machine/Exerc._____
  Weight_____ Reps _____/_____/_____
7) Machine/Exerc._____
  Weight_____ Reps _____/_____/_____
8) Machine/Exerc._____
  Weight_____ Reps _____/_____/_____

Resistance Tr. Total Time_____

CARDIO WALKING:

Treadmill: Distance _____
  Time _____ Speed _____
  Time walked without support _____
Elliptical: Distance _____Time _____
  Reversed direction every _____ minutes
  Time walked without support _____
Stepper: Distance _____Time _____
  Time walked without support _____
Track: Distance _____Time _____
  Speed or pace (if recorded) _____
  Time walked without support _____
  Fastest lap _____
  Fastest lap without support_____
Total Cardio Walking Time:_____
Max. Heart Rate Noted:_____

RECOVERY BASICS:
☐ **Were physical exercise targets (time and total no. of reps) met?**
☐ **Did I focus well on exercises?**
☐ **Did I work intensively + aggressively?**
☐ **Did I push myself to increase difficulty?**

RECOVERY PLAN: _____

Week No. _____ **Day No.:**_____

Exercises/Drills Done:
_____Time_____
_____Time_____
_____Time_____
_____Time_____
_____Time_____
_____Time_____
_____Time_____
_____Time_____
_____Time_____
_____Time_____

Total Time Spent_____

NUTRITION PLAN:
Nutrient-rich foods eaten | quantity:
BREAKFAST:
_____ | _____
_____ | _____
_____ | _____
_____ | _____
Drinks:_____
LUNCH:
_____ | _____
_____ | _____
_____ | _____
_____ | _____
_____ | _____
Drinks:_____
Snacks:_____
DINNER:
_____ | _____
_____ | _____
_____ | _____
_____ | _____
_____ | _____
_____ | _____
Drinks:_____
Snacks:_____

NOTES, SUCCESSES, BREAKTHROUGHS, PROGRESS!
_____
_____
_____
_____

RECOVERY PLAN: _____

Week No. _____ **Day No.:**_____

Exercises/Drills Done:
_____Time_____
_____Time_____
_____Time_____
_____Time_____
_____Time_____
_____Time_____
_____Time_____
_____Time_____
_____Time_____

Total Time Spent_____

SUPPLEMENTS TAKEN:
_____ | _____
_____ | _____
_____ | _____
_____ | _____
_____ | _____
_____ | _____

Supplements I Need to Buy:
_____ | _____
_____ | _____

MEDICINES TAKEN:
_____ | _____
_____ | _____
_____ | _____
_____ | _____
_____ | _____

YOGA TRAINING:
Exercises:_____
_____
_____
_____
_____
Total Yoga Time: _____
Notes:_____

Start of Week Worksheet—Week No. 9

Date: Week Beginning Monday, _____, 20___

> Whether you are thinking about the past (including the fact that you had a stroke, which you can't do anything about), or whether you are planning for the future (knowing that your best future requires you to be fully recovered from stroke), the same three words apply: GET OVER IT! Getting over what you can't control is good advice, and "getting over" stroke is a great goal!
>
> Roger Maxwell

Start of Week Statistics:

MEASUREMENTS—MEN:

Waist:_____ Chest:_____

Upper Leg: ____ Upper Arm:_____

MEASUREMENTS—WOMEN:

Waist:_____ Hips:_____

Upper Leg: ____ Upper Arm:____

WEIGHT: _____

BLOOD PRESSURE:

_____ over _____

Fill out the following information to guide you during the coming week.

Last week's successes and progress:_____

_____

_____

How well I am physically functioning right now: _____

_____

_____

Goals and expectations for this week:_____

_____

_____

Skills or exercises I want to especially focus on improving this week:_____

_____

_____

Shopping List: brain nutrient foods to add to diet this week:

_____   _____

_____   _____

If my weight or blood pressure are high, plan to reduce them (current/continuing):

_____

Daily Worksheet

Day of the Week:	Date:	Day No.	Max. Heart Rate:	A.M. Weight:	A.M. Blood Pressure: _____ OVER _____

Glasses of water drunk today (check): ○ ○ ○ ○ ○ ○ ○ ○

WALKING Plan No. _____

Week No.: _____ **Day No.:** _____

CORE WORK:

Total Time _____

RESISTANCE TRAINING:

1) Machine/Exerc. _____

   Weight _____ Reps _____/_____/_____

2) Machine/Exerc. _____

   Weight _____ Reps _____/_____/_____

3) Machine/Exerc. _____

   Weight _____ Reps _____/_____/_____

4) Machine/Exerc. _____

   Weight _____ Reps _____/_____/_____

5) Machine/Exerc. _____

   Weight _____ Reps _____/_____/_____

6) Machine/Exerc. _____

   Weight _____ Reps _____/_____/_____

7) Machine/Exerc. _____

   Weight _____ Reps _____/_____/_____

8) Machine/Exerc. _____

   Weight _____ Reps _____/_____/_____

Resistance Tr. Total Time _____

CARDIO WALKING:

Treadmill: Distance _____

   Time _____ Speed _____

   Time walked without support _____

Elliptical: Distance _____ Time _____

   Reversed direction every _____ minutes

   Time walked without support _____

Stepper: Distance _____ Time _____

   Time walked without support _____

Track: Distance _____ Time _____

   Speed or pace (if recorded) _____

   Time walked without support _____

   Fastest lap _____

   Fastest lap without support _____

Total Cardio Walking Time: _____

Max. Heart Rate Noted: _____

RECOVERY PLAN: _____

Week No. _____ **Day No.:** _____

Exercises/Drills Done:

_____ Time _____
_____ Time _____
_____ Time _____
_____ Time _____
_____ Time _____
_____ Time _____
_____ Time _____
_____ Time _____
_____ Time _____
_____ Time _____

Total Time Spent _____

NUTRITION PLAN:

Nutrient-rich foods eaten | quantity:

BREAKFAST:

_____ | _____
_____ | _____
_____ | _____
_____ | _____

Drinks: _____

LUNCH:

_____ | _____
_____ | _____
_____ | _____
_____ | _____
_____ | _____

Drinks: _____

Snacks: _____

DINNER:

_____ | _____
_____ | _____
_____ | _____
_____ | _____
_____ | _____
_____ | _____

Drinks: _____

Snacks: _____

RECOVERY PLAN: _____

Week No. _____ **Day No.:** _____

Exercises/Drills Done:

_____ Time _____
_____ Time _____
_____ Time _____
_____ Time _____
_____ Time _____
_____ Time _____
_____ Time _____
_____ Time _____
_____ Time _____

Total Time Spent _____

SUPPLEMENTS TAKEN:

_____ | _____
_____ | _____
_____ | _____
_____ | _____
_____ | _____
_____ | _____

Supplements I Need to Buy:

_____ | _____
_____ | _____

MEDICINES TAKEN:

_____ | _____
_____ | _____
_____ | _____
_____ | _____
_____ | _____
_____ | _____

YOGA TRAINING:

Exercises: _____
_____
_____
_____
_____

Total Yoga Time: _____

Notes: _____

RECOVERY BASICS:

☐ **Were physical exercise targets (time and total no. of reps) met?**

☐ **Did I focus well on exercises?**

☐ **Did I work intensively + aggressively?**

☐ **Did I push myself to increase difficulty?**

NOTES, SUCCESSES, BREAKTHROUGHS, PROGRESS!

_____
_____
_____
_____

Daily Worksheet

Day of the Week:	Date:	Day No.	Max. Heart Rate:	A.M. Weight:	A.M. Blood Pressure: _____ OVER _____

Glasses of water drunk today (check): ○ ○ ○ ○ ○ ○ ○ ○

WALKING Plan No. _____

Week No.:_____ Day No.:_____

CORE WORK:

Total Time _____

RESISTANCE TRAINING:

1) Machine/Exerc._____
   Weight_____ Reps _____/_____/_____

2) Machine/Exerc._____
   Weight_____ Reps _____/_____/_____

3) Machine/Exerc._____
   Weight_____ Reps _____/_____/_____

4) Machine/Exerc._____
   Weight_____ Reps _____/_____/_____

5) Machine/Exerc._____
   Weight_____ Reps _____/_____/_____

6) Machine/Exerc._____
   Weight_____ Reps _____/_____/_____

7) Machine/Exerc._____
   Weight_____ Reps _____/_____/_____

8) Machine/Exerc._____
   Weight_____ Reps _____/_____/_____

Resistance Tr. Total Time_____

CARDIO WALKING:

Treadmill: Distance _____
   Time _____ Speed _____
   Time walked without support _____

Elliptical: Distance _____Time _____
   Reversed direction every _____ minutes
   Time walked without support _____

Stepper: Distance _____Time _____
   Time walked without support _____

Track: Distance _____Time _____
   Speed or pace (if recorded) _____
   Time walked without support _____
   Fastest lap _____
   Fastest lap without support_____

Total Cardio Walking Time:_____
Max. Heart Rate Noted:_____

RECOVERY BASICS:

☐ **Were physical exercise targets (time and total no. of reps) met?**
☐ **Did I focus well on exercises?**
☐ **Did I work intensively + aggressively?**
☐ **Did I push myself to increase difficulty?**

RECOVERY PLAN: _____

Week No. _____ Day No.:_____

Exercises/Drills Done:

_____Time_____
_____Time_____
_____Time_____
_____Time_____
_____Time_____
_____Time_____
_____Time_____
_____Time_____
_____Time_____

Total Time Spent_____

NUTRITION PLAN:

Nutrient-rich foods eaten | quantity:

BREAKFAST:

_____ | _____
_____ | _____
_____ | _____
_____ | _____

Drinks:_____
LUNCH:

_____ | _____
_____ | _____
_____ | _____
_____ | _____
_____ | _____

Drinks:_____
Snacks:_____

DINNER:

_____ | _____
_____ | _____
_____ | _____
_____ | _____
_____ | _____
_____ | _____

Drinks:_____
Snacks:_____

RECOVERY PLAN: _____

Week No. _____ Day No.:_____

Exercises/Drills Done:

_____Time_____
_____Time_____
_____Time_____
_____Time_____
_____Time_____
_____Time_____
_____Time_____
_____Time_____
_____Time_____

Total Time Spent_____

SUPPLEMENTS TAKEN:

_____ | _____
_____ | _____
_____ | _____
_____ | _____
_____ | _____

Supplements I Need to Buy:

_____ | _____
_____ | _____

MEDICINES TAKEN:

_____ | _____
_____ | _____
_____ | _____
_____ | _____
_____ | _____
_____ | _____

YOGA TRAINING:

Exercises:_____
_____
_____
_____
_____

Total Yoga Time: _____
Notes:_____

NOTES, SUCCESSES, BREAKTHROUGHS, PROGRESS!

_____
_____
_____
_____
_____

Daily Worksheet

Day of the Week:	Date:	Day No.	Max. Heart Rate:	A.M. Weight:	A.M. Blood Pressure: _____ OVER _____

Glasses of water drunk today (check): ○ ○ ○ ○ ○ ○ ○ ○

WALKING Plan No. _____

Week No.:_____ Day No.:_____

CORE WORK:
Total Time _____

RESISTANCE TRAINING:
1) Machine/Exerc._____
 Weight_____ Reps _____/_____/_____
2) Machine/Exerc._____
 Weight_____ Reps _____/_____/_____
3) Machine/Exerc._____
 Weight_____ Reps _____/_____/_____
4) Machine/Exerc._____
 Weight_____ Reps _____/_____/_____
5) Machine/Exerc._____
 Weight_____ Reps _____/_____/_____
6) Machine/Exerc._____
 Weight_____ Reps _____/_____/_____
7) Machine/Exerc._____
 Weight_____ Reps _____/_____/_____
8) Machine/Exerc._____
 Weight_____ Reps _____/_____/_____
Resistance Tr. Total Time_____

CARDIO WALKING:
Treadmill: Distance _____
 Time _____ Speed _____
 Time walked without support _____
Elliptical: Distance _____Time _____
 Reversed direction every _____ minutes
 Time walked without support _____
Stepper: Distance _____Time _____
 Time walked without support _____
Track: Distance _____Time _____
 Speed or pace (if recorded) _____
 Time walked without support _____
 Fastest lap _____
 Fastest lap without support_____
Total Cardio Walking Time:_____
Max. Heart Rate Noted:_____

RECOVERY BASICS:
☐ **Were physical exercise targets (time and total no. of reps) met?**
☐ **Did I focus well on exercises?**
☐ **Did I work intensively + aggressively?**
☐ **Did I push myself to increase difficulty?**

RECOVERY PLAN: _____

Week No. _____ Day No.:_____

Exercises/Drills Done:
_____Time_____
_____Time_____
_____Time_____
_____Time_____
_____Time_____
_____Time_____
_____Time_____
_____Time_____
Total Time Spent_____

NUTRITION PLAN:
Nutrient-rich foods eaten | quantity:
BREAKFAST:
_____ | _____
_____ | _____
_____ | _____
_____ | _____
Drinks:_____
LUNCH:
_____ | _____
_____ | _____
_____ | _____
_____ | _____
_____ | _____
Drinks:_____
Snacks:_____
DINNER:
_____ | _____
_____ | _____
_____ | _____
_____ | _____
_____ | _____
_____ | _____
Drinks:_____
Snacks:_____

RECOVERY PLAN: _____

Week No. _____ Day No.:_____

Exercises/Drills Done:
_____Time_____
_____Time_____
_____Time_____
_____Time_____
_____Time_____
_____Time_____
_____Time_____
_____Time_____
Total Time Spent_____

SUPPLEMENTS TAKEN:
_____ | _____
_____ | _____
_____ | _____
_____ | _____
_____ | _____
Supplements I Need to Buy:
_____ | _____
_____ | _____

MEDICINES TAKEN:
_____ | _____
_____ | _____
_____ | _____
_____ | _____
_____ | _____

YOGA TRAINING:
Exercises:_____
_____
_____
_____
_____
_____
Total Yoga Time: _____
Notes:_____

NOTES, SUCCESSES, BREAKTHROUGHS, PROGRESS!
_____
_____
_____
_____
_____

Daily Worksheet

Day of the Week:	Date:	Day No.	Max. Heart Rate:	A.M. Weight:	A.M. Blood Pressure: _____ OVER _____

Glasses of water drunk today (check): ◯ ◯ ◯ ◯ ◯ ◯ ◯ ◯

WALKING Plan No. _____

Week No.:_____ Day No.:_____

CORE WORK:

Total Time _____

RESISTANCE TRAINING:

1) Machine/Exerc._____

Weight_____ Reps _____/_____/_____

2) Machine/Exerc._____

Weight_____ Reps _____/_____/_____

3) Machine/Exerc._____

Weight_____ Reps _____/_____/_____

4) Machine/Exerc._____

Weight_____ Reps _____/_____/_____

5) Machine/Exerc._____

Weight_____ Reps _____/_____/_____

6) Machine/Exerc._____

Weight_____ Reps _____/_____/_____

7) Machine/Exerc._____

Weight_____ Reps _____/_____/_____

8) Machine/Exerc._____

Weight_____ Reps _____/_____/_____

Resistance Tr. Total Time_____

CARDIO WALKING:

Treadmill: Distance _____

Time _____ Speed _____

Time walked without support _____

Elliptical: Distance _____Time _____

Reversed direction every _____ minutes

Time walked without support _____

Stepper: Distance _____Time _____

Time walked without support _____

Track: Distance _____Time _____

Speed or pace (if recorded) _____

Time walked without support _____

Fastest lap _____

Fastest lap without support_____

Total Cardio Walking Time:_____

Max. Heart Rate Noted:_____

RECOVERY BASICS:

☐ **Were physical exercise targets (time and total no. of reps) met?**

☐ **Did I focus well on exercises?**

☐ **Did I work intensively + aggressively?**

☐ **Did I push myself to increase difficulty?**

RECOVERY PLAN: _____

Week No. _____ Day No.:_____

Exercises/Drills Done:

_____Time_____

_____Time_____

_____Time_____

_____Time_____

_____Time_____

_____Time_____

_____Time_____

_____Time_____

_____Time_____

_____Time_____

Total Time Spent_____

NUTRITION PLAN:

Nutrient-rich foods eaten | quantity:

BREAKFAST:

_____ | _____

_____ | _____

_____ | _____

_____ | _____

Drinks:_____

LUNCH:

_____ | _____

_____ | _____

_____ | _____

_____ | _____

_____ | _____

Drinks:_____

Snacks:_____

DINNER:

_____ | _____

_____ | _____

_____ | _____

_____ | _____

_____ | _____

_____ | _____

Drinks:_____

Snacks:_____

RECOVERY PLAN: _____

Week No. _____ Day No.:_____

Exercises/Drills Done:

_____Time_____

_____Time_____

_____Time_____

_____Time_____

_____Time_____

_____Time_____

_____Time_____

_____Time_____

_____Time_____

Total Time Spent_____

SUPPLEMENTS TAKEN:

_____ | _____

_____ | _____

_____ | _____

_____ | _____

_____ | _____

_____ | _____

Supplements I Need to Buy:

_____ | _____

_____ | _____

MEDICINES TAKEN:

_____ | _____

_____ | _____

_____ | _____

_____ | _____

_____ | _____

_____ | _____

YOGA TRAINING:

Exercises:_____

_____

_____

_____

_____

Total Yoga Time: _____

Notes:_____

NOTES, SUCCESSES, BREAKTHROUGHS, PROGRESS!

_____

_____

_____

_____

_____

Daily Worksheet

Day of the Week:	Date:	Day No.	Max. Heart Rate:	A.M. Weight:	A.M. Blood Pressure: _____ OVER _____

Glasses of water drunk today (check): ○ ○ ○ ○ ○ ○ ○ ○

WALKING Plan No. _____

Week No.:_____ Day No.:_____

CORE WORK:
Total Time _____

RESISTANCE TRAINING:
1) Machine/Exerc._____
   Weight_____ Reps _____/_____/_____
2) Machine/Exerc._____
   Weight_____ Reps _____/_____/_____
3) Machine/Exerc._____
   Weight_____ Reps _____/_____/_____
4) Machine/Exerc._____
   Weight_____ Reps _____/_____/_____
5) Machine/Exerc._____
   Weight_____ Reps _____/_____/_____
6) Machine/Exerc._____
   Weight_____ Reps _____/_____/_____
7) Machine/Exerc._____
   Weight_____ Reps _____/_____/_____
8) Machine/Exerc._____
   Weight_____ Reps _____/_____/_____
Resistance Tr. Total Time_____

CARDIO WALKING:
Treadmill: Distance _____
   Time _____ Speed _____
   Time walked without support _____
Elliptical: Distance _____Time _____
   Reversed direction every _____ minutes
   Time walked without support _____
Stepper: Distance _____Time _____
   Time walked without support _____
Track: Distance _____Time _____
   Speed or pace (if recorded) _____
   Time walked without support _____
   Fastest lap _____
   Fastest lap without support_____
Total Cardio Walking Time:_____
Max. Heart Rate Noted:_____

RECOVERY BASICS:
☐ **Were physical exercise targets (time and total no. of reps) met?**
☐ **Did I focus well on exercises?**
☐ **Did I work intensively + aggressively?**
☐ **Did I push myself to increase difficulty?**

RECOVERY PLAN: _____

Week No. _____ Day No.:_____

Exercises/Drills Done:
_____Time_____
_____Time_____
_____Time_____
_____Time_____
_____Time_____
_____Time_____
_____Time_____
_____Time_____
_____Time_____
_____Time_____
Total Time Spent_____

NUTRITION PLAN:
Nutrient-rich foods eaten | quantity:
BREAKFAST:
_____ | _____
_____ | _____
_____ | _____
_____ | _____
_____ | _____
Drinks:_____
LUNCH:
_____ | _____
_____ | _____
_____ | _____
_____ | _____
_____ | _____
Drinks:_____
Snacks:_____
DINNER:
_____ | _____
_____ | _____
_____ | _____
_____ | _____
_____ | _____
_____ | _____
Drinks:_____
Snacks:_____

NOTES, SUCCESSES, BREAKTHROUGHS, PROGRESS!
_____
_____
_____
_____
_____

RECOVERY PLAN: _____

Week No. _____ Day No.:_____

Exercises/Drills Done:
_____Time_____
_____Time_____
_____Time_____
_____Time_____
_____Time_____
_____Time_____
_____Time_____
_____Time_____
_____Time_____
Total Time Spent_____

SUPPLEMENTS TAKEN:
_____ | _____
_____ | _____
_____ | _____
_____ | _____
_____ | _____
_____ | _____
Supplements I Need to Buy:
_____ | _____
_____ | _____

MEDICINES TAKEN:
_____ | _____
_____ | _____
_____ | _____
_____ | _____
_____ | _____
_____ | _____
_____ | _____

YOGA TRAINING:
Exercises:_____
_____
_____
_____
_____
Total Yoga Time: _____
Notes:_____

Daily Worksheet

Day of the Week:	Date:	Day No.	Max. Heart Rate:	A.M. Weight:	A.M. Blood Pressure: _____ OVER _____

Glasses of water drunk today (check): ○ ○ ○ ○ ○ ○ ○ ○

WALKING Plan No. _____

Week No.:_____ Day No.:_____

CORE WORK:

Total Time _____

RESISTANCE TRAINING:

1) Machine/Exerc._____

Weight_____ Reps _____/_____/_____

2) Machine/Exerc._____

Weight_____ Reps _____/_____/_____

3) Machine/Exerc._____

Weight_____ Reps _____/_____/_____

4) Machine/Exerc._____

Weight_____ Reps _____/_____/_____

5) Machine/Exerc._____

Weight_____ Reps _____/_____/_____

6) Machine/Exerc._____

Weight_____ Reps _____/_____/_____

7) Machine/Exerc._____

Weight_____ Reps _____/_____/_____

8) Machine/Exerc._____

Weight_____ Reps _____/_____/_____

Resistance Tr. Total Time_____

CARDIO WALKING:

Treadmill: Distance _____

Time _____ Speed _____

Time walked without support _____

Elliptical: Distance _____Time _____

Reversed direction every _____ minutes

Time walked without support _____

Stepper: Distance _____Time _____

Time walked without support _____

Track: Distance _____Time _____

Speed or pace (if recorded) _____

Time walked without support _____

Fastest lap _____

Fastest lap without support_____

Total Cardio Walking Time:_____

Max. Heart Rate Noted:_____

RECOVERY BASICS:

☐ **Were physical exercise targets (time and total no. of reps) met?**

☐ **Did I focus well on exercises?**

☐ **Did I work intensively + aggressively?**

☐ **Did I push myself to increase difficulty?**

RECOVERY PLAN: _____

Week No. _____ Day No.:_____

Exercises/Drills Done:

_____Time_____

_____Time_____

_____Time_____

_____Time_____

_____Time_____

_____Time_____

_____Time_____

_____Time_____

_____Time_____

Total Time Spent_____

NUTRITION PLAN:

Nutrient-rich foods eaten | quantity:

BREAKFAST:

_____ | _____

_____ | _____

_____ | _____

_____ | _____

Drinks:_____

LUNCH:

_____ | _____

_____ | _____

_____ | _____

_____ | _____

_____ | _____

Drinks:_____

Snacks:_____

DINNER:

_____ | _____

_____ | _____

_____ | _____

_____ | _____

_____ | _____

_____ | _____

Drinks:_____

Snacks:_____

NOTES, SUCCESSES, BREAKTHROUGHS, PROGRESS!

_____

_____

_____

_____

_____

RECOVERY PLAN: _____

Week No. _____ Day No.:_____

Exercises/Drills Done:

_____Time_____

_____Time_____

_____Time_____

_____Time_____

_____Time_____

_____Time_____

_____Time_____

_____Time_____

_____Time_____

Total Time Spent_____

SUPPLEMENTS TAKEN:

_____ | _____

_____ | _____

_____ | _____

_____ | _____

_____ | _____

_____ | _____

Supplements I Need to Buy:

_____ | _____

_____ | _____

MEDICINES TAKEN:

_____ | _____

_____ | _____

_____ | _____

_____ | _____

_____ | _____

_____ | _____

YOGA TRAINING:

Exercises:_____

_____

_____

_____

_____

Total Yoga Time: _____

Notes:_____

Daily Worksheet

Day of the Week:	Date:	Day No.	Max. Heart Rate:	A.M. Weight:	A.M. Blood Pressure: _____ OVER _____

Glasses of water drunk today (check): ○ ○ ○ ○ ○ ○ ○ ○

WALKING Plan No. _____

Week No.:_____ Day No.:_____

CORE WORK:

Total Time _____

RESISTANCE TRAINING:

1) Machine/Exerc._____

   Weight_____ Reps _____/_____/_____

2) Machine/Exerc._____

   Weight_____ Reps _____/_____/_____

3) Machine/Exerc._____

   Weight_____ Reps _____/_____/_____

4) Machine/Exerc._____

   Weight_____ Reps _____/_____/_____

5) Machine/Exerc._____

   Weight_____ Reps _____/_____/_____

6) Machine/Exerc._____

   Weight_____ Reps _____/_____/_____

7) Machine/Exerc._____

   Weight_____ Reps _____/_____/_____

8) Machine/Exerc._____

   Weight_____ Reps _____/_____/_____

Resistance Tr. Total Time_____

CARDIO WALKING:

Treadmill: Distance _____

   Time _____ Speed _____

   Time walked without support _____

Elliptical: Distance _____Time _____

   Reversed direction every _____ minutes

   Time walked without support _____

Stepper: Distance _____Time _____

   Time walked without support _____

Track: Distance _____Time _____

   Speed or pace (if recorded) _____

   Time walked without support _____

   Fastest lap _____

   Fastest lap without support_____

Total Cardio Walking Time:_____

Max. Heart Rate Noted:_____

RECOVERY PLAN: _____

Week No. _____ Day No.:_____

Exercises/Drills Done:

_____Time_____
_____Time_____
_____Time_____
_____Time_____
_____Time_____
_____Time_____
_____Time_____
_____Time_____
_____Time_____

Total Time Spent_____

NUTRITION PLAN:

Nutrient-rich foods eaten | quantity:

BREAKFAST:

_____ | _____
_____ | _____
_____ | _____
_____ | _____

Drinks:_____

LUNCH:

_____ | _____
_____ | _____
_____ | _____
_____ | _____
_____ | _____
_____ | _____

Drinks:_____
Snacks:_____

DINNER:

_____ | _____
_____ | _____
_____ | _____
_____ | _____
_____ | _____
_____ | _____

Drinks:_____
Snacks:_____

RECOVERY PLAN: _____

Week No. _____ Day No.:_____

Exercises/Drills Done:

_____Time_____
_____Time_____
_____Time_____
_____Time_____
_____Time_____
_____Time_____
_____Time_____
_____Time_____

Total Time Spent_____

SUPPLEMENTS TAKEN:

_____ | _____
_____ | _____
_____ | _____
_____ | _____
_____ | _____

Supplements I Need to Buy:

_____ | _____
_____ | _____

MEDICINES TAKEN:

_____ | _____
_____ | _____
_____ | _____
_____ | _____
_____ | _____

YOGA TRAINING:

Exercises:_____
_____
_____
_____
_____

Total Yoga Time: _____

Notes:_____

RECOVERY BASICS:

☐ **Were physical exercise targets (time and total no. of reps) met?**
☐ **Did I focus well on exercises?**
☐ **Did I work intensively + aggressively?**
☐ **Did I push myself to increase difficulty?**

NOTES, SUCCESSES, BREAKTHROUGHS, PROGRESS!

_____
_____
_____
_____
_____

Start of Week Worksheet—Week No. 10

Date: Week Beginning Monday, _____, 20___

Take some quiet time for yourself every day to enjoy the "stillness." You can meditate, listen to a relaxation CD, enjoy a beautiful view or vista, pray, sit mindfully, or whatever else you find helps rejuvenate your mind and spirit.

Kathy Maxwell

Start of Week Statistics:

MEASUREMENTS—MEN:	MEASUREMENTS—WOMEN:	WEIGHT: _____
Waist:_____ Chest:_____	Waist:_____ Hips:_____	BLOOD PRESSURE:
Upper Leg: ___ Upper Arm:____	Upper Leg: ___ Upper Arm:___	_____ over _____

Fill out the following information to guide you during the coming week.

Last week's successes and progress:_____

_____

_____

How well I am physically functioning right now: _____

_____

_____

Goals and expectations for this week:_____

_____

_____

Skills or exercises I want to especially focus on improving this week:_____

_____

_____

Shopping List: brain nutrient foods to add to diet this week:

_____   _____

_____   _____

If my weight or blood pressure are high, plan to reduce them (current/continuing):

_____

255

Daily Worksheet

Day of the Week:	Date:	Day No.	Max. Heart Rate:	A.M. Weight:	A.M. Blood Pressure: _____ OVER _____

Glasses of water drunk today (check): ○ ○ ○ ○ ○ ○ ○ ○

WALKING Plan No. _____

Week No.:_____ Day No.:_____

CORE WORK:
Total Time _____

RESISTANCE TRAINING:
1) Machine/Exerc._____
  Weight_____ Reps _____/_____/_____
2) Machine/Exerc._____
  Weight_____ Reps _____/_____/_____
3) Machine/Exerc._____
  Weight_____ Reps _____/_____/_____
4) Machine/Exerc._____
  Weight_____ Reps _____/_____/_____
5) Machine/Exerc._____
  Weight_____ Reps _____/_____/_____
6) Machine/Exerc._____
  Weight_____ Reps _____/_____/_____
7) Machine/Exerc._____
  Weight_____ Reps _____/_____/_____
8) Machine/Exerc._____
  Weight_____ Reps _____/_____/_____
Resistance Tr. Total Time_____

CARDIO WALKING:
Treadmill: Distance _____
  Time _____ Speed _____
  Time walked without support _____
Elliptical: Distance _____Time _____
  Reversed direction every _____ minutes
  Time walked without support _____
Stepper: Distance _____Time _____
  Time walked without support _____
Track: Distance _____Time _____
  Speed or pace (if recorded) _____
  Time walked without support _____
  Fastest lap _____
  Fastest lap without support_____
Total Cardio Walking Time:_____
Max. Heart Rate Noted:_____

RECOVERY BASICS:
☐ **Were physical exercise targets (time and total no. of reps) met?**
☐ **Did I focus well on exercises?**
☐ **Did I work intensively + aggressively?**
☐ **Did I push myself to increase difficulty?**

RECOVERY PLAN: _____

Week No. _____ Day No.:_____

Exercises/Drills Done:
_____Time_____
_____Time_____
_____Time_____
_____Time_____
_____Time_____
_____Time_____
_____Time_____
_____Time_____
_____Time_____
_____Time_____
Total Time Spent_____

NUTRITION PLAN:
Nutrient-rich foods eaten | quantity:
BREAKFAST:
_____ | _____
_____ | _____
_____ | _____
_____ | _____
_____ | _____
Drinks:_____
LUNCH:
_____ | _____
_____ | _____
_____ | _____
_____ | _____
_____ | _____
Drinks:_____
Snacks:_____
DINNER:
_____ | _____
_____ | _____
_____ | _____
_____ | _____
_____ | _____
_____ | _____
Drinks:_____
Snacks:_____

RECOVERY PLAN: _____

Week No. _____ Day No.:_____

Exercises/Drills Done:
_____Time_____
_____Time_____
_____Time_____
_____Time_____
_____Time_____
_____Time_____
_____Time_____
_____Time_____
_____Time_____
_____Time_____
Total Time Spent_____

SUPPLEMENTS TAKEN:
_____ | _____
_____ | _____
_____ | _____
_____ | _____
_____ | _____
Supplements I Need to Buy:
_____ | _____
_____ | _____

MEDICINES TAKEN:
_____ | _____
_____ | _____
_____ | _____
_____ | _____
_____ | _____

YOGA TRAINING:
Exercises:_____
_____
_____
_____
_____
_____
Total Yoga Time: _____
Notes:_____

NOTES, SUCCESSES, BREAKTHROUGHS, PROGRESS!
_____
_____
_____
_____
_____
_____

Daily Worksheet

Day of the Week:	Date:	Day No.	Max. Heart Rate:	A.M. Weight:	A.M. Blood Pressure: _____ OVER _____

Glasses of water drunk today (check): ○ ○ ○ ○ ○ ○ ○ ○

WALKING Plan No. _____
Week No.:_____ Day No.:_____

CORE WORK:
Total Time _____

RESISTANCE TRAINING:
1) Machine/Exerc._____
   Weight_____ Reps _____/_____/_____
2) Machine/Exerc._____
   Weight_____ Reps _____/_____/_____
3) Machine/Exerc._____
   Weight_____ Reps _____/_____/_____
4) Machine/Exerc._____
   Weight_____ Reps _____/_____/_____
5) Machine/Exerc._____
   Weight_____ Reps _____/_____/_____
6) Machine/Exerc._____
   Weight_____ Reps _____/_____/_____
7) Machine/Exerc._____
   Weight_____ Reps _____/_____/_____
8) Machine/Exerc._____
   Weight_____ Reps _____/_____/_____
Resistance Tr. Total Time_____

CARDIO WALKING:
Treadmill: Distance _____
   Time _____ Speed _____
   Time walked without support _____
Elliptical: Distance _____Time _____
   Reversed direction every _____ minutes
   Time walked without support _____
Stepper: Distance _____Time _____
   Time walked without support _____
Track: Distance _____Time _____
   Speed or pace (if recorded) _____
   Time walked without support _____
   Fastest lap _____
   Fastest lap without support_____
Total Cardio Walking Time:_____
Max. Heart Rate Noted:_____

RECOVERY BASICS:
☐ Were physical exercise targets (time and total no. of reps) met?
☐ Did I focus well on exercises?
☐ Did I work intensively + aggressively?
☐ Did I push myself to increase difficulty?

RECOVERY PLAN: _____
Week No. _____ Day No.:_____

Exercises/Drills Done:
_____Time_____
_____Time_____
_____Time_____
_____Time_____
_____Time_____
_____Time_____
_____Time_____
_____Time_____
_____Time_____
_____Time_____
Total Time Spent_____

NUTRITION PLAN:
Nutrient-rich foods eaten | quantity:
BREAKFAST:
_____ | _____
_____ | _____
_____ | _____
_____ | _____
Drinks:_____
LUNCH:
_____ | _____
_____ | _____
_____ | _____
_____ | _____
_____ | _____
Drinks:_____
Snacks:_____

DINNER:
_____ | _____
_____ | _____
_____ | _____
_____ | _____
_____ | _____
Drinks:_____
Snacks:_____

RECOVERY PLAN: _____
Week No. _____ Day No.:_____

Exercises/Drills Done:
_____Time_____
_____Time_____
_____Time_____
_____Time_____
_____Time_____
_____Time_____
_____Time_____
_____Time_____
_____Time_____
Total Time Spent_____

SUPPLEMENTS TAKEN:
_____ | _____
_____ | _____
_____ | _____
_____ | _____
_____ | _____
_____ | _____
Supplements I Need to Buy:
_____ | _____
_____ | _____

MEDICINES TAKEN:
_____ | _____
_____ | _____
_____ | _____
_____ | _____
_____ | _____
_____ | _____

YOGA TRAINING:
Exercises:_____
_____
_____
_____
_____
Total Yoga Time: _____
Notes:_____

NOTES, SUCCESSES, BREAKTHROUGHS, PROGRESS!
_____
_____
_____
_____
_____

Daily Worksheet

Day of the Week:	Date:	Day No.	Max. Heart Rate:	A.M. Weight:	A.M. Blood Pressure: _____ OVER _____

Glasses of water drunk today (check): ○ ○ ○ ○ ○ ○ ○ ○

WALKING Plan No. _____

Week No.:_____ **Day No.:**_____

CORE WORK:

Total Time _____

RESISTANCE TRAINING:

1) Machine/Exerc._____

Weight_____ Reps _____/_____/_____

2) Machine/Exerc._____

Weight_____ Reps _____/_____/_____

3) Machine/Exerc._____

Weight_____ Reps _____/_____/_____

4) Machine/Exerc._____

Weight_____ Reps _____/_____/_____

5) Machine/Exerc._____

Weight_____ Reps _____/_____/_____

6) Machine/Exerc._____

Weight_____ Reps _____/_____/_____

7) Machine/Exerc._____

Weight_____ Reps _____/_____/_____

8) Machine/Exerc._____

Weight_____ Reps _____/_____/_____

Resistance Tr. Total Time_____

CARDIO WALKING:

Treadmill: Distance _____

Time _____ Speed _____

Time walked without support _____

Elliptical: Distance _____Time _____

Reversed direction every _____ minutes

Time walked without support _____

Stepper: Distance _____Time _____

Time walked without support _____

Track: Distance _____Time _____

Speed or pace (if recorded) _____

Time walked without support _____

Fastest lap _____

Fastest lap without support_____

Total Cardio Walking Time:_____

Max. Heart Rate Noted:_____

RECOVERY PLAN: _____

Week No. _____ **Day No.:**_____

Exercises/Drills Done:

_____Time_____

_____Time_____

_____Time_____

_____Time_____

_____Time_____

_____Time_____

_____Time_____

_____Time_____

_____Time_____

Total Time Spent_____

NUTRITION PLAN:

Nutrient-rich foods eaten | quantity:

BREAKFAST:

_____ | _____

_____ | _____

_____ | _____

_____ | _____

Drinks:_____

LUNCH:

_____ | _____

_____ | _____

_____ | _____

_____ | _____

_____ | _____

Drinks:_____

Snacks:_____

DINNER:

_____ | _____

_____ | _____

_____ | _____

_____ | _____

_____ | _____

_____ | _____

Drinks:_____

Snacks:_____

RECOVERY PLAN: _____

Week No. _____ **Day No.:**_____

Exercises/Drills Done:

_____Time_____

_____Time_____

_____Time_____

_____Time_____

_____Time_____

_____Time_____

_____Time_____

_____Time_____

_____Time_____

Total Time Spent_____

SUPPLEMENTS TAKEN:

_____ | _____

_____ | _____

_____ | _____

_____ | _____

_____ | _____

Supplements I Need to Buy:

_____ | _____

_____ | _____

MEDICINES TAKEN:

_____ | _____

_____ | _____

_____ | _____

_____ | _____

_____ | _____

_____ | _____

YOGA TRAINING:

Exercises:_____

_____

_____

_____

_____

Total Yoga Time: _____

Notes:_____

RECOVERY BASICS:

☐ **Were physical exercise targets (time and total no. of reps) met?**

☐ **Did I focus well on exercises?**

☐ **Did I work intensively + aggressively?**

☐ **Did I push myself to increase difficulty?**

NOTES, SUCCESSES, BREAKTHROUGHS, PROGRESS!

_____

_____

_____

_____

_____

Daily Worksheet

Day of the Week:	Date:	Day No.	Max. Heart Rate:	A.M. Weight:	A.M. Blood Pressure: _____ OVER _____

Glasses of water drunk today (check): ○ ○ ○ ○ ○ ○ ○ ○

WALKING Plan No. _____
Week No.:_____ Day No.:_____

CORE WORK:
Total Time _____

RESISTANCE TRAINING:
1) Machine/Exerc._____
   Weight_____ Reps _____/_____/_____
2) Machine/Exerc._____
   Weight_____ Reps _____/_____/_____
3) Machine/Exerc._____
   Weight_____ Reps _____/_____/_____
4) Machine/Exerc._____
   Weight_____ Reps _____/_____/_____
5) Machine/Exerc._____
   Weight_____ Reps _____/_____/_____
6) Machine/Exerc._____
   Weight_____ Reps _____/_____/_____
7) Machine/Exerc._____
   Weight_____ Reps _____/_____/_____
8) Machine/Exerc._____
   Weight_____ Reps _____/_____/_____
Resistance Tr. Total Time_____

CARDIO WALKING:
Treadmill: Distance _____
   Time _____ Speed _____
   Time walked without support _____
Elliptical: Distance _____Time _____
   Reversed direction every _____ minutes
   Time walked without support _____
Stepper: Distance _____Time _____
   Time walked without support _____
Track: Distance _____Time _____
   Speed or pace (if recorded) _____
   Time walked without support _____
   Fastest lap _____
   Fastest lap without support_____
Total Cardio Walking Time:_____
Max. Heart Rate Noted:_____

RECOVERY PLAN: _____
Week No. _____ Day No.:_____

Exercises/Drills Done:
_____Time_____
_____Time_____
_____Time_____
_____Time_____
_____Time_____
_____Time_____
_____Time_____
_____Time_____
_____Time_____
_____Time_____
Total Time Spent_____

NUTRITION PLAN:
Nutrient-rich foods eaten | quantity:
BREAKFAST:
_____ | _____
_____ | _____
_____ | _____
_____ | _____
Drinks:_____
LUNCH:
_____ | _____
_____ | _____
_____ | _____
_____ | _____
_____ | _____
_____ | _____
Drinks:_____
Snacks:_____

DINNER:
_____ | _____
_____ | _____
_____ | _____
_____ | _____
_____ | _____
_____ | _____
Drinks:_____
Snacks:_____

RECOVERY PLAN: _____
Week No. _____ Day No.:_____

Exercises/Drills Done:
_____Time_____
_____Time_____
_____Time_____
_____Time_____
_____Time_____
_____Time_____
_____Time_____
_____Time_____
_____Time_____
Total Time Spent_____

SUPPLEMENTS TAKEN:
_____ | _____
_____ | _____
_____ | _____
_____ | _____
_____ | _____
_____ | _____
Supplements I Need to Buy:
_____ | _____
_____ | _____

MEDICINES TAKEN:
_____ | _____
_____ | _____
_____ | _____
_____ | _____
_____ | _____
_____ | _____

YOGA TRAINING:
Exercises:_____
_____
_____
_____
Total Yoga Time: _____
Notes:_____

RECOVERY BASICS:
☐ **Were physical exercise targets (time and total no. of reps) met?**
☐ **Did I focus well on exercises?**
☐ **Did I work intensively + aggressively?**
☐ **Did I push myself to increase difficulty?**

NOTES, SUCCESSES, BREAKTHROUGHS, PROGRESS!
_____
_____
_____
_____
_____

Daily Worksheet

Day of the Week:	Date:	Day No.	Max. Heart Rate:	A.M. Weight:	A.M. Blood Pressure: _____ OVER _____

Glasses of water drunk today (check): ○ ○ ○ ○ ○ ○ ○ ○

WALKING Plan No. _____

Week No.:_____ Day No.:_____

CORE WORK:

Total Time _____

RESISTANCE TRAINING:

1) **Machine/Exerc.**_____
   Weight_____ Reps _____/_____/_____
2) **Machine/Exerc.**_____
   Weight_____ Reps _____/_____/_____
3) **Machine/Exerc.**_____
   Weight_____ Reps _____/_____/_____
4) **Machine/Exerc.**_____
   Weight_____ Reps _____/_____/_____
5) **Machine/Exerc.**_____
   Weight_____ Reps _____/_____/_____
6) **Machine/Exerc.**_____
   Weight_____ Reps _____/_____/_____
7) **Machine/Exerc.**_____
   Weight_____ Reps _____/_____/_____
8) **Machine/Exerc.**_____
   Weight_____ Reps _____/_____/_____

Resistance Tr. Total Time_____

CARDIO WALKING:

Treadmill: Distance _____
   Time _____ Speed _____
   Time walked without support _____
Elliptical: Distance _____Time _____
   Reversed direction every _____ minutes
   Time walked without support _____
Stepper: Distance _____Time _____
   Time walked without support _____
Track: Distance _____Time _____
   Speed or pace (if recorded) _____
   Time walked without support _____
   Fastest lap _____
   Fastest lap without support_____

Total Cardio Walking Time:_____
Max. Heart Rate Noted:_____

RECOVERY BASICS:
☐ **Were physical exercise targets (time and total no. of reps) met?**
☐ **Did I focus well on exercises?**
☐ **Did I work intensively + aggressively?**
☐ **Did I push myself to increase difficulty?**

RECOVERY PLAN: _____

Week No. _____ Day No.:_____

Exercises/Drills Done:

_____Time_____
_____Time_____
_____Time_____
_____Time_____
_____Time_____
_____Time_____
_____Time_____
_____Time_____
_____Time_____

Total Time Spent_____

NUTRITION PLAN:

Nutrient-rich foods eaten | quantity:
BREAKFAST:

_____ | _____
_____ | _____
_____ | _____
_____ | _____

Drinks:_____
LUNCH:

_____ | _____
_____ | _____
_____ | _____
_____ | _____
_____ | _____
_____ | _____

Drinks:_____
Snacks:_____

DINNER:

_____ | _____
_____ | _____
_____ | _____
_____ | _____
_____ | _____
_____ | _____

Drinks:_____
Snacks:_____

RECOVERY PLAN: _____

Week No. _____ Day No.:_____

Exercises/Drills Done:

_____Time_____
_____Time_____
_____Time_____
_____Time_____
_____Time_____
_____Time_____
_____Time_____
_____Time_____
_____Time_____

Total Time Spent_____

SUPPLEMENTS TAKEN:

_____ | _____
_____ | _____
_____ | _____
_____ | _____
_____ | _____

Supplements I Need to Buy:

_____ | _____
_____ | _____

MEDICINES TAKEN:

_____ | _____
_____ | _____
_____ | _____
_____ | _____
_____ | _____
_____ | _____

YOGA TRAINING:

Exercises:_____
_____
_____
_____
_____
_____

Total Yoga Time: _____
Notes:_____

NOTES, SUCCESSES, BREAKTHROUGHS, PROGRESS!

_____
_____
_____
_____
_____
_____

Daily Worksheet

Day of the Week:	Date:	Day No.	Max. Heart Rate:	A.M. Weight:	A.M. Blood Pressure: _____ OVER _____

Glasses of water drunk today (check): ○ ○ ○ ○ ○ ○ ○ ○

WALKING Plan No. _____

Week No.:_____ Day No.:_____

CORE WORK:

Total Time _____

RESISTANCE TRAINING:

1) Machine/Exerc. _____
   Weight_____ Reps _____/_____/_____

2) Machine/Exerc. _____
   Weight_____ Reps _____/_____/_____

3) Machine/Exerc. _____
   Weight_____ Reps _____/_____/_____

4) Machine/Exerc. _____
   Weight_____ Reps _____/_____/_____

5) Machine/Exerc. _____
   Weight_____ Reps _____/_____/_____

6) Machine/Exerc. _____
   Weight_____ Reps _____/_____/_____

7) Machine/Exerc. _____
   Weight_____ Reps _____/_____/_____

8) Machine/Exerc. _____
   Weight_____ Reps _____/_____/_____

Resistance Tr. Total Time _____

CARDIO WALKING:

Treadmill: Distance _____
   Time _____ Speed _____
   Time walked without support _____

Elliptical: Distance _____ Time _____
   Reversed direction every _____ minutes
   Time walked without support _____

Stepper: Distance _____ Time _____
   Time walked without support _____

Track: Distance _____ Time _____
   Speed or pace (if recorded) _____
   Time walked without support _____
   Fastest lap _____
   Fastest lap without support _____

Total Cardio Walking Time: _____
Max. Heart Rate Noted: _____

RECOVERY PLAN: _____

Week No. _____ Day No.:_____

Exercises/Drills Done:

_____Time_____
_____Time_____
_____Time_____
_____Time_____
_____Time_____
_____Time_____
_____Time_____
_____Time_____
_____Time_____

Total Time Spent _____

NUTRITION PLAN:

Nutrient-rich foods eaten | quantity:

BREAKFAST:

_____ | _____
_____ | _____
_____ | _____
_____ | _____

Drinks: _____

LUNCH:

_____ | _____
_____ | _____
_____ | _____
_____ | _____
_____ | _____

Drinks: _____
Snacks: _____

DINNER:

_____ | _____
_____ | _____
_____ | _____
_____ | _____
_____ | _____
_____ | _____

Drinks: _____
Snacks: _____

RECOVERY PLAN: _____

Week No. _____ Day No.:_____

Exercises/Drills Done:

_____Time_____
_____Time_____
_____Time_____
_____Time_____
_____Time_____
_____Time_____
_____Time_____
_____Time_____
_____Time_____

Total Time Spent _____

SUPPLEMENTS TAKEN:

_____ | _____
_____ | _____
_____ | _____
_____ | _____
_____ | _____
_____ | _____

Supplements I Need to Buy:

_____ | _____
_____ | _____

MEDICINES TAKEN:

_____ | _____
_____ | _____
_____ | _____
_____ | _____
_____ | _____
_____ | _____

YOGA TRAINING:

Exercises: _____
_____
_____
_____
_____

Total Yoga Time: _____
Notes: _____

RECOVERY BASICS:

☐ **Were physical exercise targets (time and total no. of reps) met?**
☐ **Did I focus well on exercises?**
☐ **Did I work intensively + aggressively?**
☐ **Did I push myself to increase difficulty?**

NOTES, SUCCESSES, BREAKTHROUGHS, PROGRESS!

_____
_____
_____
_____
_____

Daily Worksheet

Day of the Week:	Date:	Day No.	Max. Heart Rate:	A.M. Weight:	A.M. Blood Pressure: _____ OVER _____

Glasses of water drunk today (check): ○ ○ ○ ○ ○ ○ ○ ○

WALKING Plan No. _____

Week No.:_____   Day No.:_____

CORE WORK:

Total Time _____

RESISTANCE TRAINING:

1) Machine/Exerc._____

   Weight_____ Reps ____/____/____

2) Machine/Exerc._____

   Weight_____ Reps ____/____/____

3) Machine/Exerc._____

   Weight_____ Reps ____/____/____

4) Machine/Exerc._____

   Weight_____ Reps ____/____/____

5) Machine/Exerc._____

   Weight_____ Reps ____/____/____

6) Machine/Exerc._____

   Weight_____ Reps ____/____/____

7) Machine/Exerc._____

   Weight_____ Reps ____/____/____

8) Machine/Exerc._____

   Weight_____ Reps ____/____/____

Resistance Tr. Total Time_____

CARDIO WALKING:

Treadmill: Distance _____

   Time _____ Speed _____

   Time walked without support _____

Elliptical: Distance _____Time _____

   Reversed direction every _____ minutes

   Time walked without support _____

Stepper: Distance _____Time _____

   Time walked without support _____

Track: Distance _____Time _____

   Speed or pace (if recorded) _____

   Time walked without support _____

   Fastest lap _____

   Fastest lap without support_____

Total Cardio Walking Time:_____

Max. Heart Rate Noted:_____

RECOVERY BASICS:

☐ **Were physical exercise targets (time and total no. of reps) met?**

☐ **Did I focus well on exercises?**

☐ **Did I work intensively + aggressively?**

☐ **Did I push myself to increase difficulty?**

RECOVERY PLAN: _____

Week No. _____   Day No.:_____

Exercises/Drills Done:

_____Time_____

_____Time_____

_____Time_____

_____Time_____

_____Time_____

_____Time_____

_____Time_____

_____Time_____

_____Time_____

_____Time_____

Total Time Spent_____

NUTRITION PLAN:

Nutrient-rich foods eaten | quantity:

BREAKFAST:

_____ | _____

_____ | _____

_____ | _____

_____ | _____

Drinks:_____

LUNCH:

_____ | _____

_____ | _____

_____ | _____

_____ | _____

_____ | _____

Drinks:_____

Snacks:_____

DINNER:

_____ | _____

_____ | _____

_____ | _____

_____ | _____

_____ | _____

_____ | _____

Drinks:_____

Snacks:_____

RECOVERY PLAN: _____

Week No. _____   Day No.:_____

Exercises/Drills Done:

_____Time_____

_____Time_____

_____Time_____

_____Time_____

_____Time_____

_____Time_____

_____Time_____

_____Time_____

_____Time_____

Total Time Spent_____

SUPPLEMENTS TAKEN:

_____ | _____

_____ | _____

_____ | _____

_____ | _____

_____ | _____

Supplements I Need to Buy:

_____ | _____

_____ | _____

MEDICINES TAKEN:

_____ | _____

_____ | _____

_____ | _____

_____ | _____

_____ | _____

YOGA TRAINING:

Exercises:_____

_____

_____

_____

_____

Total Yoga Time: _____

Notes:_____

NOTES, SUCCESSES, BREAKTHROUGHS, PROGRESS!

_____

_____

_____

_____

_____

Start of Week Worksheet—Week No. 11

Date: Week Beginning Monday, _____, 20___

Champions understand and believe that their limitations are governed only by their imagination. They perform and practice with a controlled intensity and never allow failure on any given day to take away from their eventual success.

Kirk Mango
from *Becoming a True Champion*

Start of Week Statistics:

MEASUREMENTS—MEN:	MEASUREMENTS—WOMEN:	WEIGHT: _____
Waist:_____ Chest:_____	Waist:_____ Hips:_____	BLOOD PRESSURE:
Upper Leg: ____ Upper Arm:____	Upper Leg: ____ Upper Arm:___	_____ over _____

Fill out the following information to guide you during the coming week.

Last week's successes and progress:_____

_____

_____

How well I am physically functioning right now: _____

_____

_____

Goals and expectations for this week:_____

_____

_____

Skills or exercises I want to especially focus on improving this week:_____

_____

_____

Shopping List: brain nutrient foods to add to diet this week:

_____   _____

_____   _____

If my weight or blood pressure are high, plan to reduce them (current/continuing):

_____

263

Daily Worksheet

Day of the Week:	Date:	Day No.	Max. Heart Rate:	A.M. Weight:	A.M. Blood Pressure: _____ OVER _____

Glasses of water drunk today (check): ○ ○ ○ ○ ○ ○ ○ ○

WALKING Plan No. _____
Week No.: _____ **Day No.:** _____

RECOVERY PLAN: _____
Week No. _____ **Day No.:** _____

RECOVERY PLAN: _____
Week No. _____ **Day No.:** _____

CORE WORK:
Total Time _____

RESISTANCE TRAINING:
1) Machine/Exerc. _____
  Weight_____ Reps _____/_____/_____
2) Machine/Exerc. _____
  Weight_____ Reps _____/_____/_____
3) Machine/Exerc. _____
  Weight_____ Reps _____/_____/_____
4) Machine/Exerc. _____
  Weight_____ Reps _____/_____/_____
5) Machine/Exerc. _____
  Weight_____ Reps _____/_____/_____
6) Machine/Exerc. _____
  Weight_____ Reps _____/_____/_____
7) Machine/Exerc. _____
  Weight_____ Reps _____/_____/_____
8) Machine/Exerc. _____
  Weight_____ Reps _____/_____/_____
Resistance Tr. Total Time _____

CARDIO WALKING:
Treadmill: Distance _____
  Time _____ Speed _____
  Time walked without support _____
Elliptical: Distance _____ Time _____
  Reversed direction every _____ minutes
  Time walked without support _____
Stepper: Distance _____ Time _____
  Time walked without support _____
Track: Distance _____ Time _____
  Speed or pace (if recorded) _____
  Time walked without support _____
  Fastest lap _____
  Fastest lap without support_____
Total Cardio Walking Time: _____
Max. Heart Rate Noted: _____

Exercises/Drills Done:
_____Time_____
_____Time_____
_____Time_____
_____Time_____
_____Time_____
_____Time_____
_____Time_____
_____Time_____
_____Time_____
_____Time_____
Total Time Spent _____

NUTRITION PLAN:
Nutrient-rich foods eaten | quantity:
BREAKFAST:
_____ | _____
_____ | _____
_____ | _____
_____ | _____
Drinks: _____
LUNCH:
_____ | _____
_____ | _____
_____ | _____
_____ | _____
_____ | _____
Drinks: _____
Snacks: _____
DINNER:
_____ | _____
_____ | _____
_____ | _____
_____ | _____
_____ | _____
_____ | _____
Drinks: _____
Snacks: _____

Exercises/Drills Done:
_____Time_____
_____Time_____
_____Time_____
_____Time_____
_____Time_____
_____Time_____
_____Time_____
_____Time_____
_____Time_____
_____Time_____
Total Time Spent _____

SUPPLEMENTS TAKEN:
_____ | _____
_____ | _____
_____ | _____
_____ | _____
_____ | _____
Supplements I Need to Buy:
_____ | _____
_____ | _____

MEDICINES TAKEN:
_____ | _____
_____ | _____
_____ | _____
_____ | _____
_____ | _____
_____ | _____

YOGA TRAINING:
Exercises: _____
_____
_____
_____
_____
Total Yoga Time: _____
Notes: _____

RECOVERY BASICS:
☐ **Were physical exercise targets (time and total no. of reps) met?**
☐ **Did I focus well on exercises?**
☐ **Did I work intensively + aggressively?**
☐ **Did I push myself to increase difficulty?**

NOTES, SUCCESSES, BREAKTHROUGHS, PROGRESS!
_____
_____
_____
_____
_____
_____

Daily Worksheet

Day of the Week:	Date:	Day No.	Max. Heart Rate:	A.M. Weight:	A.M. Blood Pressure: _____ OVER _____

Glasses of water drunk today (check): ○ ○ ○ ○ ○ ○ ○ ○

WALKING Plan No. _____

Week No.:_____ Day No.:_____

CORE WORK:

Total Time _____

RESISTANCE TRAINING:

1) Machine/Exerc._____

   Weight_____ Reps _____/_____/_____

2) Machine/Exerc._____

   Weight_____ Reps _____/_____/_____

3) Machine/Exerc._____

   Weight_____ Reps _____/_____/_____

4) Machine/Exerc._____

   Weight_____ Reps _____/_____/_____

5) Machine/Exerc._____

   Weight_____ Reps _____/_____/_____

6) Machine/Exerc._____

   Weight_____ Reps _____/_____/_____

7) Machine/Exerc._____

   Weight_____ Reps _____/_____/_____

8) Machine/Exerc._____

   Weight_____ Reps _____/_____/_____

Resistance Tr. Total Time_____

CARDIO WALKING:

Treadmill: Distance _____

   Time _____ Speed _____

   Time walked without support _____

Elliptical: Distance _____Time _____

   Reversed direction every _____ minutes

   Time walked without support _____

Stepper: Distance _____Time _____

   Time walked without support _____

Track: Distance _____Time _____

   Speed or pace (if recorded) _____

   Time walked without support _____

   Fastest lap _____

   Fastest lap without support_____

Total Cardio Walking Time:_____

Max. Heart Rate Noted:_____

RECOVERY BASICS:

☐ **Were physical exercise targets (time and total no. of reps) met?**

☐ **Did I focus well on exercises?**

☐ **Did I work intensively + aggressively?**

☐ **Did I push myself to increase difficulty?**

RECOVERY PLAN: _____

Week No. _____ Day No.:_____

Exercises/Drills Done:

_____Time_____

_____Time_____

_____Time_____

_____Time_____

_____Time_____

_____Time_____

_____Time_____

_____Time_____

_____Time_____

_____Time_____

Total Time Spent_____

NUTRITION PLAN:

Nutrient-rich foods eaten | quantity:

BREAKFAST:

_____ | _____

_____ | _____

_____ | _____

_____ | _____

Drinks:_____

LUNCH:

_____ | _____

_____ | _____

_____ | _____

_____ | _____

_____ | _____

Drinks:_____

Snacks:_____

DINNER:

_____ | _____

_____ | _____

_____ | _____

_____ | _____

_____ | _____

Drinks:_____

Snacks:_____

RECOVERY PLAN: _____

Week No. _____ Day No.:_____

Exercises/Drills Done:

_____Time_____

_____Time_____

_____Time_____

_____Time_____

_____Time_____

_____Time_____

_____Time_____

_____Time_____

_____Time_____

_____Time_____

Total Time Spent_____

SUPPLEMENTS TAKEN:

_____ | _____

_____ | _____

_____ | _____

_____ | _____

_____ | _____

Supplements I Need to Buy:

_____ | _____

_____ | _____

MEDICINES TAKEN:

_____ | _____

_____ | _____

_____ | _____

_____ | _____

_____ | _____

_____ | _____

YOGA TRAINING:

Exercises:_____

_____

_____

_____

_____

_____

Total Yoga Time: _____

Notes:_____

NOTES, SUCCESSES, BREAKTHROUGHS, PROGRESS!

_____

_____

_____

_____

_____

Daily Worksheet

Day of the Week:	Date:	Day No.	Max. Heart Rate:	A.M. Weight:	A.M. Blood Pressure: _____ OVER _____

Glasses of water drunk today (check): ○ ○ ○ ○ ○ ○ ○ ○

WALKING Plan No. _____

Week No.: _____ **Day No.:** _____

CORE WORK:

Total Time _____

RESISTANCE TRAINING:

1) Machine/Exerc. _____
   Weight _____ Reps _____/_____/_____
2) Machine/Exerc. _____
   Weight _____ Reps _____/_____/_____
3) Machine/Exerc. _____
   Weight _____ Reps _____/_____/_____
4) Machine/Exerc. _____
   Weight _____ Reps _____/_____/_____
5) Machine/Exerc. _____
   Weight _____ Reps _____/_____/_____
6) Machine/Exerc. _____
   Weight _____ Reps _____/_____/_____
7) Machine/Exerc. _____
   Weight _____ Reps _____/_____/_____
8) Machine/Exerc. _____
   Weight _____ Reps _____/_____/_____

Resistance Tr. Total Time _____

CARDIO WALKING:

Treadmill: Distance _____
   Time _____ Speed _____
   Time walked without support _____
Elliptical: Distance _____ Time _____
   Reversed direction every _____ minutes
   Time walked without support _____
Stepper: Distance _____ Time _____
   Time walked without support _____
Track: Distance _____ Time _____
   Speed or pace (if recorded) _____
   Time walked without support _____
   Fastest lap _____
   Fastest lap without support _____

Total Cardio Walking Time: _____
Max. Heart Rate Noted: _____

RECOVERY BASICS:
☐ **Were physical exercise targets (time and total no. of reps) met?**
☐ **Did I focus well on exercises?**
☐ **Did I work intensively + aggressively?**
☐ **Did I push myself to increase difficulty?**

RECOVERY PLAN: _____

Week No. _____ **Day No.:** _____

Exercises/Drills Done:

_____Time_____
_____Time_____
_____Time_____
_____Time_____
_____Time_____
_____Time_____
_____Time_____
_____Time_____
_____Time_____
_____Time_____

Total Time Spent _____

NUTRITION PLAN:

Nutrient-rich foods eaten | quantity:
BREAKFAST:
_____ | _____
_____ | _____
_____ | _____
_____ | _____
_____ | _____
Drinks: _____
LUNCH:
_____ | _____
_____ | _____
_____ | _____
_____ | _____
_____ | _____
_____ | _____
Drinks: _____
Snacks: _____

DINNER:
_____ | _____
_____ | _____
_____ | _____
_____ | _____
_____ | _____
_____ | _____
Drinks: _____
Snacks: _____

RECOVERY PLAN: _____

Week No. _____ **Day No.:** _____

Exercises/Drills Done:

_____Time_____
_____Time_____
_____Time_____
_____Time_____
_____Time_____
_____Time_____
_____Time_____
_____Time_____
_____Time_____
_____Time_____

Total Time Spent _____

SUPPLEMENTS TAKEN:

_____ | _____
_____ | _____
_____ | _____
_____ | _____
_____ | _____

Supplements I Need to Buy:
_____ | _____
_____ | _____

MEDICINES TAKEN:

_____ | _____
_____ | _____
_____ | _____
_____ | _____
_____ | _____
_____ | _____

YOGA TRAINING:

Exercises: _____
_____
_____
_____
_____

Total Yoga Time: _____
Notes: _____

NOTES, SUCCESSES, BREAKTHROUGHS, PROGRESS!
_____
_____
_____
_____
_____

Daily Worksheet

Day of the Week:	Date:	Day No.	Max. Heart Rate:	A.M. Weight:	A.M. Blood Pressure: _____ OVER _____

Glasses of water drunk today (check): ○ ○ ○ ○ ○ ○ ○ ○

WALKING Plan No. _____

Week No.:_____ Day No.:_____

CORE WORK:

Total Time _____

RESISTANCE TRAINING:

1) Machine/Exerc._____

  Weight_____ Reps _____/_____/_____

2) Machine/Exerc._____

  Weight_____ Reps _____/_____/_____

3) Machine/Exerc._____

  Weight_____ Reps _____/_____/_____

4) Machine/Exerc._____

  Weight_____ Reps _____/_____/_____

5) Machine/Exerc._____

  Weight_____ Reps _____/_____/_____

6) Machine/Exerc._____

  Weight_____ Reps _____/_____/_____

7) Machine/Exerc._____

  Weight_____ Reps _____/_____/_____

8) Machine/Exerc._____

  Weight_____ Reps _____/_____/_____

Resistance Tr. Total Time_____

CARDIO WALKING:

Treadmill: Distance _____

  Time _____ Speed _____

  Time walked without support _____

Elliptical: Distance _____Time _____

  Reversed direction every _____ minutes

  Time walked without support _____

Stepper: Distance _____Time _____

  Time walked without support _____

Track: Distance _____Time _____

  Speed or pace (if recorded) _____

  Time walked without support _____

  Fastest lap _____

  Fastest lap without support_____

Total Cardio Walking Time:_____

Max. Heart Rate Noted:_____

RECOVERY BASICS:

☐ **Were physical exercise targets (time and total no. of reps) met?**

☐ **Did I focus well on exercises?**

☐ **Did I work intensively + aggressively?**

☐ **Did I push myself to increase difficulty?**

RECOVERY PLAN: _____

Week No. _____ Day No.:_____

Exercises/Drills Done:

_____Time_____

_____Time_____

_____Time_____

_____Time_____

_____Time_____

_____Time_____

_____Time_____

_____Time_____

_____Time_____

Total Time Spent_____

NUTRITION PLAN:

Nutrient-rich foods eaten | quantity:

BREAKFAST:

_____ | _____

_____ | _____

_____ | _____

_____ | _____

Drinks:_____

LUNCH:

_____ | _____

_____ | _____

_____ | _____

_____ | _____

_____ | _____

Drinks:_____

Snacks:_____

DINNER:

_____ | _____

_____ | _____

_____ | _____

_____ | _____

_____ | _____

_____ | _____

Drinks:_____

Snacks:_____

RECOVERY PLAN: _____

Week No. _____ Day No.:_____

Exercises/Drills Done:

_____Time_____

_____Time_____

_____Time_____

_____Time_____

_____Time_____

_____Time_____

_____Time_____

_____Time_____

_____Time_____

Total Time Spent_____

SUPPLEMENTS TAKEN:

_____ | _____

_____ | _____

_____ | _____

_____ | _____

_____ | _____

_____ | _____

Supplements I Need to Buy:

_____ | _____

_____ | _____

MEDICINES TAKEN:

_____ | _____

_____ | _____

_____ | _____

_____ | _____

_____ | _____

_____ | _____

YOGA TRAINING:

Exercises:_____

_____

_____

_____

_____

Total Yoga Time: _____

Notes:_____

NOTES, SUCCESSES, BREAKTHROUGHS, PROGRESS!

_____

_____

_____

_____

_____

Daily Worksheet

Day of the Week:	Date:	Day No.	Max. Heart Rate:	A.M. Weight:	A.M. Blood Pressure: _____ OVER _____

Glasses of water drunk today (check): ○ ○ ○ ○ ○ ○ ○ ○

WALKING Plan No. _____

Week No.:_____ Day No.:_____

CORE WORK:

Total Time _____

RESISTANCE TRAINING:

1) Machine/Exerc._____

   Weight_____ Reps _____/_____/_____

2) Machine/Exerc._____

   Weight_____ Reps _____/_____/_____

3) Machine/Exerc._____

   Weight_____ Reps _____/_____/_____

4) Machine/Exerc._____

   Weight_____ Reps _____/_____/_____

5) Machine/Exerc._____

   Weight_____ Reps _____/_____/_____

6) Machine/Exerc._____

   Weight_____ Reps _____/_____/_____

7) Machine/Exerc._____

   Weight_____ Reps _____/_____/_____

8) Machine/Exerc._____

   Weight_____ Reps _____/_____/_____

Resistance Tr. Total Time_____

CARDIO WALKING:

Treadmill: Distance _____

   Time _____ Speed _____

   Time walked without support _____

Elliptical: Distance _____Time _____

   Reversed direction every _____ minutes

   Time walked without support _____

Stepper: Distance _____Time _____

   Time walked without support _____

Track: Distance _____Time _____

   Speed or pace (if recorded) _____

   Time walked without support _____

   Fastest lap _____

   Fastest lap without support_____

Total Cardio Walking Time:_____

Max. Heart Rate Noted:_____

RECOVERY BASICS:

☐ **Were physical exercise targets (time and total no. of reps) met?**

☐ **Did I focus well on exercises?**

☐ **Did I work intensively + aggressively?**

☐ **Did I push myself to increase difficulty?**

RECOVERY PLAN: _____

Week No. _____ Day No.:_____

Exercises/Drills Done:

_____Time_____

_____Time_____

_____Time_____

_____Time_____

_____Time_____

_____Time_____

_____Time_____

_____Time_____

_____Time_____

_____Time_____

Total Time Spent_____

NUTRITION PLAN:

Nutrient-rich foods eaten | quantity:

BREAKFAST:

_____ | _____

_____ | _____

_____ | _____

_____ | _____

Drinks:_____

LUNCH:

_____ | _____

_____ | _____

_____ | _____

_____ | _____

_____ | _____

_____ | _____

Drinks:_____

Snacks:_____

DINNER:

_____ | _____

_____ | _____

_____ | _____

_____ | _____

_____ | _____

_____ | _____

Drinks:_____

Snacks:_____

RECOVERY PLAN: _____

Week No. _____ Day No.:_____

Exercises/Drills Done:

_____Time_____

_____Time_____

_____Time_____

_____Time_____

_____Time_____

_____Time_____

_____Time_____

_____Time_____

_____Time_____

_____Time_____

Total Time Spent_____

SUPPLEMENTS TAKEN:

_____ | _____

_____ | _____

_____ | _____

_____ | _____

_____ | _____

_____ | _____

Supplements I Need to Buy:

_____ | _____

_____ | _____

MEDICINES TAKEN:

_____ | _____

_____ | _____

_____ | _____

_____ | _____

_____ | _____

_____ | _____

_____ | _____

YOGA TRAINING:

Exercises:_____

_____

_____

_____

_____

Total Yoga Time: _____

Notes:_____

NOTES, SUCCESSES, BREAKTHROUGHS, PROGRESS!

_____

_____

_____

_____

_____

Daily Worksheet

Day of the Week:	Date:	Day No.	Max. Heart Rate:	A.M. Weight:	A.M. Blood Pressure: _____ OVER _____

Glasses of water drunk today (check): ○ ○ ○ ○ ○ ○ ○ ○

WALKING Plan No. _____
Week No.:_____ **Day No.:**_____

CORE WORK:
Total Time _____

RESISTANCE TRAINING:

1) Machine/Exerc._____
   Weight_____ Reps _____/_____/_____
2) Machine/Exerc._____
   Weight_____ Reps _____/_____/_____
3) Machine/Exerc._____
   Weight_____ Reps _____/_____/_____
4) Machine/Exerc._____
   Weight_____ Reps _____/_____/_____
5) Machine/Exerc._____
   Weight_____ Reps _____/_____/_____
6) Machine/Exerc._____
   Weight_____ Reps _____/_____/_____
7) Machine/Exerc._____
   Weight_____ Reps _____/_____/_____
8) Machine/Exerc._____
   Weight_____ Reps _____/_____/_____

Resistance Tr. Total Time_____

CARDIO WALKING:

Treadmill: Distance _____
   Time _____ Speed _____
   Time walked without support _____
Elliptical: Distance _____ Time _____
   Reversed direction every _____ minutes
   Time walked without support _____
Stepper: Distance _____ Time _____
   Time walked without support _____
Track: Distance _____ Time _____
   Speed or pace (if recorded) _____
   Time walked without support _____
   Fastest lap _____
   Fastest lap without support_____

Total Cardio Walking Time:_____
Max. Heart Rate Noted:_____

RECOVERY BASICS:
☐ **Were physical exercise targets (time and total no. of reps) met?**
☐ **Did I focus well on exercises?**
☐ **Did I work intensively + aggressively?**
☐ **Did I push myself to increase difficulty?**

RECOVERY PLAN: _____
Week No. _____ **Day No.:**_____

Exercises/Drills Done:
_____Time_____
_____Time_____
_____Time_____
_____Time_____
_____Time_____
_____Time_____
_____Time_____
_____Time_____
_____Time_____
_____Time_____

Total Time Spent_____

NUTRITION PLAN:
Nutrient-rich foods eaten | quantity:
BREAKFAST:
_____ | _____
_____ | _____
_____ | _____
_____ | _____
_____ | _____
Drinks:_____
LUNCH:
_____ | _____
_____ | _____
_____ | _____
_____ | _____
_____ | _____
Drinks:_____
Snacks:_____

DINNER:
_____ | _____
_____ | _____
_____ | _____
_____ | _____
_____ | _____
_____ | _____
Drinks:_____
Snacks:_____

RECOVERY PLAN: _____
Week No. _____ **Day No.:**_____

Exercises/Drills Done:
_____Time_____
_____Time_____
_____Time_____
_____Time_____
_____Time_____
_____Time_____
_____Time_____
_____Time_____
_____Time_____

Total Time Spent_____

SUPPLEMENTS TAKEN:
_____ | _____
_____ | _____
_____ | _____
_____ | _____
_____ | _____
_____ | _____
_____ | _____

Supplements I Need to Buy:
_____ | _____
_____ | _____

MEDICINES TAKEN:
_____ | _____
_____ | _____
_____ | _____
_____ | _____
_____ | _____
_____ | _____
_____ | _____

YOGA TRAINING:
Exercises:_____
_____
_____
_____
_____

Total Yoga Time: _____
Notes:_____

NOTES, SUCCESSES, BREAKTHROUGHS, PROGRESS!
_____
_____
_____
_____
_____

Daily Worksheet

Day of the Week:	Date:	Day No.	Max. Heart Rate:	A.M. Weight:	A.M. Blood Pressure: _____ OVER _____

Glasses of water drunk today (check): ○ ○ ○ ○ ○ ○ ○ ○

WALKING Plan No. _____

Week No.: _____ **Day No.:** _____

CORE WORK:
Total Time _____

RESISTANCE TRAINING:
1) Machine/Exerc. _____
   Weight_____ Reps _____/_____/_____

2) Machine/Exerc. _____
   Weight_____ Reps _____/_____/_____

3) Machine/Exerc. _____
   Weight_____ Reps _____/_____/_____

4) Machine/Exerc. _____
   Weight_____ Reps _____/_____/_____

5) Machine/Exerc. _____
   Weight_____ Reps _____/_____/_____

6) Machine/Exerc. _____
   Weight_____ Reps _____/_____/_____

7) Machine/Exerc. _____
   Weight_____ Reps _____/_____/_____

8) Machine/Exerc. _____
   Weight_____ Reps _____/_____/_____

Resistance Tr. Total Time _____

CARDIO WALKING:
Treadmill: Distance _____
   Time _____ Speed _____
   Time walked without support _____
Elliptical: Distance _____Time _____
   Reversed direction every _____ minutes
   Time walked without support _____
Stepper: Distance _____Time _____
   Time walked without support _____
Track: Distance _____Time _____
   Speed or pace (if recorded) _____
   Time walked without support _____
   Fastest lap _____
   Fastest lap without support _____
Total Cardio Walking Time: _____
Max. Heart Rate Noted: _____

RECOVERY BASICS:
☐ **Were physical exercise targets (time and total no. of reps) met?**
☐ **Did I focus well on exercises?**
☐ **Did I work intensively + aggressively?**
☐ **Did I push myself to increase difficulty?**

RECOVERY PLAN: _____
Week No. _____ **Day No.:** _____

Exercises/Drills Done:
_____Time_____
_____Time_____
_____Time_____
_____Time_____
_____Time_____
_____Time_____
_____Time_____
_____Time_____
_____Time_____
Total Time Spent _____

NUTRITION PLAN:
Nutrient-rich foods eaten | quantity:
BREAKFAST:
_____ | _____
_____ | _____
_____ | _____
_____ | _____
Drinks: _____
LUNCH:
_____ | _____
_____ | _____
_____ | _____
_____ | _____
_____ | _____
Drinks: _____
Snacks: _____
DINNER:
_____ | _____
_____ | _____
_____ | _____
_____ | _____
_____ | _____
_____ | _____
Drinks: _____
Snacks: _____

RECOVERY PLAN: _____
Week No. _____ **Day No.:** _____

Exercises/Drills Done:
_____Time_____
_____Time_____
_____Time_____
_____Time_____
_____Time_____
_____Time_____
_____Time_____
_____Time_____
_____Time_____
Total Time Spent _____

SUPPLEMENTS TAKEN:
_____ | _____
_____ | _____
_____ | _____
_____ | _____
_____ | _____
_____ | _____
Supplements I Need to Buy:
_____ | _____
_____ | _____

MEDICINES TAKEN:
_____ | _____
_____ | _____
_____ | _____
_____ | _____
_____ | _____

YOGA TRAINING:
Exercises: _____
_____
_____
_____
_____
Total Yoga Time: _____
Notes: _____

NOTES, SUCCESSES, BREAKTHROUGHS, PROGRESS!
_____
_____
_____
_____
_____
_____

Start of Week Worksheet—Week No. 12

Date: Week Beginning Monday, _____, 20___

The Wright brothers' father is known to have said: "If God wanted man to fly, He would have given him wings." The Wright brothers ignored their father on this point and were the first to successfully fly. You likely know people who might argue that you can't help yourself recover from stroke—but you should ignore them. You would be much better off emulating the Wright brothers, not their father!

Roger Maxwell

Start of Week Statistics:

MEASUREMENTS—MEN:
Waist:_____ Chest:_____
Upper Leg: ____ Upper Arm:_____

MEASUREMENTS—WOMEN:
Waist:_____ Hips:_____
Upper Leg: ____ Upper Arm:____

WEIGHT: _____
BLOOD PRESSURE:
_____ over _____

Fill out the following information to guide you during the coming week.

Last week's successes and progress:_____

_____

_____

How well I am physically functioning right now: _____

_____

_____

Goals and expectations for this week:_____

_____

_____

Skills or exercises I want to especially focus on improving this week:_____

_____

_____

Shopping List: brain nutrient foods to add to diet this week:

_____   _____

_____   _____

If my weight or blood pressure are high, plan to reduce them (current/continuing):

_____

Daily Worksheet

Day of the Week:	Date:	Day No.	Max. Heart Rate:	A.M. Weight:	A.M. Blood Pressure: _____ OVER _____

Glasses of water drunk today (check): ○ ○ ○ ○ ○ ○ ○ ○

WALKING Plan No. _____

Week No.:_____ Day No.:_____

CORE WORK:

Total Time _____

RESISTANCE TRAINING:

1) Machine/Exerc._____

   Weight_____ Reps _____/_____/_____

2) Machine/Exerc._____

   Weight_____ Reps _____/_____/_____

3) Machine/Exerc._____

   Weight_____ Reps _____/_____/_____

4) Machine/Exerc._____

   Weight_____ Reps _____/_____/_____

5) Machine/Exerc._____

   Weight_____ Reps _____/_____/_____

6) Machine/Exerc._____

   Weight_____ Reps _____/_____/_____

7) Machine/Exerc._____

   Weight_____ Reps _____/_____/_____

8) Machine/Exerc._____

   Weight_____ Reps _____/_____/_____

Resistance Tr. Total Time_____

CARDIO WALKING:

Treadmill: Distance _____

   Time _____ Speed _____

   Time walked without support _____

Elliptical: Distance _____Time _____

   Reversed direction every _____ minutes

   Time walked without support _____

Stepper: Distance _____Time _____

   Time walked without support _____

Track: Distance _____Time _____

   Speed or pace (if recorded) _____

   Time walked without support _____

   Fastest lap _____

   Fastest lap without support_____

Total Cardio Walking Time:_____

Max. Heart Rate Noted:_____

RECOVERY PLAN: _____

Week No. _____ Day No.:_____

Exercises/Drills Done:

_____Time_____

_____Time_____

_____Time_____

_____Time_____

_____Time_____

_____Time_____

_____Time_____

_____Time_____

Total Time Spent_____

NUTRITION PLAN:

Nutrient-rich foods eaten | quantity:

BREAKFAST:

_____ | _____

_____ | _____

_____ | _____

_____ | _____

Drinks:_____

LUNCH:

_____ | _____

_____ | _____

_____ | _____

_____ | _____

_____ | _____

Drinks:_____

Snacks:_____

DINNER:

_____ | _____

_____ | _____

_____ | _____

_____ | _____

_____ | _____

_____ | _____

Drinks:_____

Snacks:_____

RECOVERY PLAN: _____

Week No. _____ Day No.:_____

Exercises/Drills Done:

_____Time_____

_____Time_____

_____Time_____

_____Time_____

_____Time_____

_____Time_____

_____Time_____

_____Time_____

Total Time Spent_____

SUPPLEMENTS TAKEN:

_____ | _____

_____ | _____

_____ | _____

_____ | _____

_____ | _____

Supplements I Need to Buy:

_____ | _____

_____ | _____

MEDICINES TAKEN:

_____ | _____

_____ | _____

_____ | _____

_____ | _____

_____ | _____

YOGA TRAINING:

Exercises:_____

_____

_____

_____

Total Yoga Time: _____

Notes:_____

RECOVERY BASICS:

☐ **Were physical exercise targets (time and total no. of reps) met?**

☐ **Did I focus well on exercises?**

☐ **Did I work intensively + aggressively?**

☐ **Did I push myself to increase difficulty?**

NOTES, SUCCESSES, BREAKTHROUGHS, PROGRESS!

_____

_____

_____

_____

_____

Daily Worksheet

Day of the Week:	Date:	Day No.	Max. Heart Rate:	A.M. Weight:	A.M. Blood Pressure: _____ OVER _____

Glasses of water drunk today (check): ○ ○ ○ ○ ○ ○ ○ ○

WALKING Plan No. _____
Week No.:_____ Day No.:_____

CORE WORK:
Total Time _____

RESISTANCE TRAINING:

1) **Machine/Exerc.**_____
   Weight_____ Reps _____/_____/_____
2) **Machine/Exerc.**_____
   Weight_____ Reps _____/_____/_____
3) **Machine/Exerc.**_____
   Weight_____ Reps _____/_____/_____
4) **Machine/Exerc.**_____
   Weight_____ Reps _____/_____/_____
5) **Machine/Exerc.**_____
   Weight_____ Reps _____/_____/_____
6) **Machine/Exerc.**_____
   Weight_____ Reps _____/_____/_____
7) **Machine/Exerc.**_____
   Weight_____ Reps _____/_____/_____
8) **Machine/Exerc.**_____
   Weight_____ Reps _____/_____/_____

Resistance Tr. Total Time_____

CARDIO WALKING:

Treadmill: Distance _____
   Time _____ Speed _____
   Time walked without support _____
Elliptical: Distance _____Time _____
   Reversed direction every _____ minutes
   Time walked without support _____
Stepper: Distance _____Time _____
   Time walked without support _____
Track: Distance _____Time _____
   Speed or pace (if recorded) _____
   Time walked without support _____
   Fastest lap _____
   Fastest lap without support_____

Total Cardio Walking Time:_____
Max. Heart Rate Noted:_____

RECOVERY BASICS:
☐ **Were physical exercise targets (time and total no. of reps) met?**
☐ **Did I focus well on exercises?**
☐ **Did I work intensively + aggressively?**
☐ **Did I push myself to increase difficulty?**

RECOVERY PLAN: _____
Week No. _____ Day No.:_____

Exercises/Drills Done:
_____Time_____
_____Time_____
_____Time_____
_____Time_____
_____Time_____
_____Time_____
_____Time_____
_____Time_____
_____Time_____

Total Time Spent_____

NUTRITION PLAN:
Nutrient-rich foods eaten | quantity:
BREAKFAST:
_____ | _____
_____ | _____
_____ | _____
_____ | _____
Drinks:_____
LUNCH:
_____ | _____
_____ | _____
_____ | _____
_____ | _____
_____ | _____
Drinks:_____
Snacks:_____

DINNER:
_____ | _____
_____ | _____
_____ | _____
_____ | _____
_____ | _____
_____ | _____
Drinks:_____
Snacks:_____

RECOVERY PLAN: _____
Week No. _____ Day No.:_____

Exercises/Drills Done:
_____Time_____
_____Time_____
_____Time_____
_____Time_____
_____Time_____
_____Time_____
_____Time_____
_____Time_____
_____Time_____

Total Time Spent_____

SUPPLEMENTS TAKEN:
_____ | _____
_____ | _____
_____ | _____
_____ | _____
_____ | _____

Supplements I Need to Buy:
_____ | _____
_____ | _____

MEDICINES TAKEN:
_____ | _____
_____ | _____
_____ | _____
_____ | _____
_____ | _____

YOGA TRAINING:
Exercises:_____
_____
_____
_____
_____

Total Yoga Time: _____
Notes:_____

NOTES, SUCCESSES, BREAKTHROUGHS, PROGRESS!
_____
_____
_____
_____
_____

Daily Worksheet

Day of the Week:	Date:	Day No.	Max. Heart Rate:	A.M. Weight:	A.M. Blood Pressure: _____ OVER _____

Glasses of water drunk today (check): ○ ○ ○ ○ ○ ○ ○ ○

WALKING Plan No. _____

Week No.:_____ Day No.:_____

CORE WORK:

Total Time _____

RESISTANCE TRAINING:

1) Machine/Exerc._____

Weight_____ Reps _____/_____/_____

2) Machine/Exerc._____

Weight_____ Reps _____/_____/_____

3) Machine/Exerc._____

Weight_____ Reps _____/_____/_____

4) Machine/Exerc._____

Weight_____ Reps _____/_____/_____

5) Machine/Exerc._____

Weight_____ Reps _____/_____/_____

6) Machine/Exerc._____

Weight_____ Reps _____/_____/_____

7) Machine/Exerc._____

Weight_____ Reps _____/_____/_____

8) Machine/Exerc._____

Weight_____ Reps _____/_____/_____

Resistance Tr. Total Time_____

CARDIO WALKING:

Treadmill: Distance _____

Time _____ Speed _____

Time walked without support _____

Elliptical: Distance _____Time _____

Reversed direction every _____ minutes

Time walked without support _____

Stepper: Distance _____Time _____

Time walked without support _____

Track: Distance _____Time _____

Speed or pace (if recorded) _____

Time walked without support _____

Fastest lap _____

Fastest lap without support_____

Total Cardio Walking Time:_____

Max. Heart Rate Noted:_____

RECOVERY PLAN: _____

Week No. _____ Day No.:_____

Exercises/Drills Done:

_____Time_____

_____Time_____

_____Time_____

_____Time_____

_____Time_____

_____Time_____

_____Time_____

_____Time_____

_____Time_____

Total Time Spent_____

NUTRITION PLAN:

Nutrient-rich foods eaten | quantity:

BREAKFAST:

_____ | _____

_____ | _____

_____ | _____

_____ | _____

Drinks:_____

LUNCH:

_____ | _____

_____ | _____

_____ | _____

_____ | _____

_____ | _____

_____ | _____

Drinks:_____

Snacks:_____

DINNER:

_____ | _____

_____ | _____

_____ | _____

_____ | _____

_____ | _____

_____ | _____

Drinks:_____

Snacks:_____

RECOVERY PLAN: _____

Week No. _____ Day No.:_____

Exercises/Drills Done:

_____Time_____

_____Time_____

_____Time_____

_____Time_____

_____Time_____

_____Time_____

_____Time_____

_____Time_____

_____Time_____

Total Time Spent_____

SUPPLEMENTS TAKEN:

_____ | _____

_____ | _____

_____ | _____

_____ | _____

_____ | _____

_____ | _____

Supplements I Need to Buy:

_____ | _____

_____ | _____

MEDICINES TAKEN:

_____ | _____

_____ | _____

_____ | _____

_____ | _____

_____ | _____

_____ | _____

YOGA TRAINING:

Exercises:_____

_____

_____

_____

_____

_____

Total Yoga Time: _____

Notes:_____

RECOVERY BASICS:

☐ **Were physical exercise targets (time and total no. of reps) met?**

☐ **Did I focus well on exercises?**

☐ **Did I work intensively + aggressively?**

☐ **Did I push myself to increase difficulty?**

NOTES, SUCCESSES, BREAKTHROUGHS, PROGRESS!

_____

_____

_____

_____

_____

Daily Worksheet

Day of the Week:	Date:	Day No.	Max. Heart Rate:	A.M. Weight:	A.M. Blood Pressure: _____ OVER _____

Glasses of water drunk today (check): ○ ○ ○ ○ ○ ○ ○ ○

WALKING Plan No. _____

Week No.:_____   Day No.:_____

CORE WORK:

Total Time _____

RESISTANCE TRAINING:

1) Machine/Exerc._____

  Weight_____ Reps _____/_____/_____

2) Machine/Exerc._____

  Weight_____ Reps _____/_____/_____

3) Machine/Exerc._____

  Weight_____ Reps _____/_____/_____

4) Machine/Exerc._____

  Weight_____ Reps _____/_____/_____

5) Machine/Exerc._____

  Weight_____ Reps _____/_____/_____

6) Machine/Exerc._____

  Weight_____ Reps _____/_____/_____

7) Machine/Exerc._____

  Weight_____ Reps _____/_____/_____

8) Machine/Exerc._____

  Weight_____ Reps _____/_____/_____

Resistance Tr. Total Time_____

CARDIO WALKING:

Treadmill: Distance _____

  Time _____ Speed _____

  Time walked without support _____

Elliptical: Distance _____Time _____

  Reversed direction every _____ minutes

  Time walked without support _____

Stepper: Distance _____Time _____

  Time walked without support _____

Track: Distance _____Time _____

  Speed or pace (if recorded) _____

  Time walked without support _____

  Fastest lap _____

  Fastest lap without support_____

Total Cardio Walking Time:_____

Max. Heart Rate Noted:_____

RECOVERY BASICS:

☐ **Were physical exercise targets (time and total no. of reps) met?**

☐ **Did I focus well on exercises?**

☐ **Did I work intensively + aggressively?**

☐ **Did I push myself to increase difficulty?**

RECOVERY PLAN: _____

Week No. _____   Day No.:_____

Exercises/Drills Done:

_____Time_____
_____Time_____
_____Time_____
_____Time_____
_____Time_____
_____Time_____
_____Time_____
_____Time_____
_____Time_____

Total Time Spent_____

NUTRITION PLAN:

Nutrient-rich foods eaten | quantity:

BREAKFAST:

_____ | _____
_____ | _____
_____ | _____
_____ | _____

Drinks:_____

LUNCH:

_____ | _____
_____ | _____
_____ | _____
_____ | _____
_____ | _____

Drinks:_____

Snacks:_____

DINNER:

_____ | _____
_____ | _____
_____ | _____
_____ | _____
_____ | _____
_____ | _____

Drinks:_____

Snacks:_____

RECOVERY PLAN: _____

Week No. _____   Day No.:_____

Exercises/Drills Done:

_____Time_____
_____Time_____
_____Time_____
_____Time_____
_____Time_____
_____Time_____
_____Time_____
_____Time_____
_____Time_____

Total Time Spent_____

SUPPLEMENTS TAKEN:

_____ | _____
_____ | _____
_____ | _____
_____ | _____
_____ | _____
_____ | _____

Supplements I Need to Buy:

_____ | _____
_____ | _____

MEDICINES TAKEN:

_____ | _____
_____ | _____
_____ | _____
_____ | _____
_____ | _____
_____ | _____
_____ | _____

YOGA TRAINING:

Exercises:_____

_____
_____
_____
_____
_____

Total Yoga Time: _____

Notes:_____

NOTES, SUCCESSES, BREAKTHROUGHS, PROGRESS!

_____
_____
_____
_____
_____

Daily Worksheet

Day of the Week:	Date:	Day No.	Max. Heart Rate:	A.M. Weight:	A.M. Blood Pressure: _____ OVER _____

Glasses of water drunk today (check): ○ ○ ○ ○ ○ ○ ○ ○

WALKING Plan No. _____

Week No.:_____   Day No.:_____

CORE WORK:
Total Time _____

RESISTANCE TRAINING:
1) Machine/Exerc._____
   Weight_____ Reps _____/_____/_____
2) Machine/Exerc._____
   Weight_____ Reps _____/_____/_____
3) Machine/Exerc._____
   Weight_____ Reps _____/_____/_____
4) Machine/Exerc._____
   Weight_____ Reps _____/_____/_____
5) Machine/Exerc._____
   Weight_____ Reps _____/_____/_____
6) Machine/Exerc._____
   Weight_____ Reps _____/_____/_____
7) Machine/Exerc._____
   Weight_____ Reps _____/_____/_____
8) Machine/Exerc._____
   Weight_____ Reps _____/_____/_____
Resistance Tr. Total Time_____

CARDIO WALKING:
Treadmill: Distance _____
   Time _____ Speed _____
   Time walked without support _____
Elliptical: Distance _____Time _____
   Reversed direction every _____ minutes
   Time walked without support _____
Stepper: Distance _____Time _____
   Time walked without support _____
Track: Distance _____Time _____
   Speed or pace (if recorded) _____
   Time walked without support _____
   Fastest lap _____
   Fastest lap without support_____
Total Cardio Walking Time:_____
Max. Heart Rate Noted:_____

RECOVERY BASICS:
☐ **Were physical exercise targets (time and total no. of reps) met?**
☐ **Did I focus well on exercises?**
☐ **Did I work intensively + aggressively?**
☐ **Did I push myself to increase difficulty?**

RECOVERY PLAN: _____

Week No. _____   Day No.:_____

Exercises/Drills Done:
_____Time_____
_____Time_____
_____Time_____
_____Time_____
_____Time_____
_____Time_____
_____Time_____
_____Time_____
_____Time_____
Total Time Spent_____

NUTRITION PLAN:
Nutrient-rich foods eaten | quantity:
BREAKFAST:
_____ | _____
_____ | _____
_____ | _____
_____ | _____
Drinks:_____
LUNCH:
_____ | _____
_____ | _____
_____ | _____
_____ | _____
_____ | _____
_____ | _____
Drinks:_____
Snacks:_____
DINNER:
_____ | _____
_____ | _____
_____ | _____
_____ | _____
_____ | _____
_____ | _____
Drinks:_____
Snacks:_____

RECOVERY PLAN: _____

Week No. _____   Day No.:_____

Exercises/Drills Done:
_____Time_____
_____Time_____
_____Time_____
_____Time_____
_____Time_____
_____Time_____
_____Time_____
_____Time_____
_____Time_____
Total Time Spent_____

SUPPLEMENTS TAKEN:
_____ | _____
_____ | _____
_____ | _____
_____ | _____
_____ | _____
Supplements I Need to Buy:
_____ | _____
_____ | _____
MEDICINES TAKEN:
_____ | _____
_____ | _____
_____ | _____
_____ | _____
_____ | _____
_____ | _____

YOGA TRAINING:
Exercises:_____
_____
_____
_____
_____
_____
Total Yoga Time: _____
Notes:_____

NOTES, SUCCESSES, BREAKTHROUGHS, PROGRESS!
_____
_____
_____
_____
_____
_____

Daily Worksheet

Day of the Week:	Date:	Day No.	Max. Heart Rate:	A.M. Weight:	A.M. Blood Pressure: _____ OVER _____

Glasses of water drunk today (check): ○ ○ ○ ○ ○ ○ ○ ○

WALKING Plan No. _____

Week No.:_____ Day No.:_____

CORE WORK:

Total Time _____

RESISTANCE TRAINING:

1) Machine/Exerc._____

  Weight_____ Reps _____/_____/_____

2) Machine/Exerc._____

  Weight_____ Reps _____/_____/_____

3) Machine/Exerc._____

  Weight_____ Reps _____/_____/_____

4) Machine/Exerc._____

  Weight_____ Reps _____/_____/_____

5) Machine/Exerc._____

  Weight_____ Reps _____/_____/_____

6) Machine/Exerc._____

  Weight_____ Reps _____/_____/_____

7) Machine/Exerc._____

  Weight_____ Reps _____/_____/_____

8) Machine/Exerc._____

  Weight_____ Reps _____/_____/_____

Resistance Tr. Total Time_____

CARDIO WALKING:

Treadmill: Distance _____

  Time _____ Speed _____

  Time walked without support _____

Elliptical: Distance _____Time _____

  Reversed direction every _____ minutes

  Time walked without support _____

Stepper: Distance _____Time _____

  Time walked without support _____

Track: Distance _____Time _____

  Speed or pace (if recorded) _____

  Time walked without support _____

  Fastest lap _____

  Fastest lap without support_____

Total Cardio Walking Time:_____

Max. Heart Rate Noted:_____

RECOVERY BASICS:

☐ **Were physical exercise targets (time and total no. of reps) met?**

☐ **Did I focus well on exercises?**

☐ **Did I work intensively + aggressively?**

☐ **Did I push myself to increase difficulty?**

RECOVERY PLAN: _____

Week No. _____ Day No.:_____

Exercises/Drills Done:

_____Time_____

_____Time_____

_____Time_____

_____Time_____

_____Time_____

_____Time_____

_____Time_____

_____Time_____

_____Time_____

_____Time_____

Total Time Spent_____

NUTRITION PLAN:

Nutrient-rich foods eaten | quantity:

BREAKFAST:

_____ | _____

_____ | _____

_____ | _____

_____ | _____

Drinks:_____

LUNCH:

_____ | _____

_____ | _____

_____ | _____

_____ | _____

_____ | _____

Drinks:_____

Snacks:_____

DINNER:

_____ | _____

_____ | _____

_____ | _____

_____ | _____

_____ | _____

_____ | _____

Drinks:_____

Snacks:_____

NOTES, SUCCESSES, BREAKTHROUGHS, PROGRESS!

_____

_____

_____

_____

RECOVERY PLAN: _____

Week No. _____ Day No.:_____

Exercises/Drills Done:

_____Time_____

_____Time_____

_____Time_____

_____Time_____

_____Time_____

_____Time_____

_____Time_____

_____Time_____

_____Time_____

Total Time Spent_____

SUPPLEMENTS TAKEN:

_____ | _____

_____ | _____

_____ | _____

_____ | _____

_____ | _____

_____ | _____

Supplements I Need to Buy:

_____ | _____

_____ | _____

MEDICINES TAKEN:

_____ | _____

_____ | _____

_____ | _____

_____ | _____

_____ | _____

_____ | _____

_____ | _____

YOGA TRAINING:

Exercises:_____

_____

_____

_____

_____

_____

Total Yoga Time: _____

Notes:_____

Daily Worksheet

Day of the Week:	Date:	Day No.	Max. Heart Rate:	A.M. Weight:	A.M. Blood Pressure: _____ OVER _____

Glasses of water drunk today (check): ○ ○ ○ ○ ○ ○ ○ ○

WALKING Plan No. _____

Week No.:_____ **Day No.:**_____

CORE WORK:
Total Time _____

RESISTANCE TRAINING:
1) Machine/Exerc._____
   Weight_____ Reps _____/_____/_____
2) Machine/Exerc._____
   Weight_____ Reps _____/_____/_____
3) Machine/Exerc._____
   Weight_____ Reps _____/_____/_____
4) Machine/Exerc._____
   Weight_____ Reps _____/_____/_____
5) Machine/Exerc._____
   Weight_____ Reps _____/_____/_____
6) Machine/Exerc._____
   Weight_____ Reps _____/_____/_____
7) Machine/Exerc._____
   Weight_____ Reps _____/_____/_____
8) Machine/Exerc._____
   Weight_____ Reps _____/_____/_____

Resistance Tr. Total Time_____

CARDIO WALKING:
Treadmill: Distance _____
   Time _____ Speed _____
   Time walked without support _____
Elliptical: Distance _____Time _____
   Reversed direction every _____ minutes
   Time walked without support _____
Stepper: Distance _____Time _____
   Time walked without support _____
Track: Distance _____Time _____
   Speed or pace (if recorded) _____
   Time walked without support _____
   Fastest lap _____
   Fastest lap without support_____

Total Cardio Walking Time:_____
Max. Heart Rate Noted:_____

RECOVERY PLAN: _____

Week No. _____ **Day No.:**_____

Exercises/Drills Done:
_____Time_____
_____Time_____
_____Time_____
_____Time_____
_____Time_____
_____Time_____
_____Time_____
_____Time_____
_____Time_____

Total Time Spent_____

NUTRITION PLAN:
Nutrient-rich foods eaten | quantity:
BREAKFAST:
_____ | _____
_____ | _____
_____ | _____
_____ | _____
Drinks:_____

LUNCH:
_____ | _____
_____ | _____
_____ | _____
_____ | _____
_____ | _____
Drinks:_____
Snacks:_____

DINNER:
_____ | _____
_____ | _____
_____ | _____
_____ | _____
_____ | _____
_____ | _____
Drinks:_____
Snacks:_____

RECOVERY PLAN: _____

Week No. _____ **Day No.:**_____

Exercises/Drills Done:
_____Time_____
_____Time_____
_____Time_____
_____Time_____
_____Time_____
_____Time_____
_____Time_____
_____Time_____
_____Time_____

Total Time Spent_____

SUPPLEMENTS TAKEN:
_____ | _____
_____ | _____
_____ | _____
_____ | _____
_____ | _____
_____ | _____

Supplements I Need to Buy:
_____ | _____
_____ | _____

MEDICINES TAKEN:
_____ | _____
_____ | _____
_____ | _____
_____ | _____
_____ | _____
_____ | _____

YOGA TRAINING:
Exercises:_____
_____
_____
_____
_____

Total Yoga Time: _____
Notes:_____

RECOVERY BASICS:
☐ **Were physical exercise targets (time and total no. of reps) met?**
☐ **Did I focus well on exercises?**
☐ **Did I work intensively + aggressively?**
☐ **Did I push myself to increase difficulty?**

NOTES, SUCCESSES, BREAKTHROUGHS, PROGRESS!
_____
_____
_____
_____
_____

Start of Week Worksheet—Week No. 13

Date: Week Beginning Monday, _____, 20___

Start of Week Statistics:

MEASUREMENTS—MEN:	MEASUREMENTS—WOMEN:	WEIGHT: _____
Waist:_____ Chest:_____	Waist:_____ Hips:_____	BLOOD PRESSURE:
Upper Leg: ____ Upper Arm:_____	Upper Leg: ____ Upper Arm:____	_____ over _____

Fill out the following information to guide you during the coming week.

Last week's successes and progress:_____

_____

_____

How well I am physically functioning right now: _____

_____

_____

Goals and expectations for this week:_____

_____

_____

Skills or exercises I want to especially focus on improving this week:_____

_____

_____

Shopping List: brain nutrient foods to add to diet this week:

_____   _____

_____   _____

If my weight or blood pressure are high, plan to reduce them (current/continuing):

_____

Daily Worksheet

Day of the Week:	Date:	Day No.	Max. Heart Rate:	A.M. Weight:	A.M. Blood Pressure: _____ OVER _____

Glasses of water drunk today (check): ○ ○ ○ ○ ○ ○ ○ ○

WALKING Plan No. _____

Week No.:_____ **Day No.:**_____

CORE WORK:

Total Time _____

RESISTANCE TRAINING:

1) Machine/Exerc._____

Weight_____ Reps _____/_____/_____

2) Machine/Exerc._____

Weight_____ Reps _____/_____/_____

3) Machine/Exerc._____

Weight_____ Reps _____/_____/_____

4) Machine/Exerc._____

Weight_____ Reps _____/_____/_____

5) Machine/Exerc._____

Weight_____ Reps _____/_____/_____

6) Machine/Exerc._____

Weight_____ Reps _____/_____/_____

7) Machine/Exerc._____

Weight_____ Reps _____/_____/_____

8) Machine/Exerc._____

Weight_____ Reps _____/_____/_____

Resistance Tr. Total Time_____

CARDIO WALKING:

Treadmill: Distance _____

Time _____ Speed _____

Time walked without support _____

Elliptical: Distance _____Time _____

Reversed direction every _____ minutes

Time walked without support _____

Stepper: Distance _____Time _____

Time walked without support _____

Track: Distance _____Time _____

Speed or pace (if recorded) _____

Time walked without support _____

Fastest lap _____

Fastest lap without support_____

Total Cardio Walking Time:_____

Max. Heart Rate Noted:_____

RECOVERY BASICS:

☐ **Were physical exercise targets (time and total no. of reps) met?**

☐ **Did I focus well on exercises?**

☐ **Did I work intensively + aggressively?**

☐ **Did I push myself to increase difficulty?**

RECOVERY PLAN: _____

Week No. _____ **Day No.:**_____

Exercises/Drills Done:

_____Time_____
_____Time_____
_____Time_____
_____Time_____
_____Time_____
_____Time_____
_____Time_____
_____Time_____

Total Time Spent_____

NUTRITION PLAN:

Nutrient-rich foods eaten | quantity:

BREAKFAST:

_____ | _____
_____ | _____
_____ | _____
_____ | _____

Drinks:_____

LUNCH:

_____ | _____
_____ | _____
_____ | _____
_____ | _____
_____ | _____
_____ | _____

Drinks:_____

Snacks:_____

DINNER:

_____ | _____
_____ | _____
_____ | _____
_____ | _____
_____ | _____
_____ | _____

Drinks:_____

Snacks:_____

RECOVERY PLAN: _____

Week No. _____ **Day No.:**_____

Exercises/Drills Done:

_____Time_____
_____Time_____
_____Time_____
_____Time_____
_____Time_____
_____Time_____
_____Time_____
_____Time_____

Total Time Spent_____

SUPPLEMENTS TAKEN:

_____ | _____
_____ | _____
_____ | _____
_____ | _____
_____ | _____

Supplements I Need to Buy:

_____ | _____
_____ | _____

MEDICINES TAKEN:

_____ | _____
_____ | _____
_____ | _____
_____ | _____
_____ | _____

YOGA TRAINING:

Exercises:_____
_____
_____
_____
_____

Total Yoga Time: _____

Notes:_____

NOTES, SUCCESSES, BREAKTHROUGHS, PROGRESS!

_____
_____
_____
_____
_____

Daily Worksheet

Day of the Week:	Date:	Day No.	Max. Heart Rate:	A.M. Weight:	A.M. Blood Pressure: _____ OVER _____

Glasses of water drunk today (check): ○ ○ ○ ○ ○ ○ ○ ○

WALKING Plan No. _____

Week No.:_____ Day No.:_____

CORE WORK:

Total Time _____

RESISTANCE TRAINING:

1) Machine/Exerc._____

  Weight_____ Reps _____/_____/_____

2) Machine/Exerc._____

  Weight_____ Reps _____/_____/_____

3) Machine/Exerc._____

  Weight_____ Reps _____/_____/_____

4) Machine/Exerc._____

  Weight_____ Reps _____/_____/_____

5) Machine/Exerc._____

  Weight_____ Reps _____/_____/_____

6) Machine/Exerc._____

  Weight_____ Reps _____/_____/_____

7) Machine/Exerc._____

  Weight_____ Reps _____/_____/_____

8) Machine/Exerc._____

  Weight_____ Reps _____/_____/_____

Resistance Tr. Total Time_____

CARDIO WALKING:

Treadmill: Distance _____

  Time _____ Speed _____

  Time walked without support _____

Elliptical: Distance _____Time _____

  Reversed direction every _____ minutes

  Time walked without support _____

Stepper: Distance _____Time _____

  Time walked without support _____

Track: Distance _____Time _____

  Speed or pace (if recorded) _____

  Time walked without support _____

  Fastest lap _____

  Fastest lap without support_____

Total Cardio Walking Time:_____

Max. Heart Rate Noted:_____

RECOVERY BASICS:

☐ **Were physical exercise targets (time and total no. of reps) met?**

☐ **Did I focus well on exercises?**

☐ **Did I work intensively + aggressively?**

☐ **Did I push myself to increase difficulty?**

RECOVERY PLAN: _____

Week No. _____ Day No.:_____

Exercises/Drills Done:

_____Time_____

_____Time_____

_____Time_____

_____Time_____

_____Time_____

_____Time_____

_____Time_____

_____Time_____

_____Time_____

_____Time_____

Total Time Spent_____

NUTRITION PLAN:

Nutrient-rich foods eaten | quantity:

BREAKFAST:

_____|_____

_____|_____

_____|_____

_____|_____

Drinks:_____

LUNCH:

_____|_____

_____|_____

_____|_____

_____|_____

_____|_____

Drinks:_____

Snacks:_____

DINNER:

_____|_____

_____|_____

_____|_____

_____|_____

_____|_____

Drinks:_____

Snacks:_____

NOTES, SUCCESSES, BREAKTHROUGHS, PROGRESS!

_____

_____

_____

_____

_____

RECOVERY PLAN: _____

Week No. _____ Day No.:_____

Exercises/Drills Done:

_____Time_____

_____Time_____

_____Time_____

_____Time_____

_____Time_____

_____Time_____

_____Time_____

_____Time_____

_____Time_____

_____Time_____

Total Time Spent_____

SUPPLEMENTS TAKEN:

_____|_____

_____|_____

_____|_____

_____|_____

_____|_____

Supplements I Need to Buy:

_____|_____

_____|_____

MEDICINES TAKEN:

_____|_____

_____|_____

_____|_____

_____|_____

_____|_____

_____|_____

YOGA TRAINING:

Exercises:_____

_____

_____

_____

_____

Total Yoga Time: _____

Notes:_____

Daily Worksheet

Day of the Week:	Date:	Day No.	Max. Heart Rate:	A.M. Weight:	A.M. Blood Pressure: _____ OVER _____

Glasses of water drunk today (check): ○ ○ ○ ○ ○ ○ ○ ○

WALKING Plan No. _____

Week No.:_____ **Day No.:**_____

CORE WORK:
Total Time _____

RESISTANCE TRAINING:

1) Machine/Exerc._____
  Weight_____ Reps _____/_____/_____

2) Machine/Exerc._____
  Weight_____ Reps _____/_____/_____

3) Machine/Exerc._____
  Weight_____ Reps _____/_____/_____

4) Machine/Exerc._____
  Weight_____ Reps _____/_____/_____

5) Machine/Exerc._____
  Weight_____ Reps _____/_____/_____

6) Machine/Exerc._____
  Weight_____ Reps _____/_____/_____

7) Machine/Exerc._____
  Weight_____ Reps _____/_____/_____

8) Machine/Exerc._____
  Weight_____ Reps _____/_____/_____

Resistance Tr. Total Time_____

CARDIO WALKING:

Treadmill: Distance _____
  Time _____ Speed _____
  Time walked without support _____

Elliptical: Distance _____Time _____
  Reversed direction every _____ minutes
  Time walked without support _____

Stepper: Distance _____Time _____
  Time walked without support _____

Track: Distance _____Time _____
  Speed or pace (if recorded) _____
  Time walked without support _____
  Fastest lap _____
  Fastest lap without support_____

Total Cardio Walking Time:_____

Max. Heart Rate Noted:_____

RECOVERY BASICS:
☐ **Were physical exercise targets (time and total no. of reps) met?**
☐ **Did I focus well on exercises?**
☐ **Did I work intensively + aggressively?**
☐ **Did I push myself to increase difficulty?**

RECOVERY PLAN: _____

Week No. _____ **Day No.:**_____

Exercises/Drills Done:
_____Time_____
_____Time_____
_____Time_____
_____Time_____
_____Time_____
_____Time_____
_____Time_____
_____Time_____
_____Time_____
_____Time_____

Total Time Spent_____

NUTRITION PLAN:

Nutrient-rich foods eaten | quantity:

BREAKFAST:
_____|_____
_____|_____
_____|_____
_____|_____

Drinks:_____

LUNCH:
_____|_____
_____|_____
_____|_____
_____|_____
_____|_____

Drinks:_____
Snacks:_____

DINNER:
_____|_____
_____|_____
_____|_____
_____|_____
_____|_____
_____|_____

Drinks:_____
Snacks:_____

RECOVERY PLAN: _____

Week No. _____ **Day No.:**_____

Exercises/Drills Done:
_____Time_____
_____Time_____
_____Time_____
_____Time_____
_____Time_____
_____Time_____
_____Time_____
_____Time_____
_____Time_____

Total Time Spent_____

SUPPLEMENTS TAKEN:
_____|_____
_____|_____
_____|_____
_____|_____
_____|_____
_____|_____

Supplements I Need to Buy:
_____|_____
_____|_____

MEDICINES TAKEN:
_____|_____
_____|_____
_____|_____
_____|_____
_____|_____
_____|_____

YOGA TRAINING:
Exercises:_____
_____
_____
_____
_____

Total Yoga Time: _____
Notes:_____

NOTES, SUCCESSES, BREAKTHROUGHS, PROGRESS!
_____
_____
_____
_____
_____

Daily Worksheet

Day of the Week:	Date:	Day No.	Max. Heart Rate:	A.M. Weight:	A.M. Blood Pressure: _____ OVER _____

Glasses of water drunk today (check): ◯ ◯ ◯ ◯ ◯ ◯ ◯ ◯

WALKING Plan No. _____

Week No.:_____ **Day No.:**_____

CORE WORK:
Total Time _____

RESISTANCE TRAINING:

1) Machine/Exerc._____
  Weight_____ Reps _____/_____/_____

2) Machine/Exerc._____
  Weight_____ Reps _____/_____/_____

3) Machine/Exerc._____
  Weight_____ Reps _____/_____/_____

4) Machine/Exerc._____
  Weight_____ Reps _____/_____/_____

5) Machine/Exerc._____
  Weight_____ Reps _____/_____/_____

6) Machine/Exerc._____
  Weight_____ Reps _____/_____/_____

7) Machine/Exerc._____
  Weight_____ Reps _____/_____/_____

8) Machine/Exerc._____
  Weight_____ Reps _____/_____/_____

Resistance Tr. Total Time_____

CARDIO WALKING:

Treadmill: Distance _____
  Time _____ Speed _____
  Time walked without support _____

Elliptical: Distance _____Time _____
  Reversed direction every _____ minutes
  Time walked without support _____

Stepper: Distance _____Time _____
  Time walked without support _____

Track: Distance _____Time _____
  Speed or pace (if recorded) _____
  Time walked without support _____
  Fastest lap _____
  Fastest lap without support_____

Total Cardio Walking Time:_____
Max. Heart Rate Noted:_____

RECOVERY BASICS:
☐ **Were physical exercise targets (time and total no. of reps) met?**
☐ **Did I focus well on exercises?**
☐ **Did I work intensively + aggressively?**
☐ **Did I push myself to increase difficulty?**

RECOVERY PLAN: _____

Week No. _____ **Day No.:**_____

Exercises/Drills Done:
_____Time_____
_____Time_____
_____Time_____
_____Time_____
_____Time_____
_____Time_____
_____Time_____
_____Time_____
_____Time_____
_____Time_____

Total Time Spent_____

NUTRITION PLAN:
Nutrient-rich foods eaten | quantity:

BREAKFAST:
_____|_____
_____|_____
_____|_____
_____|_____

Drinks:_____

LUNCH:
_____|_____
_____|_____
_____|_____
_____|_____
_____|_____

Drinks:_____
Snacks:_____

DINNER:
_____|_____
_____|_____
_____|_____
_____|_____
_____|_____
_____|_____

Drinks:_____
Snacks:_____

RECOVERY PLAN: _____

Week No. _____ **Day No.:**_____

Exercises/Drills Done:
_____Time_____
_____Time_____
_____Time_____
_____Time_____
_____Time_____
_____Time_____
_____Time_____
_____Time_____
_____Time_____

Total Time Spent_____

SUPPLEMENTS TAKEN:
_____|_____
_____|_____
_____|_____
_____|_____
_____|_____

Supplements I Need to Buy:
_____|_____
_____|_____

MEDICINES TAKEN:
_____|_____
_____|_____
_____|_____
_____|_____
_____|_____
_____|_____

YOGA TRAINING:
Exercises:_____
_____
_____
_____
_____
_____

Total Yoga Time: _____
Notes:_____

NOTES, SUCCESSES, BREAKTHROUGHS, PROGRESS!
_____
_____
_____
_____
_____
_____

Daily Worksheet

Day of the Week:	Date:	Day No.	Max. Heart Rate:	A.M. Weight:	A.M. Blood Pressure: _____ OVER _____

Glasses of water drunk today (check): ○ ○ ○ ○ ○ ○ ○ ○

WALKING Plan No. _____

Week No.: _____ **Day No.:** _____

CORE WORK:
Total Time _____

RESISTANCE TRAINING:
1) Machine/Exerc. _____
   Weight _____ Reps _____/_____/_____
2) Machine/Exerc. _____
   Weight _____ Reps _____/_____/_____
3) Machine/Exerc. _____
   Weight _____ Reps _____/_____/_____
4) Machine/Exerc. _____
   Weight _____ Reps _____/_____/_____
5) Machine/Exerc. _____
   Weight _____ Reps _____/_____/_____
6) Machine/Exerc. _____
   Weight _____ Reps _____/_____/_____
7) Machine/Exerc. _____
   Weight _____ Reps _____/_____/_____
8) Machine/Exerc. _____
   Weight _____ Reps _____/_____/_____
Resistance Tr. Total Time _____

CARDIO WALKING:
Treadmill: Distance _____
   Time _____ Speed _____
   Time walked without support _____
Elliptical: Distance _____ Time _____
   Reversed direction every _____ minutes
   Time walked without support _____
Stepper: Distance _____ Time _____
   Time walked without support _____
Track: Distance _____ Time _____
   Speed or pace (if recorded) _____
   Time walked without support _____
   Fastest lap _____
   Fastest lap without support _____
Total Cardio Walking Time: _____
Max. Heart Rate Noted: _____

RECOVERY BASICS:
☐ Were physical exercise targets (time and total no. of reps) met?
☐ Did I focus well on exercises?
☐ Did I work intensively + aggressively?
☐ Did I push myself to increase difficulty?

RECOVERY PLAN: _____

Week No. _____ **Day No.:** _____

Exercises/Drills Done:
_____ Time _____
_____ Time _____
_____ Time _____
_____ Time _____
_____ Time _____
_____ Time _____
_____ Time _____
_____ Time _____
_____ Time _____
Total Time Spent _____

NUTRITION PLAN:
Nutrient-rich foods eaten | quantity:
BREAKFAST:
_____ | _____
_____ | _____
_____ | _____
_____ | _____
Drinks: _____
LUNCH:
_____ | _____
_____ | _____
_____ | _____
_____ | _____
_____ | _____
Drinks: _____
Snacks: _____
DINNER:
_____ | _____
_____ | _____
_____ | _____
_____ | _____
_____ | _____
_____ | _____
Drinks: _____
Snacks: _____

RECOVERY PLAN: _____

Week No. _____ **Day No.:** _____

Exercises/Drills Done:
_____ Time _____
_____ Time _____
_____ Time _____
_____ Time _____
_____ Time _____
_____ Time _____
_____ Time _____
_____ Time _____
_____ Time _____
Total Time Spent _____

SUPPLEMENTS TAKEN:
_____ | _____
_____ | _____
_____ | _____
_____ | _____
_____ | _____
Supplements I Need to Buy:
_____ | _____
_____ | _____

MEDICINES TAKEN:
_____ | _____
_____ | _____
_____ | _____
_____ | _____
_____ | _____

YOGA TRAINING:
Exercises: _____
_____
_____
_____
_____
Total Yoga Time: _____
Notes: _____

NOTES, SUCCESSES, BREAKTHROUGHS, PROGRESS!
_____
_____
_____
_____
_____
_____

Daily Worksheet

Day of the Week:	Date:	Day No.	Max. Heart Rate:	A.M. Weight:	A.M. Blood Pressure: _____ OVER _____

Glasses of water drunk today (check): ○ ○ ○ ○ ○ ○ ○ ○

WALKING Plan No. _____
Week No.:_____ Day No.:_____

CORE WORK:
Total Time _____

RESISTANCE TRAINING:
1) Machine/Exerc._____
   Weight_____ Reps _____/_____/_____
2) Machine/Exerc._____
   Weight_____ Reps _____/_____/_____
3) Machine/Exerc._____
   Weight_____ Reps _____/_____/_____
4) Machine/Exerc._____
   Weight_____ Reps _____/_____/_____
5) Machine/Exerc._____
   Weight_____ Reps _____/_____/_____
6) Machine/Exerc._____
   Weight_____ Reps _____/_____/_____
7) Machine/Exerc._____
   Weight_____ Reps _____/_____/_____
8) Machine/Exerc._____
   Weight_____ Reps _____/_____/_____

Resistance Tr. Total Time_____

CARDIO WALKING:
Treadmill: Distance _____
   Time _____ Speed _____
   Time walked without support _____
Elliptical: Distance _____Time _____
   Reversed direction every _____ minutes
   Time walked without support _____
Stepper: Distance _____Time _____
   Time walked without support _____
Track: Distance _____Time _____
   Speed or pace (if recorded) _____
   Time walked without support _____
   Fastest lap _____
   Fastest lap without support_____
Total Cardio Walking Time:_____
Max. Heart Rate Noted:_____

RECOVERY BASICS:
☐ **Were physical exercise targets (time and total no. of reps) met?**
☐ **Did I focus well on exercises?**
☐ **Did I work intensively + aggressively?**
☐ **Did I push myself to increase difficulty?**

RECOVERY PLAN: _____
Week No. _____ Day No.:_____

Exercises/Drills Done:
_____Time_____
_____Time_____
_____Time_____
_____Time_____
_____Time_____
_____Time_____
_____Time_____
_____Time_____
_____Time_____
_____Time_____

Total Time Spent_____

NUTRITION PLAN:
Nutrient-rich foods eaten | quantity:
BREAKFAST:
_____ | _____
_____ | _____
_____ | _____
_____ | _____
Drinks:_____
LUNCH:
_____ | _____
_____ | _____
_____ | _____
_____ | _____
_____ | _____
_____ | _____
_____ | _____
Drinks:_____
Snacks:_____
DINNER:
_____ | _____
_____ | _____
_____ | _____
_____ | _____
_____ | _____
_____ | _____
Drinks:_____
Snacks:_____

NOTES, SUCCESSES, BREAKTHROUGHS, PROGRESS!
_____
_____
_____
_____
_____

RECOVERY PLAN: _____
Week No. _____ Day No.:_____

Exercises/Drills Done:
_____Time_____
_____Time_____
_____Time_____
_____Time_____
_____Time_____
_____Time_____
_____Time_____
_____Time_____
_____Time_____
_____Time_____

Total Time Spent_____

SUPPLEMENTS TAKEN:
_____ | _____
_____ | _____
_____ | _____
_____ | _____
_____ | _____

Supplements I Need to Buy:
_____ | _____
_____ | _____

MEDICINES TAKEN:
_____ | _____
_____ | _____
_____ | _____
_____ | _____
_____ | _____
_____ | _____

YOGA TRAINING:
Exercises:_____
_____
_____
_____
_____

Total Yoga Time: _____
Notes:_____

Daily Worksheet

Day of the Week:	Date:	Day No.	Max. Heart Rate:	A.M. Weight:	A.M. Blood Pressure: _____ OVER _____

Glasses of water drunk today (check): ○ ○ ○ ○ ○ ○ ○ ○

WALKING Plan No. _____

Week No.: _____ **Day No.:** _____

CORE WORK:

Total Time _____

RESISTANCE TRAINING:

1) Machine/Exerc. _____
  Weight_____ Reps _____/_____/_____

2) Machine/Exerc. _____
  Weight_____ Reps _____/_____/_____

3) Machine/Exerc. _____
  Weight_____ Reps _____/_____/_____

4) Machine/Exerc. _____
  Weight_____ Reps _____/_____/_____

5) Machine/Exerc. _____
  Weight_____ Reps _____/_____/_____

6) Machine/Exerc. _____
  Weight_____ Reps _____/_____/_____

7) Machine/Exerc. _____
  Weight_____ Reps _____/_____/_____

8) Machine/Exerc. _____
  Weight_____ Reps _____/_____/_____

Resistance Tr. Total Time _____

CARDIO WALKING:

Treadmill: Distance _____
  Time _____ Speed _____
  Time walked without support _____

Elliptical: Distance _____ Time _____
  Reversed direction every _____ minutes
  Time walked without support _____

Stepper: Distance _____ Time _____
  Time walked without support _____

Track: Distance _____ Time _____
  Speed or pace (if recorded) _____
  Time walked without support _____
  Fastest lap _____
  Fastest lap without support_____

Total Cardio Walking Time: _____

Max. Heart Rate Noted: _____

RECOVERY BASICS:

☐ **Were physical exercise targets (time and total no. of reps) met?**

☐ **Did I focus well on exercises?**

☐ **Did I work intensively + aggressively?**

☐ **Did I push myself to increase difficulty?**

RECOVERY PLAN: _____

Week No. _____ **Day No.:** _____

Exercises/Drills Done:

_____Time_____
_____Time_____
_____Time_____
_____Time_____
_____Time_____
_____Time_____
_____Time_____
_____Time_____

Total Time Spent _____

NUTRITION PLAN:

Nutrient-rich foods eaten │ quantity:

BREAKFAST:

_____ │ _____
_____ │ _____
_____ │ _____
_____ │ _____

Drinks: _____

LUNCH:

_____ │ _____
_____ │ _____
_____ │ _____
_____ │ _____
_____ │ _____
_____ │ _____

Drinks: _____

Snacks: _____

DINNER:

_____ │ _____
_____ │ _____
_____ │ _____
_____ │ _____
_____ │ _____
_____ │ _____

Drinks: _____

Snacks: _____

RECOVERY PLAN: _____

Week No. _____ **Day No.:** _____

Exercises/Drills Done:

_____Time_____
_____Time_____
_____Time_____
_____Time_____
_____Time_____
_____Time_____
_____Time_____
_____Time_____

Total Time Spent _____

SUPPLEMENTS TAKEN:

_____ │ _____
_____ │ _____
_____ │ _____
_____ │ _____
_____ │ _____
_____ │ _____

Supplements I Need to Buy:

_____ │ _____
_____ │ _____

MEDICINES TAKEN:

_____ │ _____
_____ │ _____
_____ │ _____
_____ │ _____
_____ │ _____
_____ │ _____

YOGA TRAINING:

Exercises: _____
_____
_____
_____
_____

Total Yoga Time: _____

Notes: _____

NOTES, SUCCESSES, BREAKTHROUGHS, PROGRESS!

_____
_____
_____
_____
_____

Part 4:

Retest Yourself!

Retest Yourself!

13-Week Self-Test and Abilities Assessment

This informal self-test will help you assess how much improvement you've made after 13 weeks and what areas still need work. You will summarize and review your results in the questions at the end of the form. If your improvement seems small, but it is still an improvement, do not ignore it—recognize it and congratulate yourself! If some areas did not improve, just realize they need more work. They will improve if you stay determined and persist with your recovery plans.

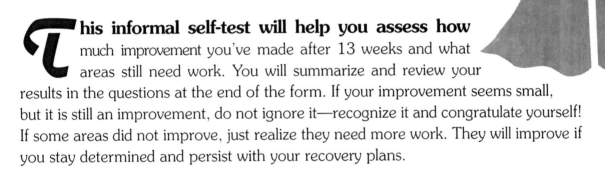

MEASUREMENTS— MEN:	MEASUREMENTS— WOMEN:	WEIGHT:
Waist:_____	Waist:_____	
Chest:_____	Hips:_____	BLOOD PRESSURE:
Upper Leg: _____	Upper Leg:_____	
Upper Arm:_____	Upper Arm:_____	_____ over _____

1. Walking

How far I can walk or run in 10 minutes (on a treadmill, a track, or the sidewalk):

_____

How far (or for how long) I can walk without any support:

_____

Compare these figures with those you wrote down on your Initial Abilities Assessment before you began your recovery plan. Based on these new numbers, has my walking improved?

O Yes   O Somewhat   O No

2. Use of Hands

Paragraph copying:

a. Copy the following paragraph in longhand on the lines provided opposite.

Taking Charge Books thinks people ARE strong enough to do just about anything and they often need to take charge of things in order to succeed. We collect all the hard-to-track-down information and put everything in one place. Taking Charge Books refuses to accept that something is a "fact" when it has not been proven to be true and we defy "authority" when it is wrong. We show you how to do something even when others have maintained it is impossible. A Taking Charge Book is practical, not theoretical. It tells the reader exactly what to do. Its plans fit into normal budgets and schedules. Taking Charge Books' recovery workbooks are written by people who have successfully recovered. *Taking Charge of Your Stroke Recovery* was designed to help stroke survivors recover even if they thought they had no other options.

My copy of this paragraph:

_____

_____

_____

_____

_____

_____

_____

_____

_____

_____

_____

_____

_____

_____

_____

b. Was the paragraph easier to write than it was when you began the recovery plan?

O Yes   O No

c. Now assign your copy a rating on its appearance:

O Excellent   O Very Good   O Good   O Fair   O Poor

3. Speaking

Answer the following questions:

a. Do I feel my speaking has improved since I began?

O Yes   O No

b. Write down the ways in which your speaking has improved. Include some of the formerly troublesome sounds, words and phrases that you have worked on and improved.

_____

_____

_____

_____

_____

c. What sounds, words, or phrases still need work?

_____

_____

_____

_____

_____

_____

d. Are there still certain circumstances that consistently make it hard for me to speak?

_____

_____

_____

e. Has my rate of speaking improved?

    O Yes   O Somewhat   O No

f. Is my ability to control how loudly and softly I speak better?

    O Yes   O Somewhat   O No

f. Is my variation of pitch better?

    O Yes   O Somewhat   O No

4. Thinking

a. Read an article in the newspaper or a magazine. A few hours later the same day or the next day, using your recall, tell your caregiver or family member about what you read so they can understand you and use the information you impart. Then answer these questions:

Am I able to understand things I read and see?

O Yes   O Somewhat   O No

Can I evaluate the information I obtain?

O Yes   O Somewhat   O No

Can I use information that I read and see?

O Yes   O Somewhat   O No

Can I convey information to others?

O Yes   O Somewhat   O No

b.   **Overall, have my thinking and understanding abilities improved?**

O Yes   O Somewhat   O No

5.   Vision

a.   **Go outside with a book to a place where you can see a street sign that is some distance away from you. Hold the book. Look at the book. Look at the street sign.**

Have your rate of focus and ability to detect details improved?

O Yes   O Somewhat   O No

b.   **Stare at the street sign. See how far to the sides of it you can see things without moving your eyes from it.**

Has your field of vision widened at all?

O Yes   O Somewhat   O No

c.   **Go to a fairly busy intersection. Look at the moving traffic. Imagine how you would react to that traffic and test yourself with two possible responses: (1) Each time a car moving in one direction passes a specific point you select beforehand, try to immediately close your hand. (2) At the same time, watch for each time a car passes a second point, and immediately make a different small movement of your hand. Do this test for about 5 minutes, then answer these questions:**

Has your rate or speed of reaction to something you see improved?

O Yes   O Somewhat   O No

Has your ability to react "properly" to it (make the correct movement) improved?

O Yes   O Somewhat   O No

6.   Eating, Drinking and Swallowing

a.   **General eating and drinking difficulties prior to beginning my swallowing recovery plan:**

O Not being able to chew items well

Has this ability improved?   O Yes   O Somewhat   O No

O Not being able to move things back and down the right "pipe"

Has this ability improved?   O Yes   O Somewhat   O No

O Not being able to keep food down

Has this ability improved?   O Yes   O Somewhat   O No

b.   Foods and drinks I had difficulty with before beginning my swallowing plan; improvements I have made with them:

Difficult foods	Improvement?		
	O Yes	O Somewhat	O No
	O Yes	O Somewhat	O No
	O Yes	O Somewhat	O No
	O Yes	O Somewhat	O No
	O Yes	O Somewhat	O No
	O Yes	O Somewhat	O No
	O Yes	O Somewhat	O No
	O Yes	O Somewhat	O No
Difficult drinks	Improvement?		
	O Yes	O Somewhat	O No
	O Yes	O Somewhat	O No
	O Yes	O Somewhat	O No
	O Yes	O Somewhat	O No
	O Yes	O Somewhat	O No
	O Yes	O Somewhat	O No

7. Single-Sided Weakness

Areas of my body that had single-sided weakness, numbness or tingling and improvements I've experienced:

Areas with Single-Sided Weakness	Improvement?		
	O Yes	O Somewhat	O No
	O Yes	O Somewhat	O No
	O Yes	O Somewhat	O No
	O Yes	O Somewhat	O No
	O Yes	O Somewhat	O No
	O Yes	O Somewhat	O No
	O Yes	O Somewhat	O No
	O Yes	O Somewhat	O No
	O Yes	O Somewhat	O No
	O Yes	O Somewhat	O No

8. Nutrition

a.   How did I do with the Nutrition Plan? Am I taking my supplements each day and eating brain-healthy foods often?

_____

_____

_____

_____

_____

_____

b. **Am I experiencing any benefits and improvements as a result of my improved nutrition? If so, what are they?**

_____

_____

_____

_____

_____

_____

_____

9. Stroke Recovery Basics

Overall, how did I do with my Stroke Recovery Basics? For each question below, assign yourself a rating. Be honest with yourself! If you accurately assess how you did, you'll more easily be able to determine what points to improve, as you continue. (The numbers after each rating are points earned for each answer that you will use in the Progress Summary.)

a. **In my walking plan exercises, did I do the suggested number of repetitions, use the recommended weights, and work the length of time suggested on the various exercises?**

O Excellent-5   O Very Good-4   O Good-3   O Fair-2   O Poor-1

b. **Did I work intensively and aggressively on my physical exercises?**

O Excellent-5   O Very Good-4   O Good-3   O Fair-2   O Poor-1

c. **On all plans, did I focus and concentrate well on my exercises as I was doing them?**

O Excellent-5   O Very Good-4   O Good-3   O Fair-2   O Poor-1

d. **On the physical exercises I did, did I push myself to keep increasing the difficulty (weight, speed, distance traveled, number of repetitions, or time spent)?**

O Excellent-5   O Very Good-4   O Good-3   O Fair-2   O Poor-1

Overall Progress Summary

To create a summary of your progress, refer back to your answers in each main numbered category in this 13-Week Self-Test and Abilities Assessment and fill in the answers to each of the summary questions below. You may also want to refer to your Weekly Worksheets to refresh yourself on your recovery progress. These summaries are for your own use and will help you determine your recovery status and what your next recovery steps should be. They will also serve as a record of your overall progress in each 13-week period.

1. Walking Progress Summary

a. **Which functions and skills in this category are progressing well? Summarize what progress has been made in each of them.**

Function/Skill: (1) _____

Progress Made: _____

_____

_____

Function/Skill: (2) _____

Progress Made: _____

_____

_____

Function/Skill: (3) _____

Progress Made: _____

_____

_____

Function/Skill: (4) _____

Progress Made: _____

_____

_____

Function/Skill: (5) _____

Progress Made: _____

Function/Skill: (6) _____

Progress Made: _____

_____

_____

Function/Skill: (7) _____

Progress Made: _____

_____

_____

Function/Skill: (8) _____

Progress Made: _____

_____

_____

b.   **Which functions and skills in this category are progressing more slowly and need more work?**

Function/Skill: (1) _____

Progress Made: _____

_____

_____

Function/Skill: (2) _____

Progress Made: _____

_____

_____

Function/Skill: (3) _____

Progress Made: _____

_____

_____

Function/Skill: (4) _____

Progress Made: _____

_____

_____

    c.   **Should I repeat this walking recovery plan or start another?**

        O Repeat Plan   O Start Another Walking Plan

2. Use of Hands Progress Summary

    a.   **Which functions and skills in this category are progressing well? Summarize what progress has been made in each of them.**

Function/Skill: (1) _____

Progress Made: _____

_____

_____

Function/Skill: (2) _____

Progress Made: _____

_____

_____

Function/Skill: (3) _____

Progress Made: _____

_____

_____

Function/Skill: (4) _____

Progress Made: _____

_____

_____

Function/Skill: (5) _____

Progress Made: _____

b. **Which functions and skills in this category are progressing more slowly and need more work?**

Function/Skill: (1) _____

Progress Made: _____

_____

_____

Function/Skill: (2) _____

Progress Made: _____

_____

_____

Function/Skill: (3) _____

Progress Made: _____

_____

_____

Function/Skill: (4) _____

Progress Made: _____

_____

_____

c. **Should I repeat this recovery plan or is this recovery complete?**

O Repeat Plan   O Recovery is Complete

3. Speaking Progress Summary

a. **Which functions and skills in this category are progressing well? Summarize what progress has been made in each of them.**

Function/Skill: (1) _____

Progress Made: _____

_____

_____

Function/Skill: (2) _____

Progress Made: _____

_____

_____

Function/Skill: (3) _____

Progress Made: _____

_____

_____

Function/Skill: (4) _____

Progress Made: _____

_____

_____

Function/Skill: (5) _____

Progress Made: _____

_____

_____

Function/Skill: (6) _____

Progress Made: _____

_____

_____

Function/Skill: (7) _____

Progress Made: _____

_____

_____

b. **Which functions and skills in this category are progressing more slowly and need more work?**

Function/Skill: (1) _____

Progress Made: _____

_____

_____

Function/Skill: (2) _____

Progress Made: _____

_____

_____

Function/Skill: (3) _____

Progress Made: _____

_____

_____

Function/Skill: (4) _____

Progress Made: _____

_____

_____

Function/Skill: (5) _____

Progress Made: _____

_____

_____

_____

c. **Should I repeat this recovery plan or is this recovery complete?**

O Repeat Plan   O Recovery is Complete

4. Thinking Progress Summary

a. **Which functions and skills in this category are progressing well? Summarize what progress has been made in each of them.**

Function/Skill: (1) _____

Progress Made: _____

_____

_____

Function/Skill: (2) _____

Progress Made: _____

_____

_____

Function/Skill: (3) _____

Progress Made: _____

_____

_____

Function/Skill: (4) _____

Progress Made: _____

_____

_____

Function/Skill: (5) _____

Progress Made: _____

_____

_____

Function/Skill: (6) _____

Progress Made: _____

_____

_____

Function/Skill: (7) _____

Progress Made: _____

_____

_____

Function/Skill: (8) _____

Progress Made: _____

_____

_____

Function/Skill: (9) _____

Progress Made: _____

_____

_____

Function/Skill: (10) _____

Progress Made: _____

_____

_____

b. **Which functions and skills in this category are progressing more slowly and need more work?**

Function/Skill: (1) _____

Progress Made: _____

_____

_____

Function/Skill: (2) _____

Progress Made: _____

_____

_____

Function/Skill: (3) _____

Progress Made: _____

_____

Function/Skill: (4) _____

Progress Made: _____

_____

_____

Function/Skill: (5) _____

Progress Made: _____

_____

_____

c.   **Should I repeat this recovery plan or is this recovery complete?**

      O Repeat Plan   O Recovery is Complete

5.   Vision Progress Summary

a.   **Which functions and skills in this category are progressing well? Summarize what progress has been made in each of them.**

Function/Skill: (1) _____

Progress Made: _____

_____

_____

Function/Skill: (2) _____

Progress Made: _____

_____

_____

Function/Skill: (3) _____

Progress Made: _____

_____

_____

Function/Skill: (4) _____

Progress Made: _____

_____

Function/Skill: (5) _____

Progress Made: _____

_____

_____

b. **Which functions and skills in this category are progressing more slowly and need more work?**

Function/Skill: (1) _____

Progress Made: _____

_____

_____

Function/Skill: (2) _____

Progress Made: _____

_____

_____

Function/Skill: (3) _____

Progress Made: _____

_____

_____

Function/Skill: (4) _____

Progress Made: _____

_____

_____

Function/Skill: (5) _____

Progress Made: _____

_____

_____

c. **Should I repeat this recovery plan or is this recovery complete?**

O Repeat Plan   O Recovery is Complete

6. Eating, Drinking and Swallowing Progress Summary

a. **Which functions and skills in this category are progressing well? Summarize what progress has been made in each of them.**

Function/Skill: (1) _____

Progress Made: _____

_____

_____

Function/Skill: (2) _____

Progress Made: _____

_____

_____

Function/Skill: (3) _____

Progress Made: _____

_____

_____

Function/Skill: (4) _____

Progress Made: _____

_____

_____

Function/Skill: (5) _____

Progress Made: _____

_____

_____

b. **Which functions and skills in this category are progressing more slowly and need more work?**

Function/Skill: (1) _____

Progress Made: _____

_____

Function/Skill: (2) _____

Progress Made: _____

_____

_____

Function/Skill: (3) _____

Progress Made: _____

_____

_____

Function/Skill: (4) _____

Progress Made: _____

_____

_____

c.   Should I repeat this recovery plan or is this recovery complete?

○ Repeat Plan   ○ Recovery is Complete

7. Single-Sided Weakness Progress Summary

a.   **Which functions and skills in this category are progressing well? Summarize what progress has been made in each of them.**

Function/Skill: (1) _____

Progress Made: _____

_____

_____

Function/Skill: (2) _____

Progress Made: _____

_____

_____

Function/Skill: (3) _____

Progress Made: _____

_____

_____

Function/Skill: (4) _____

Progress Made: _____

_____

_____

Function/Skill: (5) _____

Progress Made: _____

_____

_____

Function/Skill: (6) _____

Progress Made: _____

_____

_____

Function/Skill: (7) _____

Progress Made: _____

_____

_____

Function/Skill: (8) _____

Progress Made: _____

_____

_____

b. **Which functions and skills in this category are progressing more slowly and need more work?**

Function/Skill: (1) _____

Progress Made: _____

_____

_____

Function/Skill: (2) _____

Progress Made: _____

_____

_____

Function/Skill: (3) _____

Progress Made: _____

_____

_____

Function/Skill: (4) _____

Progress Made: _____

_____

_____

Function/Skill: (5) _____

Progress Made: _____

_____

_____

c. **Should I repeat this recovery plan or is this recovery complete?**

O Repeat Plan   O Recovery is Complete

8. Nutrition Progress Summary

a. **Summarize how I did with my nutrition plan:**

O Excellent   O Very Good   O Good   O Fair   O Poor

If you did well, congratulations! You are giving your brain and body the "raw materials" that they need to recover fully.

9.   Stroke Recovery Basics Progress Summary

Add up your Recovery Basics scores from the ratings you assigned yourself on page 297. Your total number of points shows you how you did with your Recovery Basics:

20 = Outstanding

16-19 = Very good

12-15 = Good

8-11 = Fair

4-7 = Poor

Keep working to improve your Recovery Basics as you continue with new recovery plans. The better you hold to these principles, the faster your recovery will be!

To continue with your recovery plans, be sure to order a new workbook now for your next 13 weeks, if you don't already have one. When you are ready, you can put a check mark by each recovery plan you intend to do next in the selection chart in your new workbook. We look forward to having you continue *Taking Charge of Your Stroke Recovery!*

Recommended Books and Other Resources

Helpful and Interesting Books

10-Fold Origami, by Peter Engel (New York: Sterling Publishing, October 7, 2008)

The Better Brain Book, by David Perlmutter, M.D. (New York: Riverhead Books, 2004).

Collins COBUILD English Dictionary for Advanced Learners (London, UK: HarperCollins Publishers, 2003).

Dental Floss for the Mind: A Complete Program for Boosting Your Brain Power, by Michel Noir, Ph.D., and Bernard Croisile, M.D., Ph.D. (New York: McGraw-Hill, 2005).

The Great Origami Book & Kit, by Zulal Ayture-Scheele (New York: Sterling Publishing, 2000).

Hypothyroidism Type 2: The Epidemic, by Mark Starr, M.D. (Columbia, MO: Mark Starr Trust, 2007). Website at www.type2hypothyroidism.com/.

Kirigami, by Jeffrey Rutzky (book and kit) (New York: Metro Books, 2007).

Light on Yoga: The classic guide to yoga from the world's foremost authority, by B.K.S. Iyengar (Thorsons, 2001).

Macmillan English Dictionary for Advanced Learners of American English (Oxford, UK: Macmillan Education, 2002).

The New Oxford American Dictionary (New York and Oxford, UK: Oxford University Press, 2001).

Survival of the Fattest: The Key to Human Brain Evolution, by Stephen C. Cunnane (Singapore: World Scientific Publishing Co. Pte. Ltd., 2005).

Websites & Companies

Bayho.com. Huge selection of supplements and nutritional products, including NutriWest products, at www.bayho.com.

Broda O. Barnes M.D. Research Foundation Inc. The Broda O. Barnes, M.D. Research Foundation, Inc. is a not-for-profit organization dedicated to education, research and training in the field of thyroid and metabolic balance. The Foundation works nationally and internationally to disseminate the work of Dr. Barnes and other pioneers in the field of thyroid and other endocrine dysfunctions through lectures, seminars, consultations, and publications to physicians, medical research personnel, health professionals, clinics and the lay public. Website at www. brodabarnes.org.

EasierLiving.com. This website provides a very large selection of medical, health and home convenience ("life issue problems") type products which can be purchased by individuals as well as organizations. They also sell food preparation and eating supplies for those with swallowing or hand-function difficulties. Their company description: "Easierliving.com is part of the Alimed, Inc. Family of Web Sites. AliMed is a leading manufacturer and supplier of high quality products—everything from pre-formed orthoses, alarms for fall management, cushions, diagnostic imaging and operating room accessories, orthopedic rehabilitation equipment, ergonomic workplace solutions and now our latest endeavor into Emergency Preparedness. For over 35 years, we have served a broad range of manufacturing and service industries including all segments of the healthcare market... hospitals, nursing homes, HMO's outpatient clinics, and private medical practices." Website at www.easierliving.com.

RosettaStone™ language software. Learning a new language can be stimulating, fun, and mind-expanding. This company's method is recommended by many people as being the easiest and fastest way to learn a new language. Their website reads, "Rosetta Stone Inc. is a leading provider of language-learning software. Acclaimed for the speed, power and effectiveness of its Dynamic Immersion® method, Rosetta Stone is a revolutionary language-learning software program.... A comprehensive product demonstration of Rosetta Stone is available online at www.RosettaStone.com and at retail kiosks located in select malls and airports throughout the United States … To obtain more information or to purchase the program, call (800) 788-0822 or visit www.RosettaStone.com."

Spectrum Organics. Healthful oils for eating and cooking. Spectrum's website description reads, "Explore Spectrum's select organic and artisan vegetable oils from around the world. Discover healthy, delicious dressings, vinegars and spreads. Our Organic Coconut Oil and Shortening give you crisp crusts and chewy cookies -- and even buttery soft skin and hair! And, as always, they're trans-fat free." www. spectrumorganics.com.

Vitacost.com. Huge selection of supplements and nutritional products, available at well-discounted prices. Excellent service in our experience.

YES-Supplements.com. Manufactures innovative proprietary formula of essential fatty acids called PEOs (Parent Essential Oils) that are especially effective in improving cellular oxygenation and many other aspects of health. Helps support brain and nerve functions. Visit www.yes-supplements.com.

References

[i] David Perlmutter, M.D. *The Better Brain Book* (New York: Riverhead Books, 2004), p. 193.

[ii] Katzman R, et al., "Clinical, Pathological, and Neurochemical Changes in Dementia: A Subgroup With Preserved Mental Status and Numerous Neocortical Plaques," *Annals of Neurology* (1988), vol. 23(2), pp. 8-144.

[iii] American Heart Association, "Extended, Progressive Physical Therapy Aids Stroke Survivors' Mobility," *ScienceDaily* (August 22, 2003), "Science News" column. http://www.sciencedaily.com/releases/2003/08/030821073013.htm# (accessed May 2008).

[iv] American Heart Association, "Extended, Progressive Physical Therapy Aids Stroke Survivors' Mobility," *ScienceDaily* (August 22, 2003), Science News column; Pohl M., et al., "Speed-dependent Treadmill Training in Ambulatory Hemiparetic Stroke Patients: A Randomized Controlled Trial," *Stroke* (2002), vol. 33, pp. 553-58; Pamela Duncan, et al. "Randomized Clinical Trial of Therapeutic Exercise in Subacute Stroke," *Stroke* (September 2003), http://www.strokeaha.org.

[v] Pohl M., Mehrholz J., et al., "Speed-dependent Treadmill Training in Ambulatory Hemiparetic Stroke Patients: A Randomized Controlled Trial," *Stroke*, 2002, vol. 33, pp. 553-58.

[vi] Mark Starr, M.D. *Hypothyroidism Type 2: The Epidemic* (Columbia, MO: Mark Starr Trust, 2007).

[vii] Barnes, B.O., M.D. *Heart Attack Rareness in Thyroid-Treated Patients* (Springfield, IL: Charles C. Thomas, 1972).

[viii] Cunnane, Stephen C. *Survival of the Fattest: The Key to Human Brain Evolution* (Singapore: World Scientific Publishing Co. Pte. Ltd., 2005).

[ix] The Weston A. Price Foundation for Wise Traditions in Food, Farming, and the Health Arts website, "Confused About Fats?" http://www.westonaprice.org/knowyourfats/index.html (accessed July 2008).

[x] Sally Fallon and Mary G. Enig, PhD, "The Great Con-ola," posted 28 July 2002, Miscellaneous articles, The Weston A. Price Foundation for Wise Traditions in Food, Farming, and the Health Arts website. http://www.westonaprice.org/knowyourfats/index.html (accessed July 2008).

[xi] "Serrapeptase, also known as serratia peptidase is [an] enzyme…. Clinical studies show that serrapeptase induces fibrinolytic, anti-inflammatory and anti-edemic (prevents swelling and fluid retention) activity in a number of tissues, and that its anti-inflammatory effects are superior to other proteolytic enzymes.(n.17) Besides reducing inflammation, one of serrapeptase's most profound benefits is reduction of pain, due to its ability to block the release of pain-inducing amines from inflamed tissues.(n.18) Physicians throughout Europe and Asia have recognized the anti-inflammatory and pain-blocking benefits of this naturally occurring substance and are using it in treatment as an alternative to salicylates, ibuprofen, and other NSAIDs." (n.19)

[References: Note 17, Mazzone A, Catalani M, Costanzo M, Drusian A, Mandoli A, Russo S, Guarini E, Vesperini G. "Evaluation of Serratia peptidase in acute or chronic inflammation of otorhinolaryngology pathology: a multicentre, double-blind, randomized trial versus placebo." *Journal of International Medical Research* 1990; 18(5):379-88. Note 18, Mazzone A, et al. "Evaluation of Serratia peptidase in acute or chronic inflammation of otorhinolaryngology pathology: a multicentre, double-blind, randomized trial versus placebo." *Journal of International Medical Research* 1990; 18(5):379-88. Note 19, Aso T, et al. "Breast engorgement and its treatment: Clinical effects of Danzen an anti-inflammatory enzyme preparation." *The World of Obstetrics and Gynecology* (Japanese). 1981; 33:371-9.] From SmartNutrition.com, at http://smart-drugs.net/serrapeptase-research.htm (accessed April 10, 2008).

[xii] Peskin, Brian Scott and Habib, Amid, M.D. *The Hidden Story of Cancer* (Houston, TX: Pinnacle Press, 2007), pp. 195, 199-201.

[xiii] Dr. Jane Durga, Martin P.J. van Boxtel, Prof. Evert G. Schouten, Prof. Frans J. Kok, Prof. Jelle Jolles, Martijn B. Katan, and Petra Verhoef. "Effect of 3-year folic acid supplementation on cognitive function in older adults in the FACIT trial: a randomised, double blind, controlled trial." *The Lancet* 2007; 369:208-216.

Date	Notes

Notes, Progress, Successes

Notes, Progress, Successes	
Date	**Notes**

Notes, Progress, Successes

Date	Notes

Printed in the United States
!06304BV00002B/26/P